RADIATION PRO

RADIATION PROTECTION

Euclid Seeram, RTR, B.Sc., M.Sc.
Medical Imaging Advanced Studies
British Columbia Institute of Technology
Burnaby, British Columbia
Canada

WITH A CONTRIBUTION BY

Elizabeth L. Travis, Ph.D.
Department of Experimental Radiotherapy
University of Texas M.D. Anderson Cancer Center
Houston, Texas

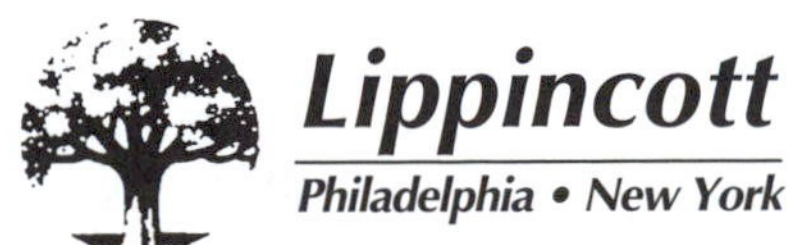

Acquisitions Editor: Kathleen P. Lyons
Editorial Assistant: Stephanie Harold
Production Editor: Molly E. Connors

Library of Congress Cataloging-in-Publications Data

Seeram, Euclid.
Radiation protection / Euclid Seeram ; with a contribution by Elizabeth L. Travis.
p. cm.
Includes bibliographical references and index.
ISBN 0–397–55032–4
1. Radiation—Safety measures. 2. Radiologic technologists.
I. Travis, Elizabeth Latorre. II. Title.
RC78.3.S44 1997
616.07′54′0289—dc20 96–25440
CIP

Care has been taken to confirm the accuracy of the information presented and to describe generally accepted practices. However, the authors, editors, and publisher are not responsible for errors or omissions or for any consequences from application of the information in this book and make no warranty, express or implied, with respect to the contents of the publication.

The authors, editors and publisher have exerted every effort to ensure that drug selection and dosage set forth in this text are in accordance with current recommendations and practice at the time of publication. However, in view of ongoing research, changes in government regulations, and the constant flow of information relating to drug therapy and drug reactions, the reader is urged to check the package insert for each drug for any change in indications and dosage and for added warnings and precautions. This is particularly important when the recommended agent is a new or infrequently employed drug.

Some drugs and medical devices presented in this publication have Food and Drug Administration (FDA) clearance for limited use in restricted research settings. It is the responsibility of the health care provider to ascertain the FDA status of each drug or device planned for use in their clinical practice.

9 8 7 6 5 4 3 2 1

This book is dedicated with love and sincere appreciation to my mother-in-law, Joan Penner, the most well-informed person I know, and to my father-in-law, Edward Penner, retired research scientist extraordinaire.

Reviewers

Thomas J. Beck, ScD
Assistant Professor
Department of Radiology
The Johns Hopkins Hospital
Baltimore, Maryland

Charles Collins, Jr.
Professor of Radiation Technology
San Diego Mesa College
San Diego, California

Dawn Couch Moore, MMSc, RT(R)
Assistant Professor
Program of Radiologic Technology
Emory University
Atlanta, Georgia

William Hachman, BS, RTR
Midland College
Midland, Texas

Wynn Harrison, MEd
Weber State University
Ogden, Utah

Elwin R. Tilson, EdD, RTR
Radiologic Technologies
School of Allied Health Professions
Armstrong State College
Savannah, Georgia

Rebecca Waters, BS, ARRT(R)
Medical Imaging Program Director
Minnesota Riverland Technical College
Austin, Minnesota

Foreword

"Superb" is the best word I can think of to describe this textbook. This text provides an up-to-date account of the newest and latest radiation protection recommendations for radiation technologists all over the world.

Euclid Seeram, a true educator, has provided comprehensive coverage of all aspects of radiation protection, written in his usual clear and concise manner. The content of this text certainly fulfills the author's desire to produce a textbook with features that set it apart from other current texts. One look through the chapter contents will assure the reader that the author has met his objective.

Mr. Seeram is to be commended for the educationally sound principles employed in the writing of this book. Each chapter begins with a statement of learning objectives and an outline of the material to be covered, followed by easy-to-read text. Review questions and references are also provided with each chapter. To assist the reader, pertinent information has been highlighted.

The author's continual quest for knowledge and his ability to share this knowledge succinctly with his readers will continue to make him a successful author and a sought-after guest lecturer across the Americas.

Shirley Hundvik, MEd, RT
Program Head, Medical Radiography
British Columbia Institute of Technology
Burnaby, British Columbia, Canada, *and*
Education Chairman
International Society of Radiographers
and Radiological Technologists

PREFACE

There are few books on radiation protection for radiologic technologists. Several recent issues make the appearance of this text timely: (1) the Committee on Bioeffects of Ionizing Radiation (BEIR) now estimates the risk of radiation injury to the population to be greater than they had previously estimated; (2) current studies are now concerned with the bioeffects of low-level radiation, which is characteristic of diagnostic radiology; (3) based on a close examination of the radiation data on the Hiroshima and Nagasaki atom bomb survivors, the International Commission of Radiological Protection (ICRP) recently revised its recommendations on radiation protection and lowered the annual dose limit to the whole body for radiation workers from 50 mSv to 20 mSv; (4) the introduction of new imaging techniques, such as magnetic resonance imaging (MRI), requires an understanding of the bioeffects of exposure to magnetic fields and radio waves, as well as a thorough knowledge of the safety issues surrounding the use of these techniques to image the human body; and (5) quality control is an effective dose reduction tool and is now considered an essential element of radiation protection programs.

Keeping these recent developments in mind, the purpose of this book is to:

1. Provide a current and thorough overview of the bioeffects of radiation.
2. Provide comprehensive coverage of the physical principles and technical aspects of radiation protection in diagnostic radiology.
3. Explore the hazards and safety considerations of MRI.
4. Explain the role of quality assurance/quality control in radiation protection.
5. Describe the recent recommendations and new developments in radiation protection for patients undergoing diagnostic X-ray examinations.
6. Summarize the results of various dose studies in X-ray imaging, including computed tomography and mammography.

With these goals in mind, this book can be used as an introduction to radiation protection in radiography courses, as a reference for the professional technologist, and as a supplement for applied fields such as biomedical engineering technology and dental hygiene programs.

The book is organized into five sections. Part I provides background material intended to orient the reader to the nature and scope of radiation protection, and it includes three chapters. Chapter 1 introduces the reader to radiation protection and presents a comprehensive overview of the fundamentals of radiation protection. As such, it should be considered a pivotal chapter that can be used as a roadmap to the rest of the book. Chapter 2 reviews the basic physics necessary for a clear understanding of radiation protection. It assumes that the reader has a background in high school physics. Chapter 3 details the nature of radiation exposure.

Part II (Chapter 4) is an introduction to the bioeffects of radiation, material that provides the basis for radiation protection.

The seven chapters in Part III describe the general principles and technical aspects of radiation protection. Chapter 5 presents an explanation of radiation protection concepts, Chapter 6 describes dose limits, and Chapter 7 outlines radiation protection organizations. Chapter 8 should also be considered a pivotal chapter because it explains the factors that affect dose in radiography, fluoroscopy, mammography, and computed tomography. The results of various dose studies in radiography, fluoroscopy, mammography, and computed tomography are presented in Chapter 9 as a means of motivating technologists to explore this area of radiation protection. Chapter 10 provides the guidelines and recommendations for dose reduction. It is important to note that in this chapter some of the recommendations are cited verbatim from government radiation protection reports. For example, with regard to the exposure switch on mobile equipment, the National Council on Radiation Protection Measurements (NCRP) in Report No. 102 (1989) recommends that "the exposure switch on mobile radiography units shall be so arranged that the operator can stand at least 2 m (6 ft) from the patient, the tube and the useful beam" (p 25). The purpose of these references is to motivate the student to refer to these reports so that they can capture a glimpse of the original wording of the recommendations, rather than reading summaries of the recommendations provided by others, myself included. Finally, Chapter 11 completes Part III, and it addresses concepts of shielding diagnostic X-ray facilities.

Parts IV and V are each single-chapter parts that cover the safety aspects of MRI (Chapter 12) and the role of quality assurance/quality control in radiation protection of both patients and personnel (Chapter 13).

In addition, the book contains a few appendices and a glossary of terms.

In writing this text, an important challenge was to meet the varied requirements of its users, both students and instructors alike. In doing so, I have written the material in a concise manner in order to maintain the student's interest and attention. This includes the addition of pedagogical features such as detailed chapter outlines, learning objectives, and the various review boxes scattered throughout the chapters. These boxes might reasonably be seen as a replacement for conventional end of chapter summaries. Finally, a set of multiple choice review questions are included at the end of each chapter so that students can test their understanding of the material. There are 300 multiple choice questions included in the book.

The content of this book is intended to meet the educational requirements (for entry to practice radiography) of the following professional associations: the American Society of Radiologic Technologists (ASRT), the Canadian Association of Medical Radiation Technologists (CAMRT), the College of Radiographers in the United Kingdom, and radiography societies and associations in Asia/Australasia and Europe-Africa regions. One should note, however, that the guidelines and recommendations of all countries could not be included in the textbook and readers must consult radiation protection reports of their respective national radiation protection agencies and organizations.

Radiation protection is an integral part of the education of radiologic technologists, who play a significant role in the limitation of radiation exposure to the population. This book offers a small step toward achieving that goal.

Best wishes in your pursuit of the study of radiation protection.

Euclid Seeram, RTR, BSc MSc

ACKNOWLEDGMENTS

The single most important and satisfying task in writing a textbook of this nature is to acknowledge the help and encouragement of those individuals who perceive the value of the contribution to the literature.

The content of this book is built around the work and expertise of several noted physicists, radiobiologists, and radiologists who have done the original research. In reality, they are the tacit authors of this text, and I am truly grateful to all of them. I owe a good deal of thanks to Dr. Elizabeth Travis, a radiobiologist at the University of Texas M.D. Anderson Cancer Center, who took the time out of her busy schedule to write Chapter 4, "Bioeffects of Radiation." In addition, the reviewers deserve a special word of gratitude for their time and effort in not only offering positive comments but also constructive feedback, which helped to shape the manuscript to its present form.

I am indebted to the following companies and their representatives, who provided me with technical information, illustrations, and photographs for use in the text: Elscint, Landauer, Nuclear Associates, and Siemens. Equally important are the numerous authors and publishers who generously gave permission from their original publications, most notably, the Radiological Society of North America (RSNA), the International Commission on Radiological Protection (ICRP), the National Council on Radiation Protection and Measurements (NCRP), Mosby-YearBook, Williams & Wilkins, CRC Press, Appleton & Lange, and Lippincott–Raven Publishers. In this regard, I am also grateful to Stewart Bushong, ScD, Perry Sprawls, PhD, Jerrold Bushberg, PhD, and Anthony Wolbarst, PhD, for the use of several illustrations from their excellent radiologic physics textbooks. Two other individuals who deserve mention here are my good friends Randy Ross, MSc, and Francine Anselmo, RTR, MBA, both radiation protection officers with the Radiation Protection and Tobacco Enforcement Branch of the British Columbia Ministry of Health, who kept providing me with the most up-to-date information on radiation protection. Thanks to both of you for your willingness to share this material, and for your efficiency in responding to my needs.

The typing of this manuscript was done by Betty Fowler, medical stenographer. Thanks, Betty, for a job well done.

My gratitude also extends to those individuals at Lippincott–Raven for their excellent work on the manuscript from its initial stages to the final product. First, thanks to Dr. Andrew Allen, PhD, Executive Editor, for considering the proposal and finalizing the details. Second, the following individuals continued the communications and work where Andrew left off: Laura Dover, Editorial Assistant, Kathleen Lyons, Associate Editor, and Stephanie Harold, Editoral Assistant, all of the Nursing and Allied Health Division of Lippincott–Raven. Thanks to all of you for your hard work and dedication to this project, especially Stephanie for the never ending e-mail, phone calls, and letters. I would also like to thank the design, production, and marketing teams for their wonderful efforts in getting this book out to the world. In addition, the individuals at P.M. Gordon Associates deserve special mention for their efforts in the production process, particularly Darrin Kiessling who kept the production schedule right on target. Thanks Darrin for your efficient and careful work on the manuscript.

One individual who read the entire manuscript on behalf of the publisher, and to whom I am extremely thankful, is Crystal Norris, a freelance developmental editor. Crystal's skills have helped shape the manuscript into the final product.

I extend my sincere gratitude to my family for their help, love, support, and encouragement as I worked on this book: my wife, Trish, radiographer extraordinaire and a very special person in my life, provided me with the motivation needed to complete this project; and my son David, a very special young man, who is currently studying mathematics and music—thanks for your love, pride, and encouragement. I love you both.

I must not forget my dear parents. Thank you for your love and encouragement and thanks for having me. In this regard, I am also grateful to my mother-in-law and father-in-law, Joan and Edward Penner. This book is dedicated to you both for all the good things you've done for me and my family.

Finally, to all the students who have passed through my radiobiology and radiation protection classes throughout the years: Thanks for the questions.

Contents

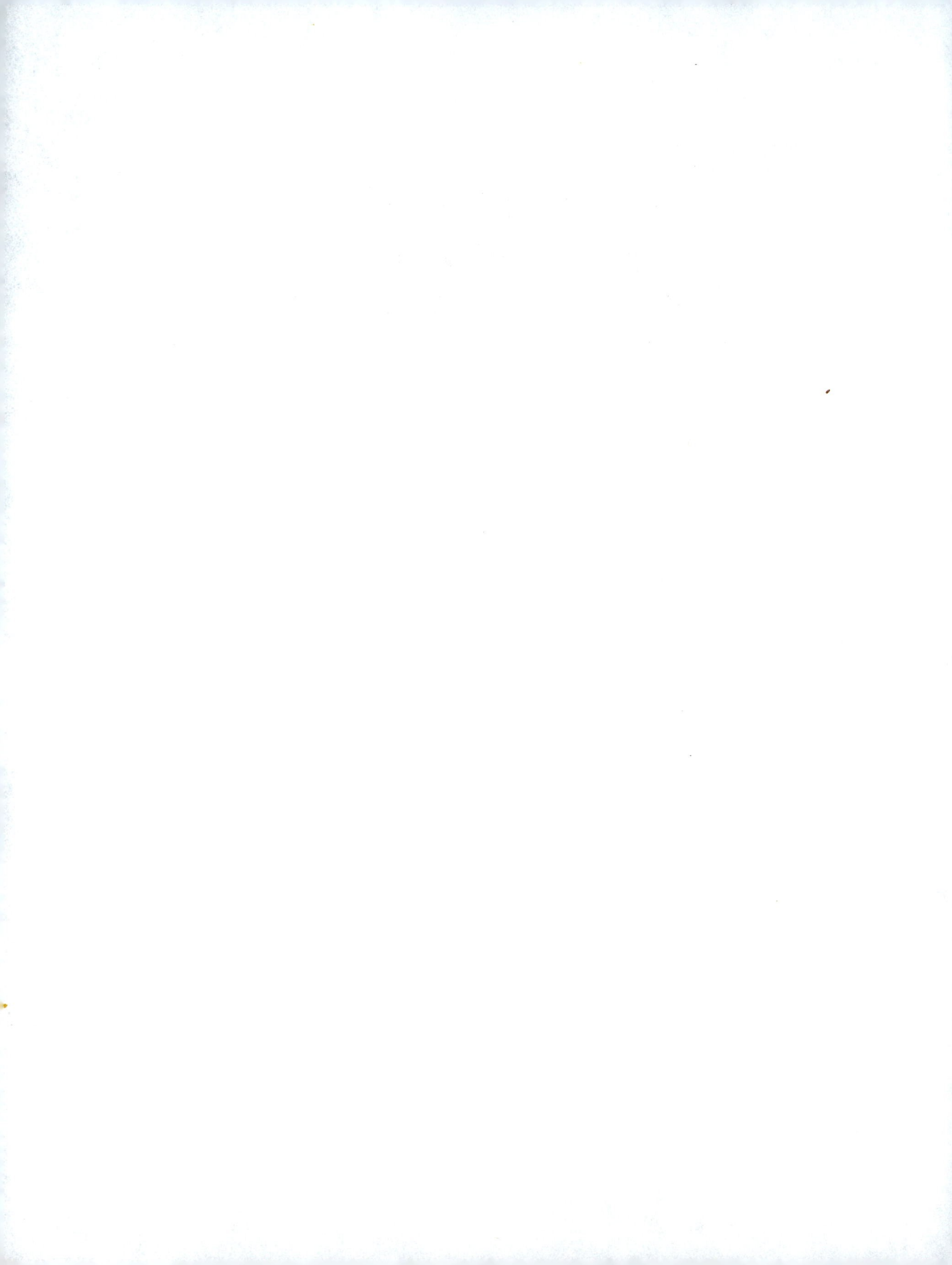

Part I
An Overview of Radiation Protection

CHAPTER ONE

Introduction to Radiation Protection

Learning Objectives

Upon completion of this chapter, the reader should be able to:

1 ■ State several reasons why protection of the patient undergoing a radiology examination is of primary concern to the technologist.

2 ■ List the sources of data on the biological effects of radiation on humans.

3 ■ State the meaning of the term "dose-response model" and list three dose-response models.

(continued)

4 ■ Identify two categories of biological effects of radiation.

5 ■ Describe briefly the International Commission on Radiological Protection (ICRP) framework for radiation protection.

6 ■ Identify the various factors affecting dose in radiography, fluoroscopy, mammography (breast imaging), computed tomography, and magnetic resonance imaging.

7 ■ Identify the types of radiation to which patients and technologists are exposed.

8 ■ Identify the essential features of four periods in the history of radiation protection.

9 ■ Explain the three fundamental principles of radiation protection.

10 ■ State the meaning of technical aspects of radiation protection and procedural aspects of radiation protection.

11 ■ List three radiation protection quantities and their respective units.

12 ■ Define the term "quality assurance" and explain its role in radiation protection of patients and personnel.

13 ■ List international and national radiation protection organizations.

14 ■ Explain the responsibilities of the technologist in protecting the patient from radiation.

Introduction

Radiation protection in diagnostic radiology is concerned with the physical, technical, and procedural factors involved in protecting both patients and personnel from unnecessary radiation exposure. In addition, radiation protection requires an understanding of the biological effects of radiation because recommendations for the safe use of radiation are based on the risks of radiation exposure.

As pointed out by the International Commission on Radiological Protection (ICRP):

> . . . the primary aim of radiological protection is to provide an appropriate standard of protection for man without unduly limiting the beneficial practices giving rise to radiation exposure. This aim cannot be achieved on the basis of scientific concepts alone. All those concerned with radiological protection have to make value judgments about the relative importance of different kinds of risk and about the balancing of risks and benefits (ICRP, 1991, p. 3).

Radiation protection of the patient in radiology is of primary concern to the radiologic technologist for several reasons:

1. There is a great deal of evidence to suggest that radiation is harmful not only to exposed individuals but to their descendants as well.
2. The patient receives more radiation from diagnostic examinations than from any other source of radiation.
3. A number of dose–response models (relationships between different levels of dose and the biological reaction that is observed in the irradiated individual) suggest that no dose of radiation is safe.
4. There is evidence to suggest that some radiologic procedures deliver high doses of radiation.
5. The radiologic technologist is responsible for the technical aspects of examination that influence the radiation exposure to the patient. Radiation protection of the patient and other individuals will depend on the technical expertise of the technologist.

This chapter introduces a number of ideas and concepts necessary for an understanding of radiation protection in diagnostic radiology. The sources of data on biological effects of radiation and the rationale for protection are introduced at the beginning of the chapter. This is followed by an overview of the basic framework for radiation protection and exposure schemes in radiology, as well as by a discussion of how individuals are exposed. Our third topic deals with the fundamental principles and objectives of radiation protection as well as the technical considerations relating to protection in diagnostic radiology. The chapter concludes with an overview of agencies responsible for radiation protection standards and recommendations and the responsibilities of the technologist as a radiation worker.

A Rationale for Radiation Protection

As stated earlier, radiation protection deals with the protection of humans from the harmful effects of radiation. These harmful effects have been studied extensively, and information regarding the kinds of injury stems from several sources of data.

Sources of Data on Biological Effects

Radiation protection guides, standards, and recommendations are based on knowledge of the biological effects of radiation. The data on these radiation biological effects are derived from both animal and human studies.[1] The data for the human exposure come from the following:

1. Early radiation workers who were exposed to high doses, such as physicists and radiologists.
2. The atomic bomb explosions at Hiroshima and Nagasaki.
3. Nuclear reactor accidents such as the catastrophe at Three Mile Island and, more recently, at Chernobyl.
4. Patient exposure in radiation therapy.
5. Patient exposure in diagnostic radiology.

An important concept that has emerged from these studies is the dose–risk relationship. This has also been referred to as a dose–response model (defined earlier). The model shows what happens to the risk of radiation injury as the dose increases.

Dose–Response Models

The three dose–response models shown in Figure 1-1 will be addressed in greater detail in Chapter 4. They are introduced here only to make the following points:

1. The straight line portion above the curved dotted line, which starts from about 0.5 Sv (see Chapter 3 for a discussion of the various units of measure), indicates the biological effects of high doses of radiation, for example, those received as a result of an atomic bomb explosion.
2. The effects at low doses have been extrapolated from the high-dose effects because it is not possible to irradiate humans with low doses of radiation directly and study the effects. Three relationships are shown in the region where the dose is < 0.5 Sv. Scientists believe that these are the relationships for low-dose effects, and in 1990, they suggested that, for diagnostic radiology, the linear model is applicable because it represents a conservative estimate of the risks of radiation used to image humans.
3. Note that all three of the lines in the low-dose region start at 0. This means that no dose of radiation is thought to be safe, and there is some risk associated even with small doses. In this regard, these models are called *nonthreshold models*.
4. A *threshold model* is also seen in Figure 1-1. In this case, the model indicates that below a certain dose, referred to as the threshold dose, no effect is observed. It is only when

[1] *It is not within the scope of this chapter to discuss the details of these studies; however, they have been documented in several major reports of the Committee on the Biological Effects of Ionizing Radiation (BEIR) and the United Nations Scientific Committee on the Effects of Atomic Radiations (UNSCEAR). The interested student should refer to the BEIR V Report (1990) and the UNSCEAR Report (1988) for further details of these studies.*

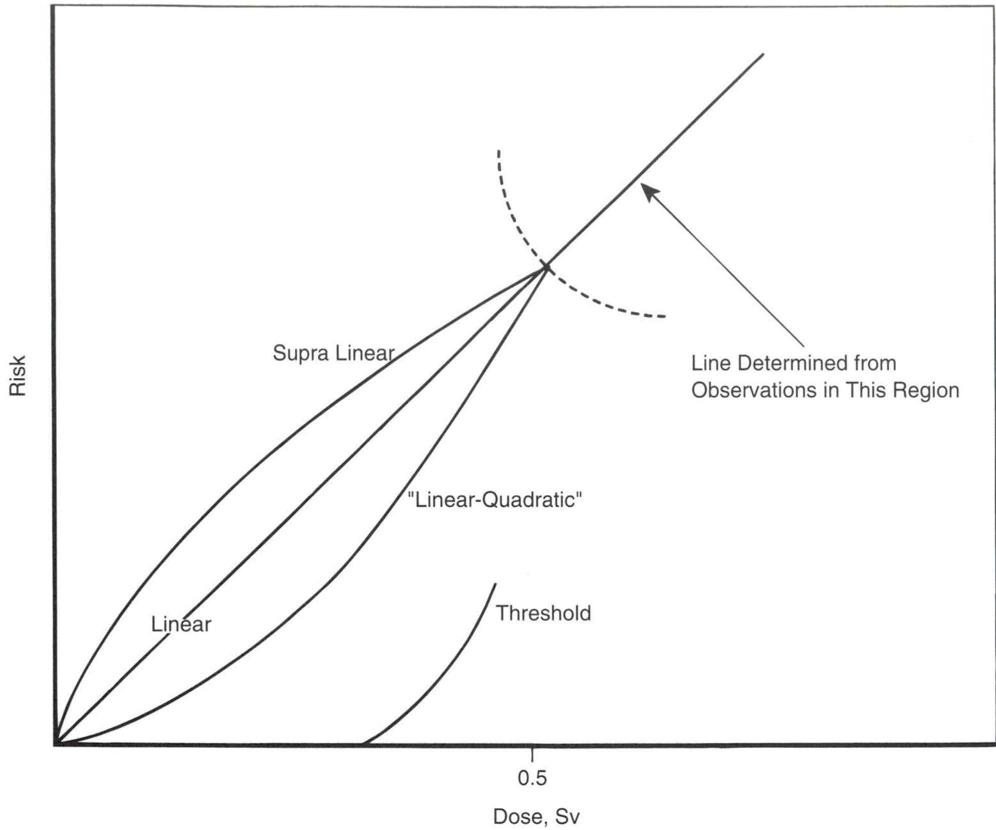

FIGURE 1-1. Three dose–response relationships. [From Southwood, Sir R. (1987). In Jones, R.R. & Southwood, R., eds. *Radiation and Health*. New York: John Wiley & Sons. Reproduced by permission.]

the threshold dose is reached that we begin to observe a biological effect.

Biological Effects

Biological effects can be placed into two categories: (1) *somatic effects*, those effects that appear in the individual exposed to radiation; and (2) *genetic effects*, those effects occurring in future descendants of the exposed individual.

Later, another system of classification of biological effects was introduced. This system is referred to as the stochastic/nonstochastic classification system.

The basic differences between stochastic and nonstochastic effects, which will be described in detail in Chapter 4, are: *Stochastic effects*, which are random in nature, are those in which the probability of the effect occurring depends on the amount of radiation dose. The effect increases as the dose increases. In addition, there is no threshold dose for stochastic effects.

Nonstochastic effects, however, are those effects for which the severity of the effect in the exposed individual increases as the radiation dose increases, and for which there is a threshold. Today nonstochastic effects are referred to as *deterministic effects* (ICRP, 1991).

Framework for Radiation Protection

Because exposure to radiation can be attributed to natural as well as man-made sources, radiation protection considerations must encompass some sort of framework within which we can operate. One comprehensive radiation protection framework is that of the ICRP, a framework subscribed to by various national radiation protection organizations including the National Council on Radiation Protection and Measurements (NCRP) in the United States, and the Radiation Protection Bureau (RPB), in Canada.

Framework of the ICRP

The framework adopted by the ICRP (1991) "is intended to prevent the occurrence of deterministic effects, by keeping doses below relevant thresholds and to ensure that all reasonable steps are taken to reduce the induction of stochastic effects" (p. 25). The framework encompasses a number of concepts, only two of which will be discussed here. The first is the types of exposure from which individuals can receive radiation doses: occupational exposure, medical exposure, and public exposure. Whereas occupational exposure refers to exposure due to work activities, medical exposure refers to exposure due to diagnostic examinations and radiation therapy procedures and does not include occupational exposure. Public exposure, on the other hand, constitutes all other exposures such as exposure to natural sources of radiation (see Chapter 3).

The second concept of the framework of importance to the radiologic technologist is what the ICRP refers to as "the system of radiological protection," which is guided by three fundamental principles:

1. *Justification* for exposing individuals to radiation. This gives rise to what has been referred to as a benefit–risk analysis.
2. That exposures be kept as low as reasonably achievable, taking into consideration economic and social factors. This is known as *the ALARA concept*, and it has become an important standard in radiation protection.
3. Establishment of *dose limits* to individuals exposed to radiation. These limits are numerical standards that are deemed to be acceptable and no greater than other risks, in light of the current knowledge of the biological effects of radiation.

These principles will be discussed further in Chapter 5.

Reduction of Dose Limits

Radiation dose limits have undergone several reductions throughout the years (Fig. 1-2). In 1990, the BEIR Committee revised its previously documented radiation risk estimates. The most recent report of the BEIR, Report V (1990), estimates the risk of radiation to be about three to four times greater than was previously estimated. This result is based on new risk models, revised dosimetry techniques, and better follow-up of those individuals who were exposed as a result of the atomic bomb explosions at Hiroshima and Nagasaki.

This major revision has led the ICRP to change its previously recommended dose limit for individuals who are occupationally exposed (technologists), from 50 millisieverts (5 rem) per year to 20 millisieverts (2 rem) per year (ICRP, 1991).

Exposure Factors in Diagnostic Radiology

There are several imaging modalities in radiology (diagnostic radiography, nuclear medicine, ultrasound, and magnetic resonance imaging) that deliver radiation exposures to patients and personnel. In this book, only conventional radiography and fluoroscopy, mammography, computed to-

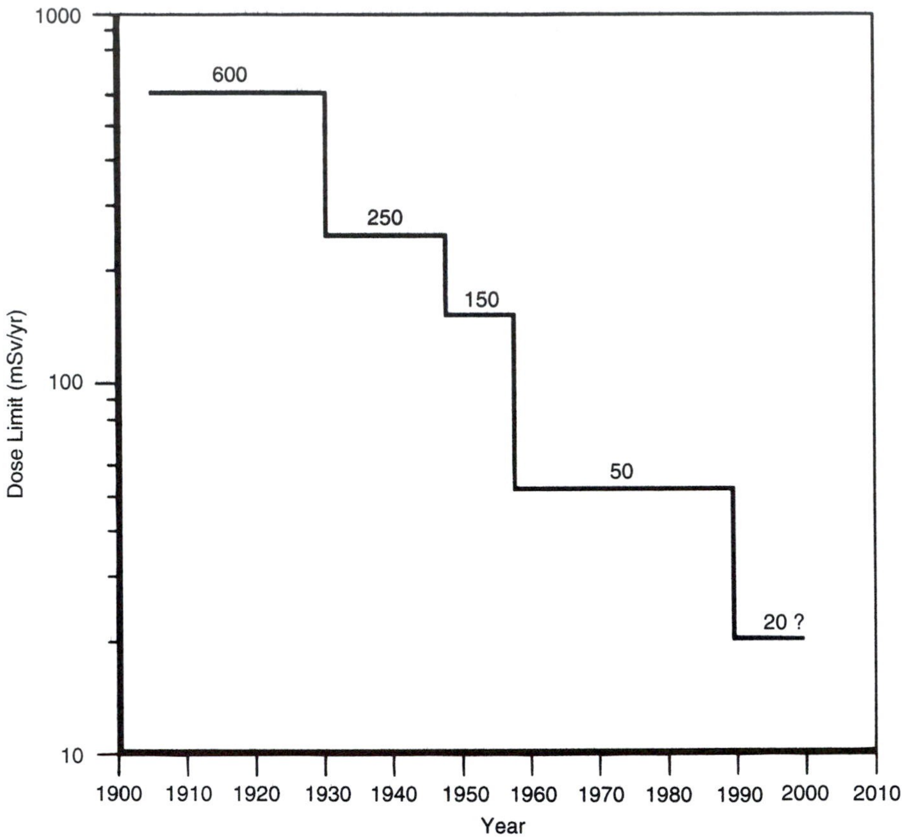

FIGURE 1-2. Trends in the annual whole body dose limit. [From Edwards, M. (1991). Development of radiation protection standards. *Radiographics, 11*, 699–705. Reproduced by permission.]

mography, and magnetic resonance imaging will be discussed. These will only be reviewed here with the goal of introducing some of the major factors affecting exposure in radiology.

Radiography

The basic scheme for patient exposure in radiography is illustrated in Figure 1-3. Several factors affecting patient exposure are shown, some of which are under the direct control of the technologist (such as the kVp, distance, beam area, grid, and screens) and some of which are not (waveform, thickness, and density of the patient and the tabletop). One of the major factors affecting patient exposure is that of the beam area incident on the patient. The technologist can limit this area, hence reducing patient dose by collimating the beam only to the anatomy of interest.

In addition to the factors shown in Figure 1-3 are *technique factors*, which determine the density and contrast of the radiographic image. These factors are the kilovoltage (kVp), the milliamperes (mA), and the exposure time, in seconds (s). Whereas the milliamperes (product of mA and time in seconds) determine the density of the radiograph, the kilovoltage primarily

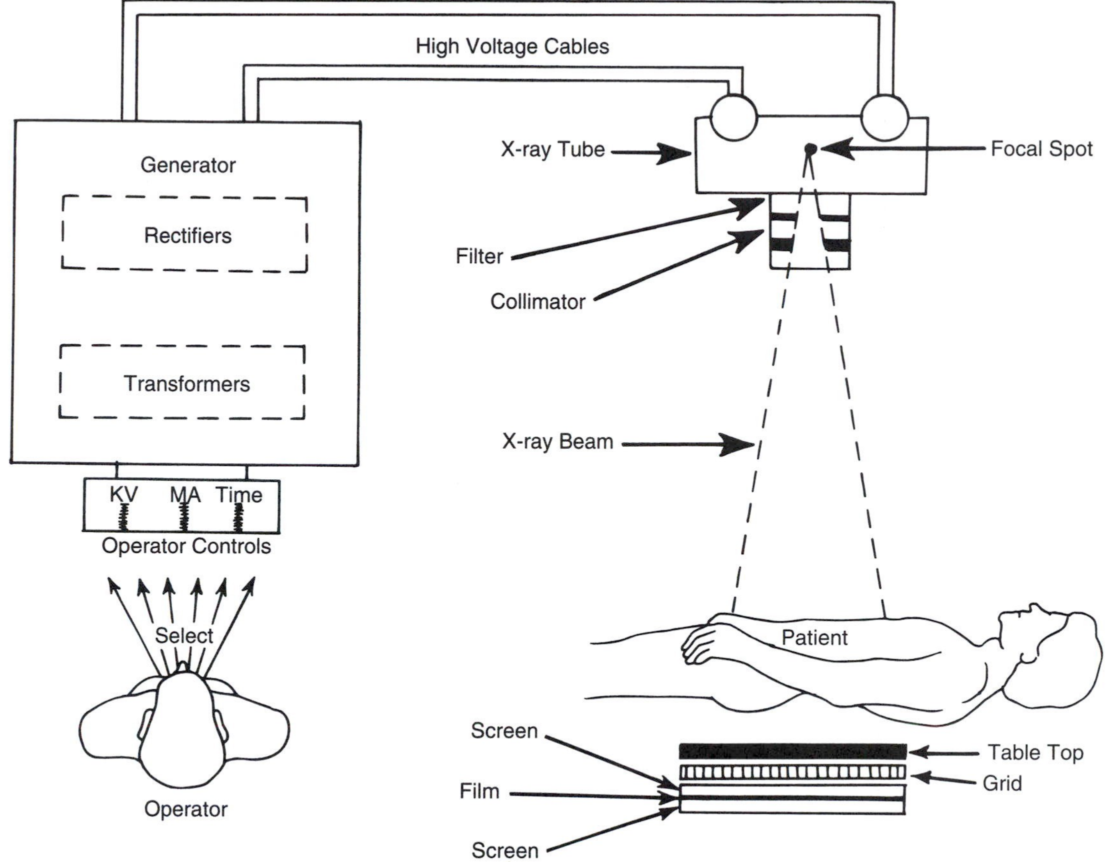

FIGURE 1-3. The basic scheme for patient exposure in conventional radiography. Several factors affecting patient exposure are shown as well. [From Sprawls, P. (1990). *Principles of radiography for technologists.* Rockville, MD: Aspen Publishers. Reproduced by permission.]

affects the contrast. It is important to realize that these factors also affect the dose to the patient in that the kilovoltage affects the penetration of the radiation beam, whereas the number of amperes affects the quantity of radiation falling on the patient.

High kilovoltage techniques with low milliamperes result in less dose to the patient (because more radiation is transmitted through the patient rather than being absorbed by the tissues) compared with low kilovoltage and high milliampere techniques, which result in more dose to the patient because more radiation is absorbed rather than being transmitted.

These factors will be discussed in detail when we deal with the factors affecting patient dose, which will be covered in Chapter 8.

Fluoroscopy

The same factors that affect patient exposure in radiographic procedures apply to fluoroscopy as well, except for a few minor differences. Fluoroscopy (Fig. 1-4) is governed by fluoroscopic technique factors, which include both kilovoltage and low tube currents (about 1–3 mA), which provide the image on the television monitor. In fluoroscopy the exposure to the pa-

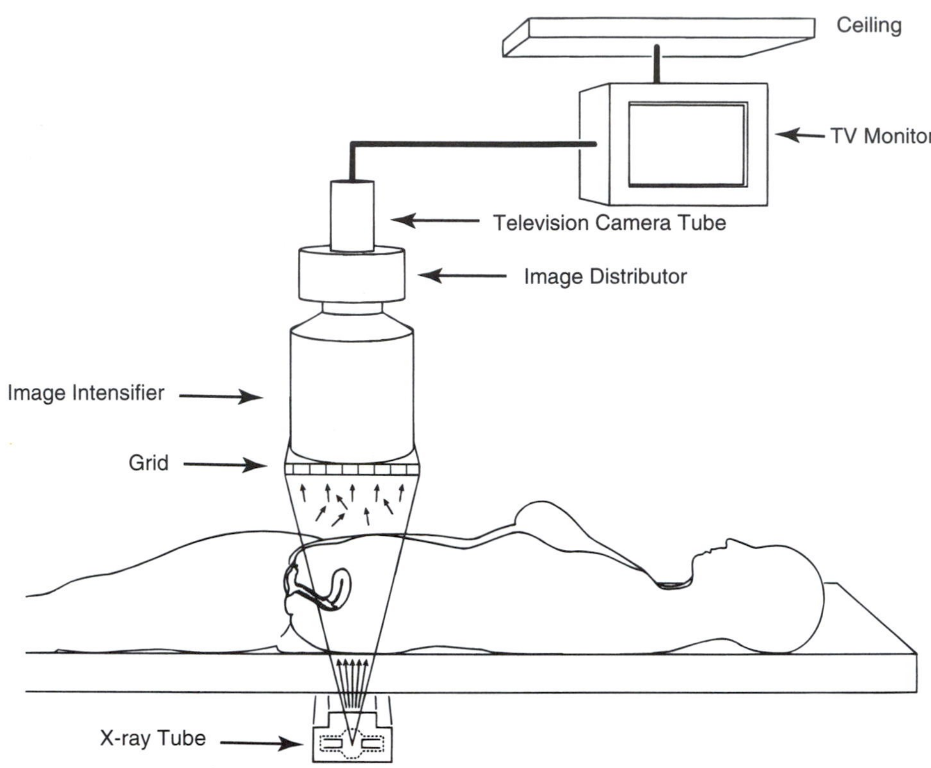

FIGURE 1-4. A generalized scheme for fluoroscopy. [From Wagner, L.K. (1985). *Exposure of the pregnant patient to diagnostic radiations*. Philadelphia: J.B. Lippincott. Reproduced by permission.]

tient lasts for several minutes (so that the radiologist has enough time to examine the television image).

During fluoroscopy the radiologist records images on film, and in this situation the machine is capable of switching from fluoroscopic factors to radiographic technique factors. In addition to these *spot film images*, as they are called, "overhead" radiographic images are also taken by the technologist after the fluoroscopic examination.

Another important point about patient exposure in fluoroscopy relates to the movement of the beam. Whereas the beam in radiography remains fixed and exposes one small region of the body, the beam in fluoroscopy may cover a greater region of the body because the nature of the examination dictates that the beam be made to scan the anatomy under consideration. For example, for an upper gastrointestinal fluoroscopic examination, the beam is moved from the neck, along the midline of the chest and subsequently along the upper abdominal area to examine the esophagus, stomach, and duodenum.

Patient exposure in fluoroscopy is of primary importance not only to the radiologist but also to the technologist for several reasons:

1. The beam may cover a wider area of the patient's body.
2. Fluoroscopic exposure factors are used during the fluoroscopic examination. The x-ray tube is energized for longer periods of time compared with the extremely short exposure times in radiography.
3. Radiographic exposure factors are used when the radiologist records a spot film and when the technologist records radiographic

images ("overheads") after the fluoroscopic portion of the procedure.

These factors will be discussed further in Chapter 8.

Mammography—Breast Imaging

Mammography, now referred to as breast imaging, is radiography of the breast. Because the breast is soft tissue, mammography is considered soft tissue radiography. The physical requirements for mammography are thus fundamentally different from those of conventional radiography. The major difference relates to the x-ray spectrum needed to image soft tissues. The spectrum is obtained using a molybdenum target with low kilovoltage techniques to obtain good differential absorption by the soft tissues. With low kilovoltage techniques, the number of milliamperes required in mammography is considerably high. Radiation protection in mammography is of vital importance not only because of the high doses (Bushong, 1993) but also because the breast is sensitive to radiation (Bushong, 1993). For these reasons, mammography is discussed further in Chapters 8, 9, and 10.

Computed Tomography

Computed tomography (CT) is a mathematically based technique that uses a computer to reconstruct images of the body based on x-ray transmission measurements recorded by special detectors. The beam geometry is significantly different from that used in radiography and fluoroscopy in that a highly collimated beam of radiation passes through very thin slices of the body. The anatomy can be scanned slice-by-slice or in large volumes. The basic scheme for patient exposure in conventional CT is shown in Figure 1-5. The x-ray tube rotates around the patient to image cross-sectional slices of the body. The radiation beam falls onto detectors that have several different properties compared with film.

The patient dose in CT varies depending on the nature of the examination. In general, the dose is affected by a number of image parame-

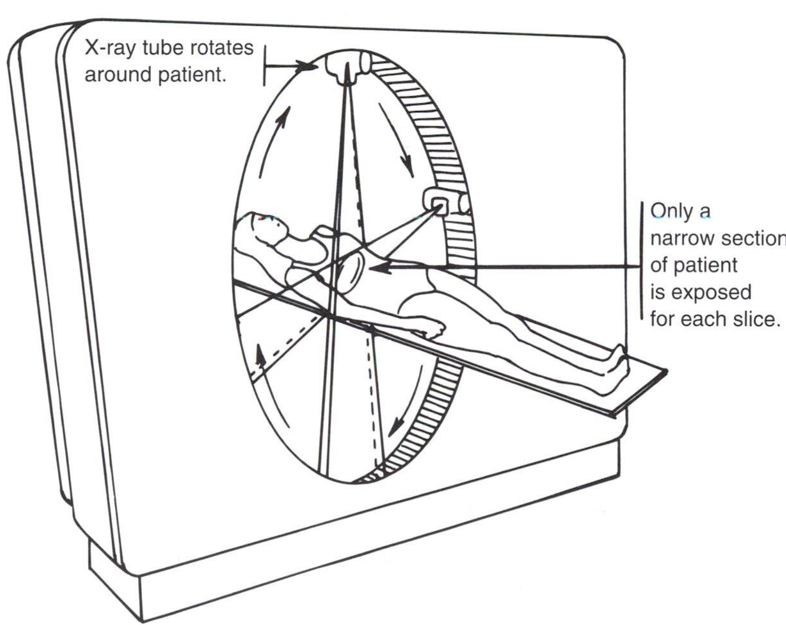

FIGURE 1-5. Exposure of the patient in computed tomography. A highly collimated beam of x-rays passes through a thin cross section of the anatomy. [From Wagner, L.K. (1985). *Exposure of the pregnant patient to diagnostic radiations*. Philadelphia: J.B. Lippincott. Reproduced by permission.]

ters and x-ray beam parameters. Whereas the beam parameters include kilovoltage, milliamperage, filtration, collimation, and detection efficiency, image parameters are related to dose through the following relationship:

$$\text{Dose} \propto \frac{1}{\sigma e^3 h}, \tag{1-1}$$

where σ = noise, e = spatial resolution, and h = slice thickness. From this relationship, if we wanted to improve spatial resolution by a factor of 2, the dose must be increased by a factor of 8. These factors will be discussed in Chapter 8.

Magnetic Resonance Imaging

Magnetic resonance imaging (MRI) is yet another diagnostic imaging technique that exposes the patient to forms of physical energy other than ionizing radiation (x-rays). MRI has become a useful tool in diagnostic radiology, and its applications have become increasingly commonplace. Equally important are the biological effects of the exposure fields operating in MRI.

The basic scheme for MRI is shown in Figure 1-6. First, the patient is placed in a strong stationary magnetic field, which causes magnetic nuclei in the body to become aligned with this field. The patient is then irradiated with radiowaves of a specific frequency. When the radiowaves are turned off, the patient emits radiowaves of the same frequency. These radiowaves are collected by a receiver and they are digitized for subsequent processing by a computer, which reconstructs an image of the internal anatomy. The third field operating in MRI is a moving magnetic field referred to as a gradient field. The purpose of this field is to isolate the signals coming from a particular region of the body; hence, it determines slice localization.

The biological effects of MRI have been studied by several investigators who have conducted research on the degree of harm posed by the three fields operating in MRI, that is, the static magnetic field, the time-varying magnetic field (gradient field), and radiofrequency (radiowaves) exposure.

MRI is a relatively new area of study in radiology in terms of biological effects, and protection and guidelines for the safe use of this modality have already been established. These

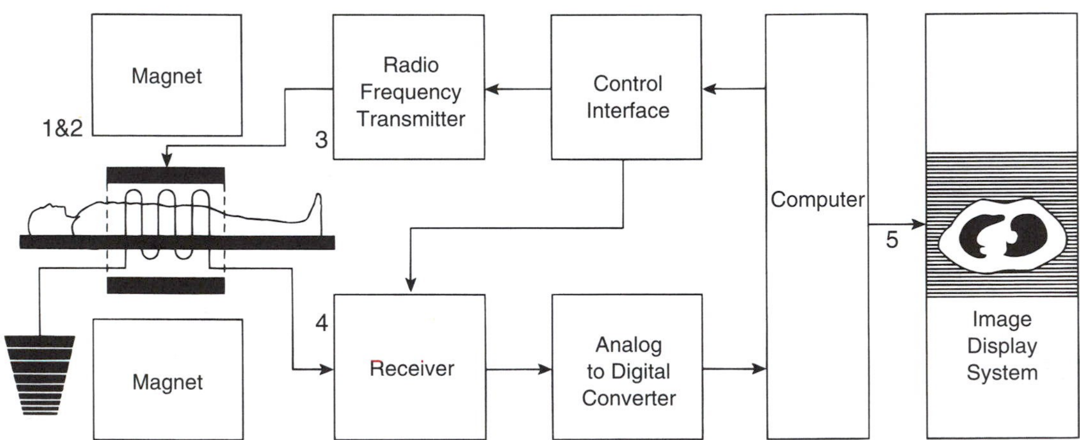

FIGURE 1-6. In magnetic resonance imaging, the patient is exposed to three fields: a static magnetic field, a moving magnetic field, and a radiofrequency field (radiowaves). [From NCRP. (1983). *Proceedings of the Eighteenth Annual Meeting. Radiation Protection and New Medical Diagnostic Approaches.* NCRP. Reproduced by permission.]

guidelines will change as the technology develops. MRI safety considerations will be discussed in Chapter 12.

Patient and Technologist Exposure

A knowledge of the ways in which the patient and technologist are exposed to radiation in the radiology department will serve as a guide to radiation protection. The three types of radiation to which patients and technologists are exposed are shown in Figure 1-7. These are *primary radiation* (radiation that emanates from the x-ray tube and passes through the patient to form the x-ray image), *leakage radiation* (radiation that penetrates the protective housing of the x-ray tube), and *scattered radiation* (radiation scattered by the patient as a result of Compton interactions).

Patient Exposure

The patient is always exposed to the primary beam or useful beam (as it is sometimes referred). The beam is shaped in such a manner as to image only the anatomy of interest. This is accomplished by collimation, which is under the direct control of the technologist. In pregnant patients, the conceptus (a term used "to

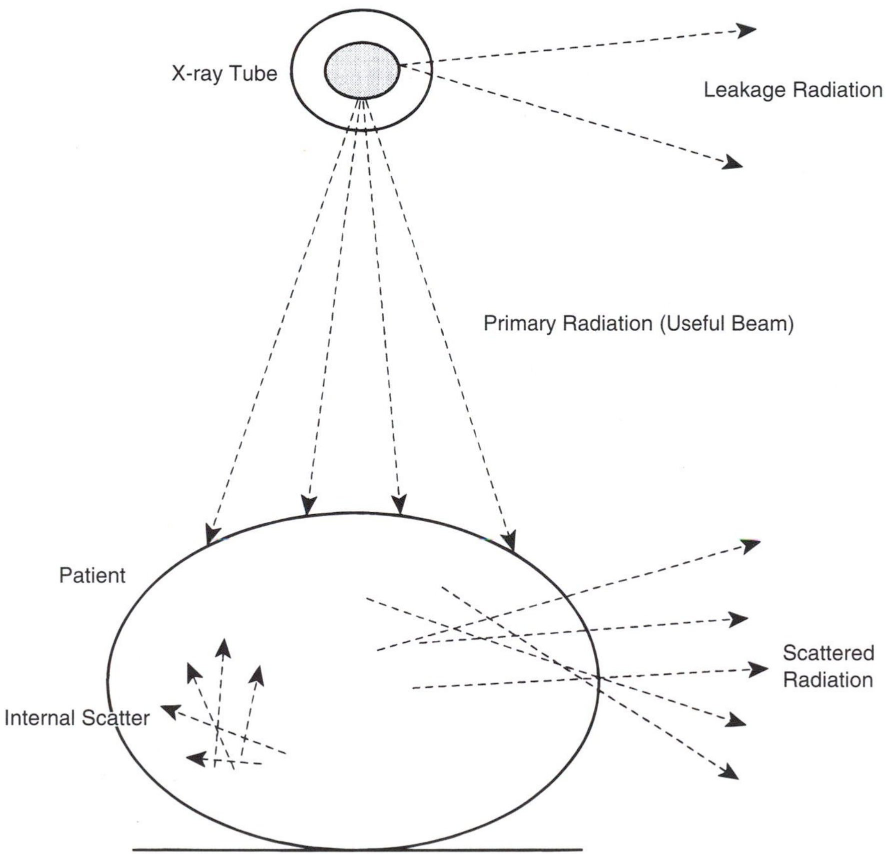

FIGURE 1-7. The three types of radiation to which patients and technologists are exposed in diagnostic radiology.

describe all the prenatal tissues from the moment of conception until birth" (Wagner, 1985, p. ix), is subject to exposure not only from scattered rays (Fig. 1-8) but also from the primary beam as well, as shown in Figure 1-9.

Technologist Exposure

The technologist is subject to exposure from leakage and scattered radiation if proper operational practices are not maintained. For example, if the technologist stands in the x-ray room outside the protective control booth, and without a protective lead apron during an exposure, she or he will be exposed to radiation scattered from the patient. Even in situations in which an apron is worn, such as in fluoroscopy, certain body regions of the technologist (the head, neck, and extremities, for example) are subject to exposure from scattered radiation. Patient and technologist exposure can be minimized only if the technologist pays careful attention to radiation protection concepts and practices and maintains the highest safety standards.

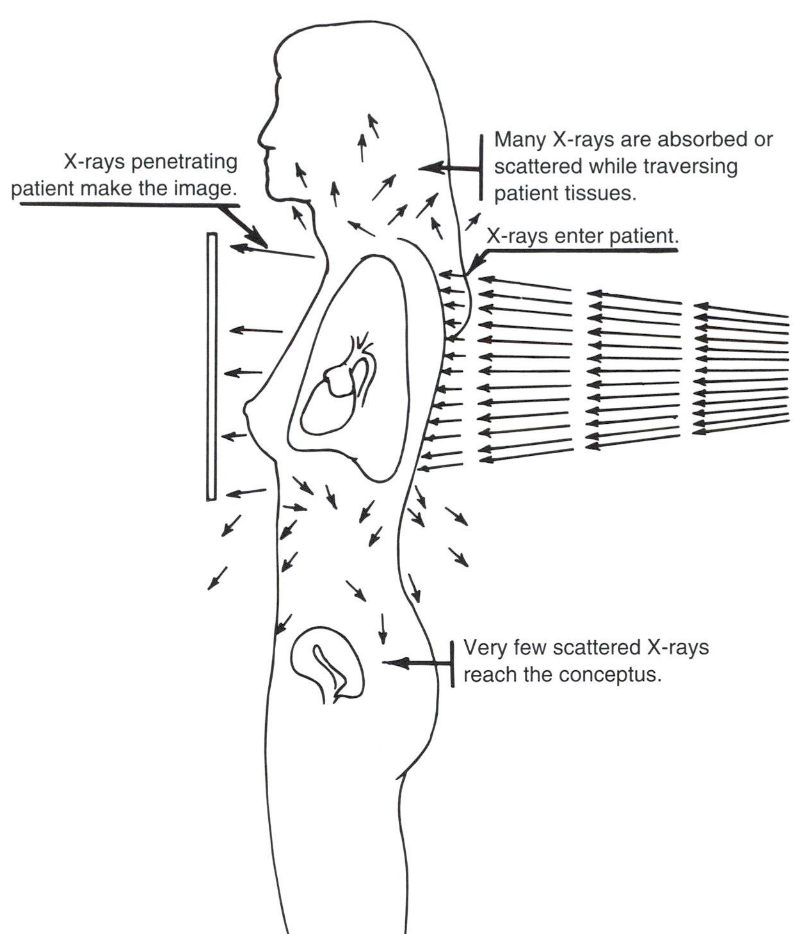

FIGURE 1-8. In radiography, while the patient is exposed by the useful beam (primary beam), the conceptus is exposed to radiation that is scattered in the patient. [From Wagner, L.K. (1985). *Exposure of the pregnant patient to diagnostic radiations*. Philadelphia: J.B. Lippincott. Reproduced by permission.]

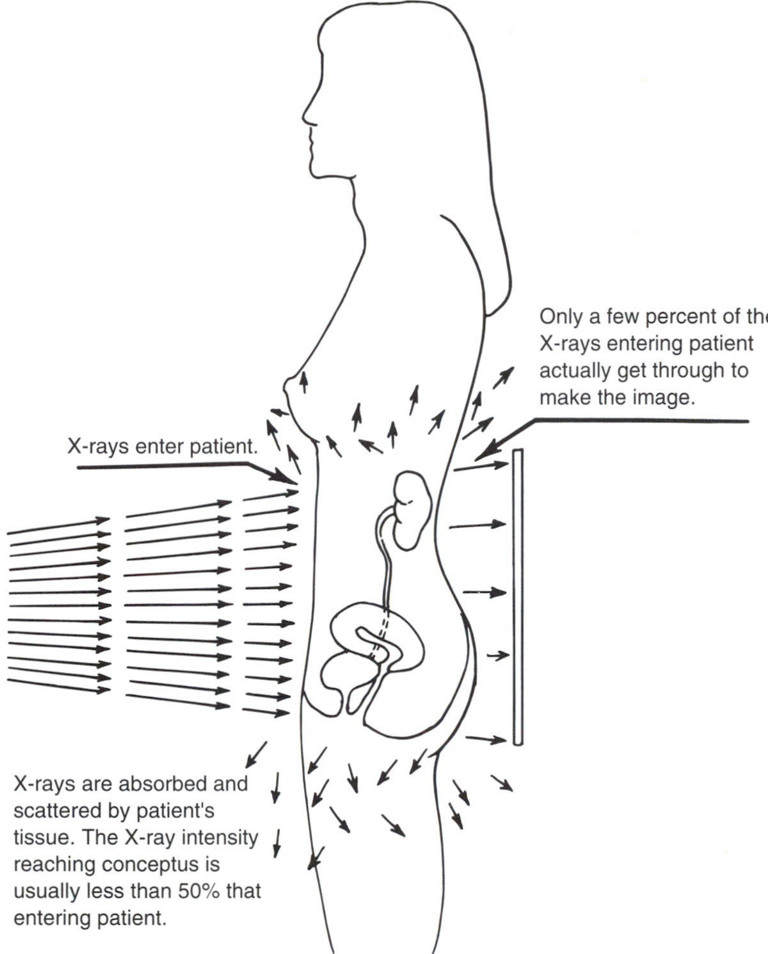

FIGURE 1-9. The conceptus can also be exposed to primary beam radiation. [From Wagner, L.K. (1985). *Exposure of the pregnant patient to diagnostic radiations*. Philadelphia: J.B. Lippincott. Reproduced by permission.]

Radiation Protection Concepts

The development of radiation protection concepts is guided by history, and in this section we begin our discussion by taking a cursory glance at what took place after W.C. Roentgen discovered x-rays in 1895.

Historical Perspectives

The need for radiation protection was recognized during the early 1900s, when early radiation workers observed skin changes as a result of long exposure to radiation. The history of radiation protection can be broken down into the four periods shown in Table 1-1. During these periods several concepts emerged that were particularly intended to reduce the amount of radiation to both the patient and the radiation worker. These concepts relate to various models of biologic injury, technical aspects of protection, the formation of scientific organizations whose function is solely dedicated to the field of radiation protection (for example, the Radiation Research Society and the Health Physics Society), and standards of practice for which vari-

TABLE 1-1. THE HISTORY OF THE DEVELOPMENT OF RADIATION PROTECTION METHODS

Era of the protection pioneers (1895–1915)
Marked by the initial recognition of the hazard of radiation and the development of the earliest protective measures by a small cadre of prescient pioneers.

Golden age of radiology (1915–1940)
Noteworthy not only as a time of great progress in the medical application of x-rays and radioactivity, but for the beginnings of established units of measurement and organized efforts in radiation protection.

Golden age of radiation protection (1940–1960)
The scientific and technical bases of modern protection were developed and the profession of health physics was born.

Modern era (1960 to present)
Characterized by great growth and complexity in the medical applications of x-rays, radioactivity, and new modalities. Intensified concern and regulation of all things radiological.

SOURCE: Brodsky, A., & Kathren, R. (1989). Historical development of radiation safety practices in radiology. *Radiographics*, 9, 1267–1275. Reproduced by permission.

ous guidelines and recommendations have been established. For example, current radiation protection standards are guided by three principles: net benefit of the exposure, ALARA, and a system of dose limitation.

The development of the concept of dose limits is an interesting topic to be explored from a historical perspective. For example, following early reports of radiation injury, soon after the discovery of x-rays, the idea of limiting the amount of radiation exposure an individual received began to emerge. This was marked by the introduction of the *erythema dose* (a certain amount of radiation needed to produce a reddening of the skin), followed by other concepts that experienced change to the present time.

The erythema dose, which was proposed by A. Mutscheller and R.M. Sievert, was followed by the use of the *tolerance dose*, a term used to refer to an acceptable level of radiation. Later, the ICRP replaced the term tolerance dose with the term *maximum permissible dose* (MPD), which was subsequently changed around 1977 to a concept referred to as the *dose equivalent limit*. These changes were attributed to the results of various studies on biological effects of radiation, such as studies by Müller (1928) and the Committee on the Biological Effects of Atomic Radiation (BEAR) (1960), which provided information on the risks of radiation.

Finally, the most recent change to the concept of dose limitation came about in 1990, when the ICRP, in Publication 60, once again made several changes to their radiation protection recommendations. One such change was the replacement of the term "dose equivalent limit" with the term "equivalent dose." In addition, the dose limit for occupationally exposed workers was reduced from 50 to 20 mSv per year. This revision was based on new information regarding the risks of radiation published in the BEIR V Report (1990), which concluded that the risks of radiation are three to four times greater than had been previously estimated in the BEIR III Report (1980).

These biological effects data serve to contribute to the development of radiation protection concepts and procedures. As researchers find out more about the biological effects of radiation, radiation protection guidelines and recommendations will continue to evolve.

Three Fundamental Principles

Anyone who works with radiation or who might be subject to radiation exposure should be familiar with what Bushong (1993) called "the cardinal principles of radiation protection." These principles are related to time, shielding, and distance, and they are intended to reduce the radiation exposure an individual may receive. Essentially, radiation exposure can be minimized if:

1. The time of the exposure is kept as short as possible because the exposure is directly proportional to time. In radiography, if we

increase the time by a factor of 2, then the dose is also increased by a factor of 2.

2. A protective shield is placed between the x-ray tube and the individuals exposed (patient and technologist). The shield, which is usually made of lead, can be placed on top of the patient's gonads to absorb unnecessary radiation.
3. The distance from the radiation source and the individual exposed is kept as great as possible. When the distance increases, the radiation exposure decreases according to a physical law referred to as the *inverse square law.* The mathematical expression for this law is:

$$I \propto \frac{1}{d^2}, \quad (1\text{-}2)$$

where I = intensity of the radiation and d = distance. The expression is read as follows: the intensity of radiation is inversely proportional to the square of the distance.

These principles will be discussed further in Chapter 5.

Technical and Procedural Considerations

In addition to the fundamental principles, radiation protection involves technical and procedural considerations. Whereas *technical* considerations refer to equipment design intended to minimize and control radiation exposure, and the design of radiation facilities to provide a safe environment in which to work (such as the design of protective shielding), *procedural* aspects refer to the ways in which activities are performed to reduce the exposure to individuals. For example, the technologist should always conduct a radiographic examination such that:

1. Patient positioning is accurate, so as to avoid repeats due to poor positioning.
2. The technique factors (kilovoltage and milliamperage) are optimized to reduce the dose to the patient and maintain acceptable image quality.
3. The appropriate film-screen combination is used.
4. Only the minimal number of views is taken.
5. The patient's gonads are protected by using a lead shield.
6. The useful beam is collimated to the anatomy of interest.
7. The technologist always remains in the protective control booth in the x-ray room during the exposure or wears a lead apron when standing outside the control booth, as is the case in fluoroscopy.
8. The technologist ensures that the patient understands all instructions with respect to respiration and motion.
9. The patient is observed during the exposure.
10. The patient is free of any foreign objects (such as necklaces, watches, buttons, or hairpins) that may result in a repeat examination because these objects will appear as image artifacts and interfere with diagnosis.
11. The patient is properly immobilized if required.

Patient Exposure and Image Quality

The goal of radiology is to contribute to restoring the patient's well-being through diagnosis and therapy. Diagnosis is dependent upon optimum image quality, which requires adequate radiation exposure. Image quality factors such as contrast, blur, density, and noise all depend on the patient exposure. "Within certain limits, increasing image quality requires an increase in patient exposure" (Sprawls, 1990, p. 254). On the other hand, the objectives of radiation protection require that to prevent biological effects, the radiation dose to an individual should be kept as low as reasonably achievable. Therefore, it is essential that a compromise be maintained between image quality and radiation dose.

Radiation Quantities and Units

Another important radiation protection concept is that of radiation quantities and their units. There are three fundamental radiation quantities of importance to the technologist. These are *exposure, absorbed dose,* and *dose equivalent.* Whereas *exposure* refers to the quantity of radiation falling on the patient, *absorbed dose* is the amount of energy absorbed by the patient per unit mass of tissue. *Dose equivalent,* on the other hand, refers to occupational exposure, the radiation received by radiation workers. In 1990 the ICRP recommended that the term "dose equivalent" be replaced by the term "equivalent dose."

The new unit of exposure (international system of units = SI units) is the *coulomb per kilogram* (C/kg), which replaced the old unit, the roentgen (R) where $1 \text{ R} = 2.58 \times 10^{-4}$ C/kg. The unit of absorbed dose is the *gray* (Gy), which refers to 1 joule (J) of energy deposited in 1 kg of material. Finally, the unit of equivalent dose is the *sievert* (Sv), which is equal to the absorbed dose multiplied by the quality factor for the particular radiation.

These terms and their units will be explained in greater detail in Chapter 3.

Quality Assurance/Total Quality Management/Continuous Quality Improvement

The idea and concepts of *quality assurance* (QA) have become mandatory and commonplace in radiology departments. QA programs are intended to ensure the production of optimum diagnostic information with minimum cost to the institution and minimal dose to patients. QA includes both *quality control* (QC) and *quality administration.* Whereas QC pertains to the technical aspects of instrumentation, quality administration addresses management aspects that ensure that QC monitoring is carried out judiciously.

The technologist plays an important role in QC programs, and with adequate training the technologist may even assume the role of "quality control technologist." The QC technologist is viewed as an individual who carries out QC test procedures, records the results, and, in some cases, interprets and makes recommendations for corrective action.

One of the goals of QC programs is to ensure that diagnostic images are obtained with minimal radiation dose to the patient. In doing so, the QC program is designed to monitor all the appropriate variables in the imaging chain that affect dose. For example, QC in diagnostic radiography would ensure that the kilovoltage, milliamperage, and exposure time are accurate and that the radiation output from the x-ray tube corresponds to the correct value for the appropriate technique selection.

QC tests that check the radiation dose in fluoroscopy, mammography, and CT have now become routine in institutions where these procedures are done. In Chapter 13, we elaborate on QC concepts only as they relate to radiation protection.

More recently, two other concepts have emerged to relate to the idea of quality assurance. These are *total quality management* (TQM) and *continuous quality improvement* (CQI), and they are beginning to receive attention in the radiology literature (Evans, 1993; Nelson, 1994; Hynes, 1994).

The TQM system essentially involves the notion that the entire staff of a facility should participate in the review of both the paradigm and the procedures that contribute to the delivery of quality patient care services (Evans, 1993). It is recommended that those institutions undergoing accreditation by the Joint Commission for Accreditation of Healthcare Organizations (JCAHO) make use of the TQM system for such reviews.

The concept of CQI, initially developed for use in industry, is now being applied to the health care industry. As pointed out by Hynes (1994), CQI "dictates that every activity in an imaging facility be identified and clear standards (indicators) set and measured to allow development of policies amenable to evaluation and review, with the aim of yet further improvement" (p. 354).

Radiation Protection Organizations and Reports

In our discussion so far, we have been referring to one important radiation protection organization, that is, the ICRP. There are a number of other organizations, committees, and agencies that play major roles in the development and implementation of radiation protection guides and control procedures.

Organizations

Essentially, organizations can be classified as either international or national. There are several international groups including the following: International Commission on Radiological Protection (ICRP), International Commission on Radiological Units and Measurements (ICRU), International Atomic Energy Agency (IAEA), and International Radiation Protection Association (IRPA).

The ICRP's recommendations are usually adapted by several countries to meet their own needs. For example, in the United States, one such organization includes the National Council on Radiation Protection and Measurements (NCRP). In Canada, the main agency is the Radiation Protection Bureau (RPB). In Great Britain, the organization is the National Radiological Protection Board (NRPB). The NRPB has been instrumental in establishing guidelines for MRI.

Radiation protection organizations will be discussed in Chapter 6.

Reports and Publications

Radiation protection guides, standards, and control procedures are officially documented in various reports and publications. Several of these, which are particularly important to the radiologic technologist, include the following:

1. ICRP Publication 34: *Protection of the Patient in Diagnostic Radiology.*
2. ICRP Publication 60: *1990 Recommendations of the International Commission on Radiological Protection.*
3. NCRP Report No. 99: *Quality Assurance for Diagnostic Imaging Equipment.*
4. NCRP Report No. 100: *Exposure of the U.S. Population from Diagnostic Medical Radiation.*
5. NCRP Report No. 102: *Medical X-Ray, Electron Beam and Gamma-Ray Protection for Energies up to 50 MeV (Equipment Design, Performance and Use).*
6. NCRP Report No. 105: *Radiation Protection for Medical and Allied Health Personnel.*
7. NCRP Report No. 107: *Implementation of the Principle of as Low as Reasonably Achievable (ALARA) for Medical and Dental Personnel.*
8. NCRP Report No. 116: *Limitation of Exposure to Ionizing Radiation.*
9. Safety Code 20A: *X-Ray Equipment in Medical Diagnosis Part A: Recommended Safety Procedures for Installation and Use. Health and Welfare Canada.*
10. Safety Code 26: *Guidelines on Exposure to Electromagnetic Fields from Magnetic Resonance Clinical Systems. Health and Welfare Canada.*

Radiation Protection and the Technologist

Ultimately, the radiologist in charge of the department has the responsibility of ensuring radiation protection of patients and personnel. The radiologist must be trained in radiation protection theory and practice as well as keep up-to-date with changes in radiation protection recommendations as imaging technologies continue to evolve and as we obtain more information on the biological effects of radiation. The radiologist, however, may assign this particular responsibility to another individual depending on the size of the radiology facility. Usually, this task (radiation safety) is assigned to a person specifically trained in health physics or to a person trained in medical physics. The health physicist, as Bushong (1993) indicated, "is a radiation scientist, engineer or physician concerned with the research, teaching, or operational aspects of radiation safety." This person is generally referred to as a radiation safety officer (RSO) or simply a safety officer.

In cases in which hospitals and/or radiology departments cannot support such officers, other individuals are appointed to facilitate radiation protection practices. It is also important that these individuals be trained in radiation protection.

The radiologic technologist receives training in radiation protection (hence, the need for this book) as well as education in radiological physics, radiographic technique, and radiation biology. The technologist is therefore prepared to assume a fundamental and significant role in radiation protection.

Responsibilities

The technologist conducts the radiographic examination of the patient and is therefore ultimately responsible for the direct radiation protection measures applied to the patient. The first responsibility, therefore, is to the patient. In doing so, the technologist also has a responsibility to the population because medical radiation represents the largest man-made source of radiation exposure to the population. As a conscientious radiation worker, the technologist plays a significant role in minimizing the radiation risks to the population.

The technologist also has a responsibility to herself or himself and to other personnel who work in radiology or those who may be subject to exposure where radiological examinations are conducted. For example, when an examination is conducted with mobile equipment in the emergency department, the technologist "should be cognizant of orientation of the beam with respect to any other patients, employees or other individuals in the room" (NCRP, 1989, p. 50). In addition, "a female operator should be encouraged to notify her employer if she believes herself to be pregnant, in order that appropriate steps may be taken to ensure that her work duties during the remainder of the pregnancy are compatible with accepted maximum radiation exposure . . ." (Health and Welfare Canada, 1992, p. 13).

The fourth area of responsibility falls within the domain of continuing education. It is mandatory that the technologist keep current with the changes and developments not only in radiation protection but also in related topics as well, such as radiation risks.

Radiation protection is an integral part of the curriculum of radiologic technology programs. It is significant to the daily activities of the technologist for reasons highlighted in this chapter. The concepts and principles of radiation protection relevant to the radiologic technologist will be elaborated in the chapters to follow.

REVIEW QUESTIONS

1. The factors involved in protecting patients and personnel from unnecessary radiation in diagnostic radiology include:
   A. Physical factors.
   B. Technical factors.
   C. Procedural factors.
   D. All of the above.

2. Recommendations for the safe use of radiation are based on the:
   A. Patient's clinical problem.
   B. Technical factors used in the examination.
   C. Risks of radiation exposure.
   D. Value judgments of the staff conducting the examination.

3. Which of the following represents the data from which human exposure to radiation is derived?
   A. Atomic bomb explosion at Hiroshima and Nagasaki.
   B. Nuclear reactor accidents.
   C. Patient exposure in radiation therapy and diagnostic radiology.
   D. All of the above.

4. In a nonthreshold dose–response model:
   A. No dose of radiation is safe.
   B. No effect is observed below a certain dose of radiation referred to as the threshold dose.
   C. A biological effect is observed when the threshold dose is exceeded.
   D. All of the above.

5. Which of the following dose–response models is best applicable to diagnostic radiology?
   A. Supralinear model.
   B. Linear quadratic model.
   C. Linear model.
   D. Threshold model.

6. Which of the following refers to the somatic effects of radiation exposure?
   A. Effects appear in the offspring of the individual exposed.
   B. Effects appear in the genes of the offspring's children.
   C. There is no threshold dose for somatic effects.
   D. Effects appear in the individual exposed and there is a threshold dose for such effects.

7. The framework of the ICRP for radiation protection is intended to:
   A. Prevent deterministic effects (nonstochastic effects) from appearing.
   B. Keep doses below relevant thresholds.
   C. Minimize the induction of stochastic effects.
   D. All of the above.

8. Which of the following refers to exposures received during diagnostic and therapeutic examinations?
   A. Medical exposure.
   B. Occupational exposure.
   C. Public exposure.
   D. All of the above.

9. Which of the following concepts deals with keeping exposures to a minimum?
   A. Benefit–risk analysis.
   B. ALARA.
   C. Dose limitation.
   D. Justification.

10. The current annual dose limit for radiologic technologists is:
    A. 50 Sv.
    B. 50 mSv.
    C. 20 mSv.
    D. 20 Sv.

11. Exposure technique factors include all of the following except:
    A. Collimation.
    B. kVp.
    C. mA.
    D. Seconds.

12. Which of the following uses a computer to build up an image of the patient?
    A. Radiography.
    B. Computed tomography.
    C. Fluoroscopy.
    D. Mammography.

13. Which of the following uses radiowaves to produce images of patients?
    A. Magnetic resonance imaging.
    B. Computed tomography.
    C. Digital radiography.
    D. Digital fluoroscopy.

14. Which of the following delivers the radiation dose needed to produce the image of the patient?
    A. Primary radiation.
    B. Secondary radiation.
    C. Scattered radiation.
    D. Leakage radiation.

15. Which of the following terms is currently used to refer to an acceptable level of radiation for technologists?
    A. Erythema dose.
    B. Tolerance dose.
    C. Maximum permissible dose.
    D. Dose equivalent limit.

16. In radiography, if the exposure time is increased by a factor of 4, the dose will:
    A. Increase by a factor of 2.
    B. Increase by a factor of 4.
    C. Decrease by a factor of 4.
    D. Decrease by a factor of 8.

17. The inverse square law states that the intensity of radiation:
    A. Decreases inversely as the square of the distance.
    B. Is directly proportional to the square of the distance.
    C. Increases as the distance increases.
    D. Is directly proportional to the mAs.

18. The technical aspects of radiation protection refer to all of the following except:
    A. Observation of the patient during the examination.
    B. Equipment design to minimize radiation exposure.
    C. Shielding the facilities to protect workers and patients and members of the public from unnecessary radiation exposure.
    D. Equipment specifications to control radiation exposure.

19. The SI unit of radiation exposure is the:
    A. Gray (Gy).
    B. Sievert (Sv).
    C. Coulombs per kilogram (C/kg).
    D. Roentgen.

20. Absorbed dose is the:
    A. Quantity of radiation falling on the patient.
    B. Radiation received by the radiation worker during work activities.
    C. Amount of energy absorbed by the individual per unit mass of tissue.
    D. All of the above.

21. The unit of absorbed dose is the:
    A. C/kg.
    B. gray.
    C. sievert.
    D. rem.

22. The unit of equivalent dose is the:
    A. C/kg.
    B. gray.
    C. sievert.
    D. rad.

23. Quality control deals with all of the following except:
    A. Equipment performance.
    B. Quality control tests.
    C. Corrective action.
    D. Management of human resources.

24. In the United States, which of the following is most significant in the development of radiation protection standards?
    A. ICRP.
    B. NCRP.
    C. NRPB.
    D. IRPA.

25. Who plays a major role in protecting patients from unnecessary radiation exposure during radiographic examinations?

A. The technologist.
B. The medical physicist.
C. The radiologist.
D. The patient's physician.

REFERENCES

Bushong, S. (1993). *Radiologic science for technologists* (5th ed.). St Louis: Mosby-Year Book.

Committee on the Biological Effects of Ionizing Radiations: *Health Effects of Low Levels of Ionizing Radiation* (BEIR V). National Academy Press. 1990.

Evans, K.D. (1993). In Total quality management for the ultrasound department. *Journal of Diagnostic Medical Sonography, 9,* 202–205.

Health and Welfare Canada. (1992). *Safety code 20A: X-ray equipment in medical diagnosis. Part a: Recommended safety procedures for installation and use.* Ottawa: Radiation Protection Bureau.

Hynes, D.M. (1994). Quality management. *Journal of the Canadian Association of Radiologists, 45,* 353–354.

International Commission on Radiological Protection. (1991). *1990 recommendations of the International Commission on Radiological Protection.* [ICRP Publication 60. Annals of the ICRP 21 (1–3)]. Elsmford, NY: Pergamon Press.

Müller, HJ (1927). Artificial transmutation of the gene. *Science* 66: p 84–86.

National Council on Radiation Protection and Measurements. (1989). *Radiation protection for medical and allied health personnel* (NCRP Report No. 105). Bethesda, MD: NCRP.

Nelson, M.T. (1994). Continuous quality improvement (CQI) in radiology: An overview. *Applied Radiology,* Vol 23. No. 7 p. 11–16.

Sprawls, P. (1990). *Principles of radiography for technologists.* Rockville, MD: Aspen Publishers.

Travis, E. (1989). *Primer of medical radiobiology* (2nd ed.). Chicago: Year Book Medical.

United Nations Scientific Committee on the Effects of Atomic Radiation: *Sources, Effects and Risks of Ionizing Radiation. Report to the General Assembly.* United Nations, New York. 1988

Wagner, L.K. (1985). *Exposure of the pregnant patient to diagnostic radiations.* Philadelphia: J.B. Lippincott.

SUGGESTED READINGS

Evans, K.D. (1993). Total quality management for the ultrasound department. *Journal of Diagnostic Medical Sonography, 9,* 202–205.

Hynes, D.M. (1994). Quality management. *Journal of the Canadian Association of Radiologists, 45,* 353–354.

Nelson, M.T. (1994). Continuous quality improvement (CQI) in radiology: An overview. *Applied Radiology,* 23, 11–16.

CHAPTER TWO

Essential Physics for Radiation Protection: An Overview

Learning Objectives

Upon completion of this chapter, the reader should be able to:

1. Describe the basic structure of the atom.
2. Explain two processes by which energy is dissipated in matter.
3. Identify two types of radiation and describe the essential characteristics of each.
4. List the properties of x-rays and describe how x-rays are produced in an x-ray tube.
5. Explain the production of bremsstrahlung radiation and characteristic radiation.
6. Define the term x-ray emission spectrum.
7. Define the terms x-ray quality and x-ray quantity and discuss the factors affecting each of them.
8. Explain the following three mechanisms of x-ray interaction with matter: classical scattering, Compton effect, and photoelectric absorption.
9. Define each of the following terms: radiation attenuation, linear attenuation coefficient, mass attenuation coefficient, and half value layer.
10. Explain the following two classes of radiation interaction that lead to biological responses in living things: direct action and indirect action.
11. Describe the basic chemical reactions that occur when radiation interacts with water.
12. Define the terms linear energy transfer (LET) and relative biological effectiveness (RBE) and briefly describe the relationship between LET and RBE.

Introduction

Protecting patients from unnecessary radiation in diagnostic radiology requires that the radiologic technologist possess an understanding of certain fundamental principles in physics. Without such an understanding, the radiologic technologist would have neither a foundation for understanding the nature of radiation-induced biological effects nor an appreciation of the steps necessary to prevent them.

The purpose of this chapter is to describe, with little mathematics, the essential physics of how radiation is absorbed in tissue. The topics addressed range from atomic structure, energy dissipation in matter, and the nature of electromagnetic radiations. Also examined are the interactions of radiation with matter, radiation attenuation, and other physical factors, such as linear energy transfer and relative biological effectiveness.

Atomic Structure

When a beam of x-rays passes through the body, x-ray photons interact with the electrons of the atoms making up the various tissues. For this reason, it is important to review the structure of the atom.

All matter consists of atoms, the building blocks of the universe. The modern picture of the atom is based on the theoretical work of Niels Bohr, who presented his planetary model of the atom in 1913. In this model, the atom is shown as consisting of a dense nucleus surrounded by electrons. This model is used to depict the helium atom in Figure 2-1.

Atomic Nucleus

The *nucleus*, which forms the focal point around which the rest of the atom is gathered, is positively charged and consists of two particles, protons and neutrons. These nuclear particles are collectively known as *nucleons*. Whereas *protons* are positively charged, *neutrons* are electrically neutral. When the number of protons equals the number of orbital electrons, the atom is said to be electrically neutral.

The number of protons within the nucleus is called the *atomic number* (Z) and the total

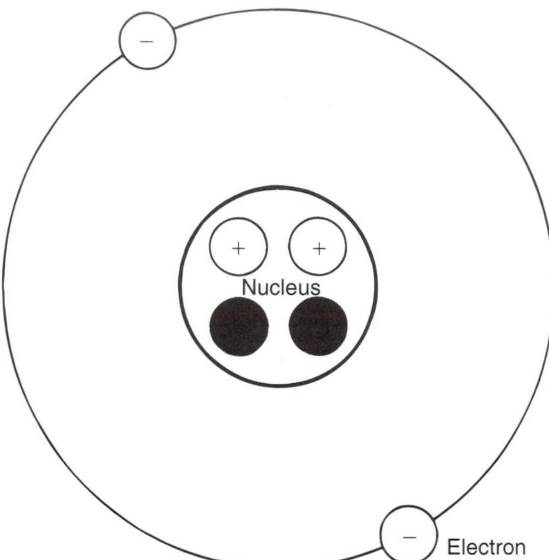

FIGURE 2-1. Bohr's planetary model of the atom shows a dense nucleus surrounded by orbiting electrons.

number of nucleons (protons and neutrons) is called the *mass number* (A). The mass number must not be confused with the *atomic mass*, the actual mass of the atom.

Electrons

Electrons are the negatively charged particles that orbit the central nucleus. Depending on the atom, electrons orbit the nucleus at fixed distances in different orbital levels referred to as *quantum levels*. These levels, or shells (so called because the orbits are three-dimensional), are represented by the letters K, L, M, N, O . . . , with the K shell being the innermost shell (closest to the nucleus). These shells are also assigned corresponding *quantum numbers* (1, 2, 3, 4, 5 . . .) with the K shell being assigned the quantum number of 1. The number of electrons contained in each shell is given by the expression $2(n)^2$, where n is the quantum number of the shell. For example, the K shell can contain only two electrons $[2 \times (1)^2]$, while the M shell can have only 18 electrons $[2 \times (3)^2] = 2 \times 9$. Figure 2-2 illustrates the arrangement of electrons in various shells, or orbital levels, around the nucleus.

Electrons that are closer to the nucleus have greater binding energies than those that are farther away. This means that it will take more energy to remove a K-shell electron than to remove an electron in the O-shell, for example.

As the number of protons in the nucleus increases, the binding energy increases as well. This means that the binding energy for a hydrogen (Z = 1) K-shell electron is less than that of the K-shell electron of tungsten (Z = 74).

Electrons can be transferred to other orbits within the atom or they can be completely removed from the atom. The removal of an electron from its orbit creates a vacancy, or hole, in that orbit. This prompts a cascading effect, in which the hole is immediately filled by an electron from an outer orbit, and so on down through successively affected orbits. In other words, if an electron from a K-shell is ejected, an electron from the L-shell may fill the vacancy in the K-shell; the L-shell vacancy may be filled by an electron from the M-shell, and so on. The energy released by these electron transitions is expressed in one of two ways: as electromagnetic or particulate radiation. The characteristics of each of these types of radiation will be reviewed subsequently.

Energy Dissipation in Matter

Excitation

In *excitation* a fraction of the energy of the radiation is transferred to the electrons of the absorbing material. Electrons respond by jumping to another orbital level farther away from the nucleus. They are not ejected from the atom. This process is shown in Figure 2-3, where the K-shell electron is raised to the L-shell as the

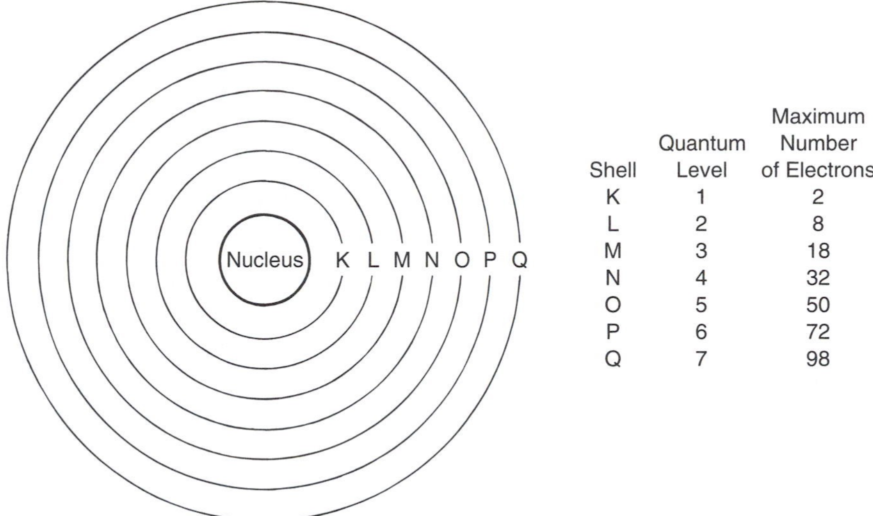

Shell	Quantum Level	Maximum Number of Electrons
K	1	2
L	2	8
M	3	18
N	4	32
O	5	50
P	6	72
Q	7	98

FIGURE 2-2. The arrangement of electrons in various shells or orbital levels around the nucleus.

positive charge passes the atom. As the positive charge moves away from the atom, the electron falls back into its original orbit.

Ionization

In contrast to excitation, *ionization* occurs when the radiation has enough energy to eject the electron completely from the atom. In other words, the amount of energy is greater than the binding energy of the electron. In this case, the radiation is referred to as ionizing radiation. Every ionization results in an energy dissipation of ~33 electron volts (eV), the amount of energy needed to break chemical bonds.

Ionization results in *ion pairs*, which are made up of the ejected electron (negative ion) and the portion of the atom that remains after loss of the electron (positive ion). See Figure 2-4 for a depiction of just such an ion pair. Depending on its energy, the ejected electron can cause further ionizations along the length of the path it travels in the absorbing material. This process, referred to as *secondary ionization*, gives rise to secondary electrons, or "delta rays."

Types of Radiation

Earlier reference was made to both *electromagnetic* and *particulate radiations*, the types of radiation that appear as a result of the energy released by electron transitions. In this section, the essential characteristics of each will be briefly reviewed. The student who is interested in a more thorough treatment of these topics should refer to a radiologic physics text.

Radiation is the propagation of energy through space or matter, in the form of waves or particles. In general, there are two types of radiation: *natural background radiation* and *man-made radiation*. An example of the former type is cosmic radiation, which consists of high speed particles that originate in space. There is nothing that can be done to stop this form of natural radiation from arriving here on earth. The earth itself consists of various sources of natural radiation, such as rocks, water, granite, natural gas, the air, and phosphates. Even our bodies emit some form of radiation. Man-made radiation arises from nuclear reactors, nuclear fall-out, and artificially produced radioactive materials. In diagnostic x-ray imaging, the source of x-rays is the x-ray tube.

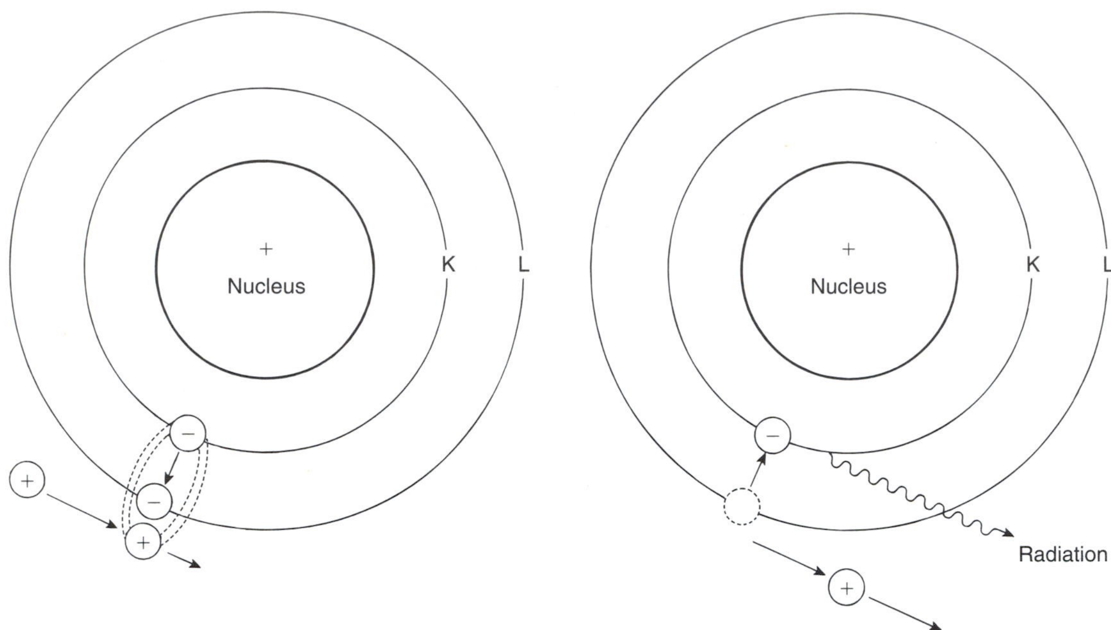

FIGURE 2-3. During excitation of the atom, electrons are not ejected, but rather they are moved into orbital levels farther away from the central nucleus.

Radiation, whether it be natural background or man-made, can be classified as electromagnetic radiation or particulate radiation.

Electromagnetic Radiation

Electromagnetic radiation consists of both an electric and a magnetic field, which propagate through space at right angles to each other, as shown in Figure 2-5. These fields are capable of energy transfer from point to point and have physical properties that are similar to those of visible light.

Electromagnetic radiation includes cosmic rays (high energy, short wavelength), gamma rays, x-rays, ultraviolet radiation, visible light, infrared (heat) radiation, microwaves, and radiowaves (low energy, long wavelength). These are arranged systematically to show the range of their frequencies, wavelengths, and energies (see Fig. 2-6). This arrangement is known as the *electromagnetic spectrum.*

The different types of electromagnetic radiation can be described in terms of their energy and wavelength. The energy of the radiation is inversely proportional to the wavelength. This means that the higher the energy of the radiation, the shorter its wavelength and the more penetrating its radiation. For example, x-rays and gamma rays are more penetrating than ultraviolet light, which can penetrate the human skin to a depth of only about 1 mm.

X-rays and gamma rays are both classified as ionizing radiation. That is to say, each type of radiation interacts with matter so as to eject electrons completely from the atom, thus leaving behind ion pairs. Ultraviolet radiation, visible light, infrared radiation, microwaves, and radiowaves, however, are forms of nonionizing radiation, which means that they do not have enough energy to eject electrons from the atom.

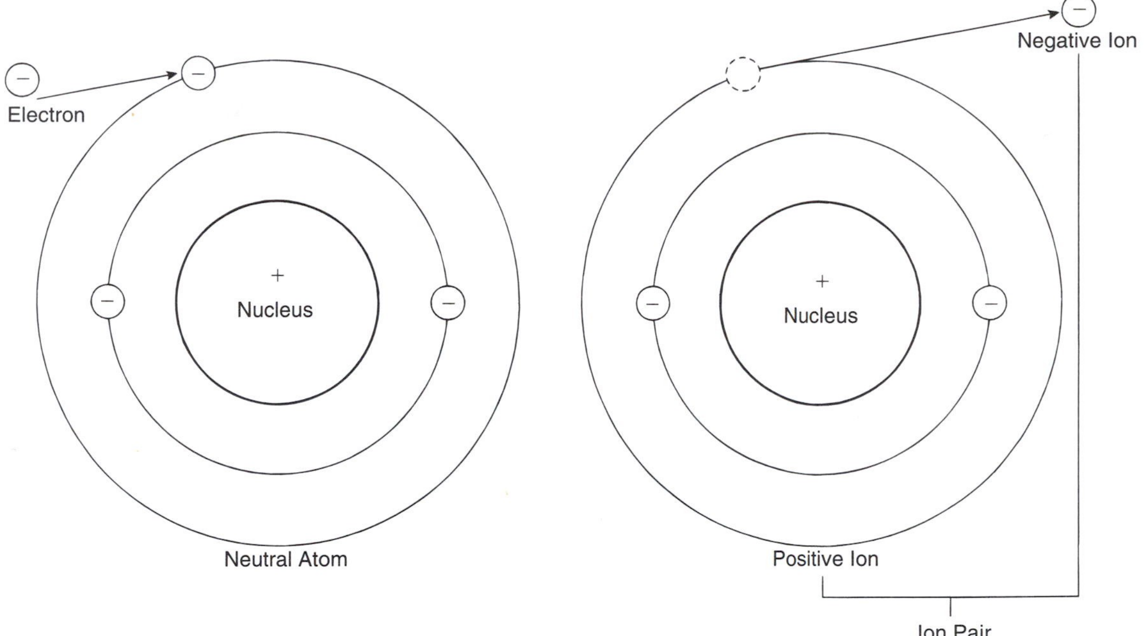

FIGURE 2-4. During ionization of the atom, electrons are ejected from the atom. The resulting ion pairs are made up of the ejected electron (negative ion) and the remaining atom, which has lost an electron (positive ion).

WAVE-PARTICLE THEORY OF ELECTROMAGNETIC RADIATION

Electromagnetic radiation can be thought of as having a *wave-particle duality.* This means that the radiation can behave either as a wave or as a particle. A *wave* is a disturbance that carries energy from point to point. A *particle* is a discrete "packet" of energy, referred to as a photon. Photons are responsible for ejecting electrons from atoms, thus causing ionization.

A wave is characterized by its velocity, wavelength, and frequency. The *frequency* (f) refers to the number of vibrations per second and its unit of measure is cycles per second (cps); it can also be given in hertz (Hz), where 1 Hz = 1 cps. The wavelength (λ) is the distance taken up by one cycle of a wave. The unit of wavelength is the meter (m).

The fundamental *wave equation* relates the wavelength (λ) and frequency (f) of a wave to its speed or velocity (c) via the following equation:

$$c = \lambda f \qquad (2\text{-}1)$$

An x-ray can behave as a wave, or it can behave as a particle. It was Max Planck who suggested that these photons had an energy (E) related to the frequency (υ), as captured in the expression:

$$E = h\upsilon \qquad (2\text{-}2)$$

where h is a constant, known as Planck's constant ($h = 6.626 \times 10^{-34}$ joule-seconds). The relationship between photon energy (E) and wavelength (λ) is given by the expression:

$$\lambda = \frac{12.4}{E} \qquad (2\text{-}3)$$

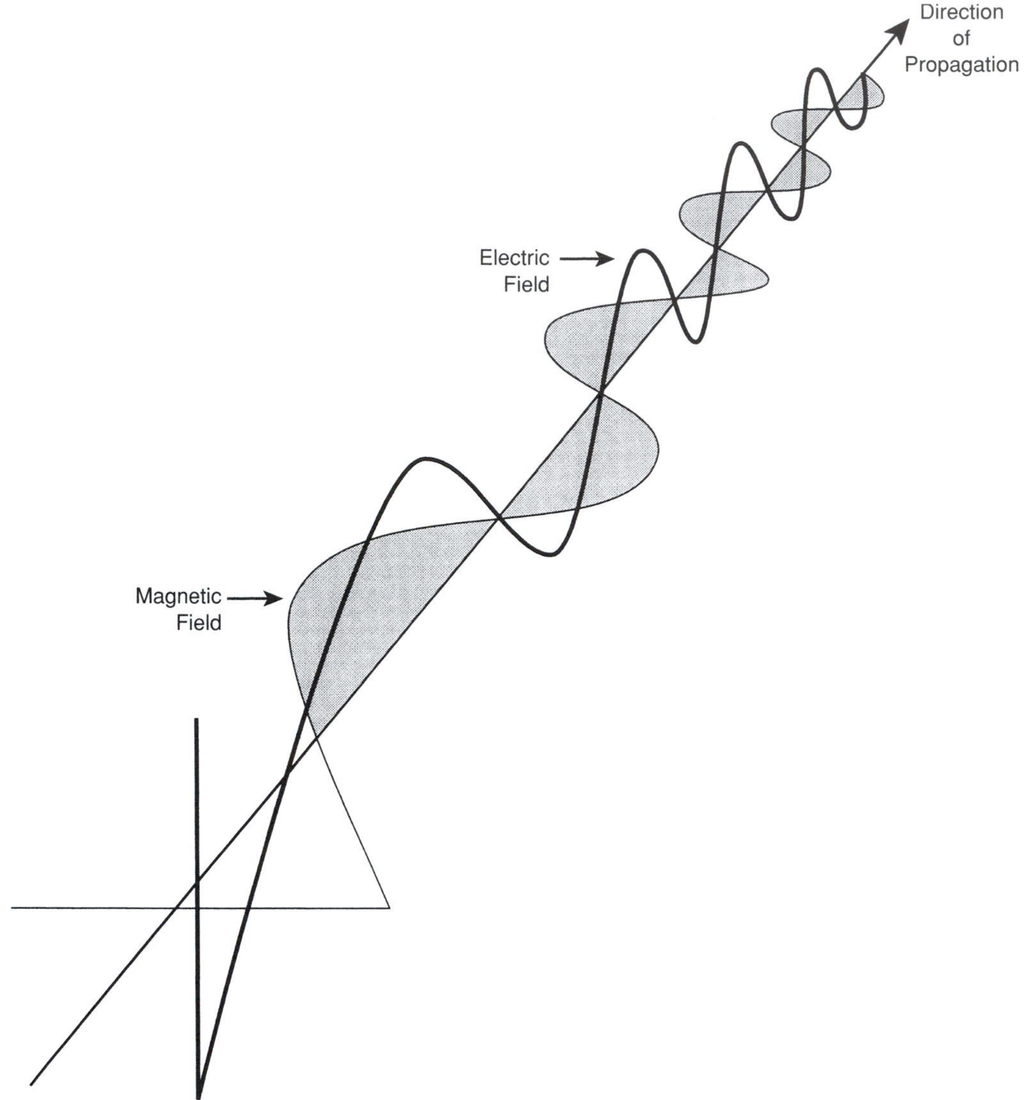

FIGURE 2-5. The propagation of an electromagnetic wave. The wave consists of an electric field and a magnetic field oscillating at right angles to each other in the direction of propagation.

The unit of energy, E, is the kiloelectron volt (keV), which is the energy of an electron accelerated through 1000 volts. In Eq. 2–3, the unit of wavelength (λ) is the angstrom (Å), which is equal to 10^{-8} cm.

The notion of x-rays behaving as "packets of energy," or photons, is relevant to radiobiology. Hall (1994) explained this relevance as follows:

> When x-rays are absorbed in living material, energy is deposited in the tissues and cells. This

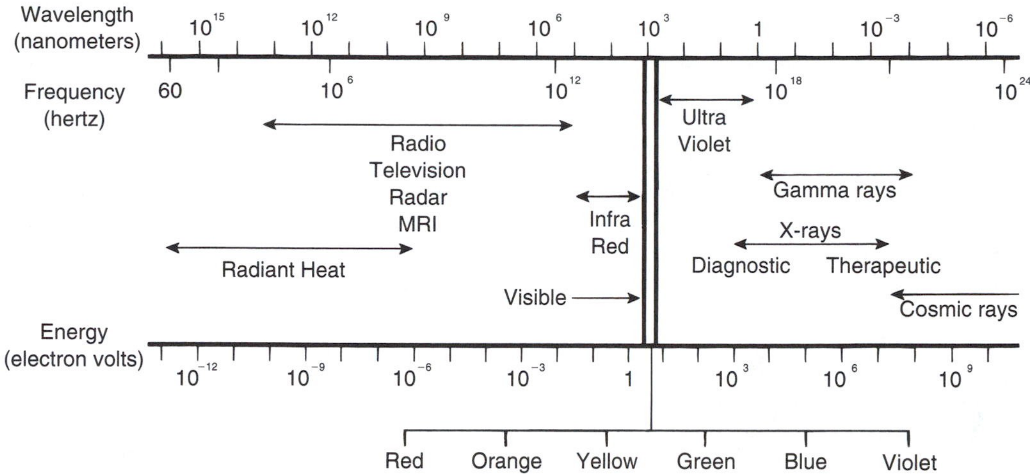

FIGURE 2-6. The electromagnetic spectrum. [From Bushberg, J.T., Seibert, J.A., Leidholdt, Jr, E.M., & Boone, J.M. (1994). *The essential physics of medical imaging.* Baltimore: Williams & Wilkins. Reproduced by permission.]

> energy is deposited unevenly in discrete packets. The energy of a beam of x-rays is quantized into large individual packets, each of which is big enough to break a chemical bond and initiate the change of events that culminates in a biological change. (p. 4).

Particulate Radiation

Particulate radiation refers to particles that are ejected from atoms at very high speeds and have, in most cases, extremely high energies. Particulate radiation may include one or more components of the atom, such as an electron, a proton, or a neutron. Examples of particulate radiation are alpha particles (helium nuclei), beta particles (high-speed electrons), protons (positively charged particles), energetic neutrons (atomic particles with no charge), and cosmic rays.

The various kinds of particulate radiation also have different penetrating abilities. For example, alpha particles are less penetrating than beta particles, which in turn are less penetrating than gamma or x-rays (Fig. 2-7). A thin sheet of paper will shield against alpha particles, whereas beta particles will penetrate the paper but may be shielded by a block of wood.

Characteristics of X-Rays

X-rays were discovered by Professor W.C. Roentgen in 1895, while he was investigating the nature of cathode rays (electrons). During his experiments, he noticed the fluorescence of a barium-platinocyanide screen located near the cathode ray tube with which he was working. He attributed this fluorescence to something (that was invisible) coming from the tube. He called this something *x-rays.* Further experiments led him to see the bones of his hand, as well as others, when he placed them between the tube and the screen. Not only were these rays invisible, they were penetrating as well.

Properties of X-Rays

Roentgen's early experiments led him to several conclusions about the properties of x-rays, a few of which include the following:

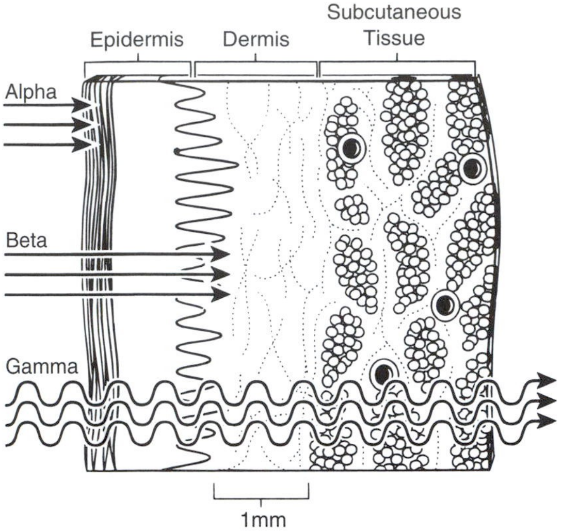

FIGURE 2-7. The penetrating ability of particulate (alpha and beta) and electromagnetic (gamma) radiations. [From Wootton, R. (Ed.). (1993). *Radiation protection of patients*. Cambridge, England: Cambridge University Press. Reproduced by permission.]

1. X-rays can affect photographic plates.
2. X-rays are not affected by magnetic or electrical fields.
3. X-rays can cause certain materials to fluoresce.
4. X-rays can cause ionization.
5. X-rays can be absorbed by high atomic number elements, such as lead.
6. X-rays can penetrate most substances including soft tissues and bone.

These properties make x-rays particularly suitable for use in diagnostic radiology.

The X-Ray Tube

X-rays are produced when high speed electrons collide with a target. In diagnostic radiology, an *x-ray tube* is used to produce x-rays needed for imaging patients. A schematic representation of a rotating-anode x-ray tube and its associated power supply (generator) is shown in Figure 2-8. The major components of the tube include two electrodes, an *anode* (positive electrode) and a *cathode* (negative electrode), positioned as shown in Figure 2-8 and enclosed in an evacuated glass envelope.

The cathode consists of a tungsten filament (coil of wire), which is heated by the filament power supply. At a certain temperature (≥2000°C) electrons are "boiled off" (*thermionic emission*) the filament and are subsequently accelerated across the tube to strike a small area on the anode disk referred to as the *target*. The target is usually made of tungsten alloyed with other elements (rhenium and molybdenum, for example). Tungsten has a high atomic number, a high melting point, and dissipates heat very rapidly; all of these properties are important for the efficient production of x-rays.

When the electrons from the filament collide with the target of the anode, about ≥99% of the energy of the electrons is converted into heat and the other ≤1% is converted into x-rays. These x-rays arise from the two physical processes resulting in the production of Bremsstrahlung radiation and characteristic x-rays. These two processes will be described later in this chapter; they are important to the radiologic technologist.

In preparation for x-ray production, the technologist sets up exposure *technique factors* for a particular examination. These factors are kilovolts (kVp), milliamperes (mA), and the exposure time in seconds (s). During the exposure, the ejected electrons from the filament are accelerated across the tube because of the voltage (kVp) between the cathode and the anode. The higher the kilovoltage, the faster the electrons will travel, and the greater the penetrating power (or quality) of the x-ray beam emitted from the target. The flow of electrons across the tube is referred to as the tube current, or mA. The greater the mA, the greater the number of electrons flowing across the tube and the greater the quantity of the photons emitted from the target (see page 35 for a definition of photon quantity). The exposure time determines the

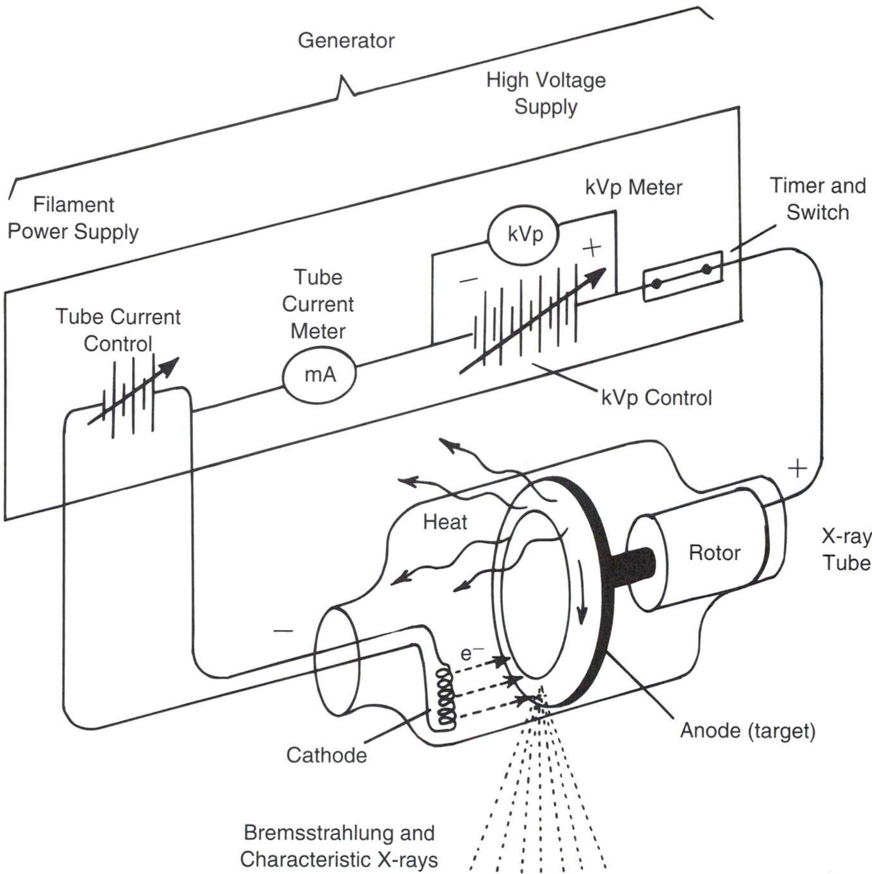

FIGURE 2-8. A basic schematic of the major components of an x-ray tube and its associated power supply. [From Wolbarst, A.B. (1993). *Physics of radiology*. Norwalk, CT: Appleton & Lange. Reproduced by permission.]

duration of the flow of electrons across the tube. The product of mA and time in seconds is the mAs. The greater the mAs, the greater the quantity of photons emitted from the target and the greater the dose to the patient. The concepts of beam quality and quantity will be elaborated later in this chapter.

Origin of X-Rays

X-rays are produced when high-speed electrons interact with electrons and nuclei of target atoms. When the interaction is between high-speed electrons and the inner shell electrons of target atoms, *characteristic x-rays* are produced. When the interaction is between high-speed electrons and the charged nuclei of target atoms, *Bremsstrahlung* x-rays are produced.

CHARACTERISTIC X-RAYS

The production of characteristic x-rays is illustrated in Figure 2-9. When high-speed electrons interact with inner shell electrons of target atoms to cause ionization, characteristic radiation results.

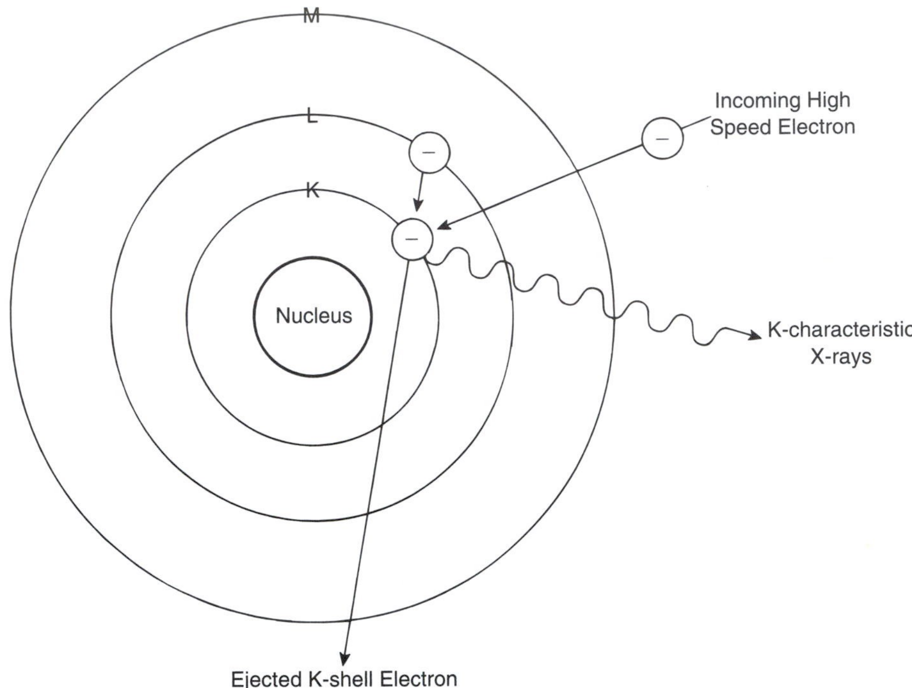

FIGURE 2-9. The production of characteristic x-rays.

> **REVIEW BOX:**
> In ionization, electrons are ejected completely from atoms, thus leaving vacancies in the electron shells, which are filled immediately by electrons in outer shells.

As the electrons move from any of the outer shells to replace electrons ejected from inner shells, x-ray photons are produced. In Figure 2-9, the electron from the L-shell fills the K-shell vacancy, resulting in the production of x-rays. Characteristic x-rays are only useful in diagnostic radiology if they have enough energy to penetrate body tissues and get to the film.

The x-rays emitted as a result of the K-shell being filled are called K-characteristic x-rays. Similarly, L-characteristic x-rays, M-characteristic x-rays, etc., can be produced. These emissions are called characteristic because the x-rays produced are characteristic of target elements and differ as a function of their binding energy. For example, the energy of the K-characteristic x-rays of tungsten will be different from the energy of the K-characteristic x-rays of lead.

BREMSSTRAHLUNG RADIATION

Bremmstrahlung is the German word for "braking" or "slowing down." Brems (for short) radiation is produced when a high-speed electron is decelerated in an interaction with the charged nuclei of target atoms (and not the electrons). As an electron approaches the nucleus, it slows down, loses its initial kinetic energy (KE), and changes its direction of travel, with less KE. This difference in KE reappears in the form of Bremsstrahlung radiation, as illustrated in Figure 2-10. Brems radia-

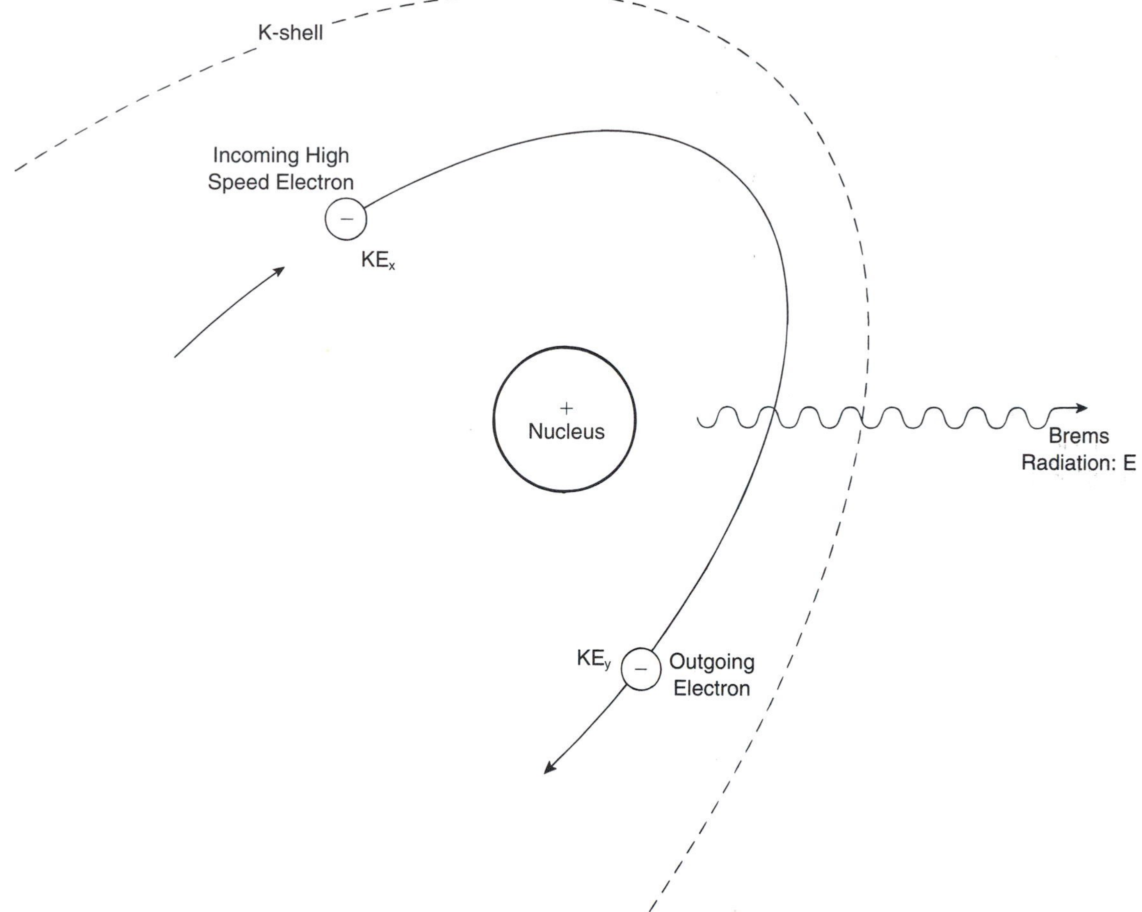

FIGURE 2-10. Bremsstrahlung radiation is produced when a high-speed electron is decelerated in an interaction with the charged nuclei of target atoms.

tion can have a wide range of energies (Fig. 2-11) because the incoming high-speed electrons can lose varying amounts of KE as they pass by the nucleus (some may be closer to the nucleus while others may be farther away). For example, a high-speed electron with a KE of 70 keV can result in Brems radiation having energies ranging from 0 to 70 keV. (Recall that characteristic x-rays can be produced only at specific energies, equal to the difference in the binding energies of the electrons in the inner and outer shells.)

X-Ray Emission Spectrum

The emission of characteristic and Brems radiation is illustrated in Figure 2-12. This is referred to as the *x-ray emission spectrum,* a plot of the number of x-ray photons per unit energy (intensity) as a function of x-ray energy.

An understanding of the x-ray emission spectrum will provide the technologist with a further insight into how various technical factors affect the radiation dose to the patient. These

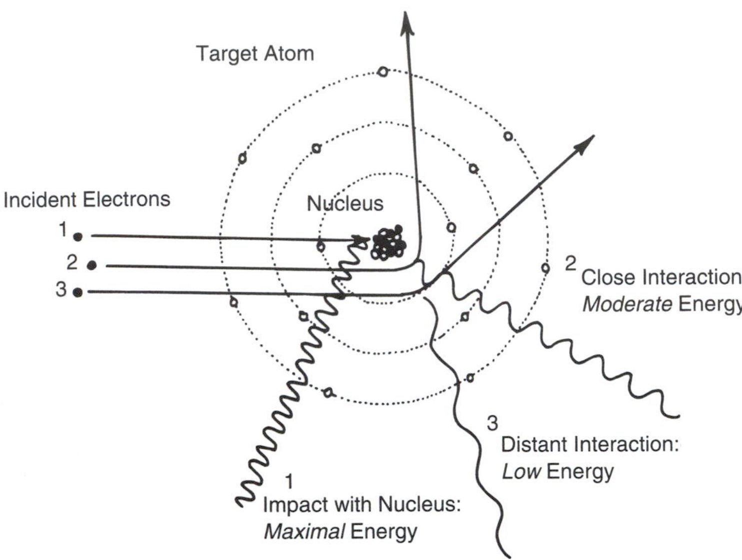

FIGURE 2-11. Bremsstrahlung radiation can have a wide range of energies depending on how close the incident electrons get to the nucleus. [From Bushberg, J.T., Seibert, J.A., Leidholdt, Jr, E.M., & Boone, J.M. (1994). *The essential physics of medical imaging*. Baltimore: Williams & Wilkins. Reproduced by permission.]

factors include mA, kVp, filtration, waveform, and target material of the x-ray tube, to be reviewed subsequently.

Two spectra are shown in Figure 2-12, the characteristic, or *discrete emission spectrum*, and the Brems, or *continuous x-ray spectrum*. Whereas the discrete spectrum shows that characteristic x-rays are emitted only at specific photon energies (characteristic x-ray spectrum, from K-x-rays on up for tungsten, for example, consists of 15 different energies), the continuous spectrum shows that the energies of Brems radiation range from zero to some maximum. According to Bushong (1993, p. 154), "the maximum energy that an x-ray can have is numerically equal to the kVp of the operation. This is why it is called the kVp(eak). The greatest number of x-ray photons is emitted with energy approximately one-third of the maximum photon energy. The number of x-rays emitted decreases rapidly at very low photon energies and below 5 keV nearly reaches zero."

X-Ray Quantity and Quality

The number of x-ray photons in the beam per unit energy is referred to as the *quantity*. The quantity of x-rays is increased when the current to the filament of the x-ray tube is increased; this, of course, translates into an increase in filament temperature. As the filament temperature increases, more electrons are produced. More electrons simply means more x-rays, that is, an increase in quantity. Other factors affecting x-ray quantity include the tube current (mA), the tube voltage (kVp), beam filtration, the distance from the target of the tube and the image receptor, and the atomic number of the target material. These factors influence the size and relative position of the x-ray emission spectrum.

The *quality* of an x-ray beam refers to the energy of the beam. In this case the energy of the beam is sometimes discussed in terms of its "hardness" or "penetrating power." Quality is controlled by the voltage applied between the anode and cathode of the x-ray tube. Increasing the voltage (kVp) across the tube increases the beam energy (because the electrons are accelerated across the tube with more kinetic energy). Other factors that affect x-ray quality include the target material, voltage waveform, and filtration. These will be discussed briefly in the next subsection.

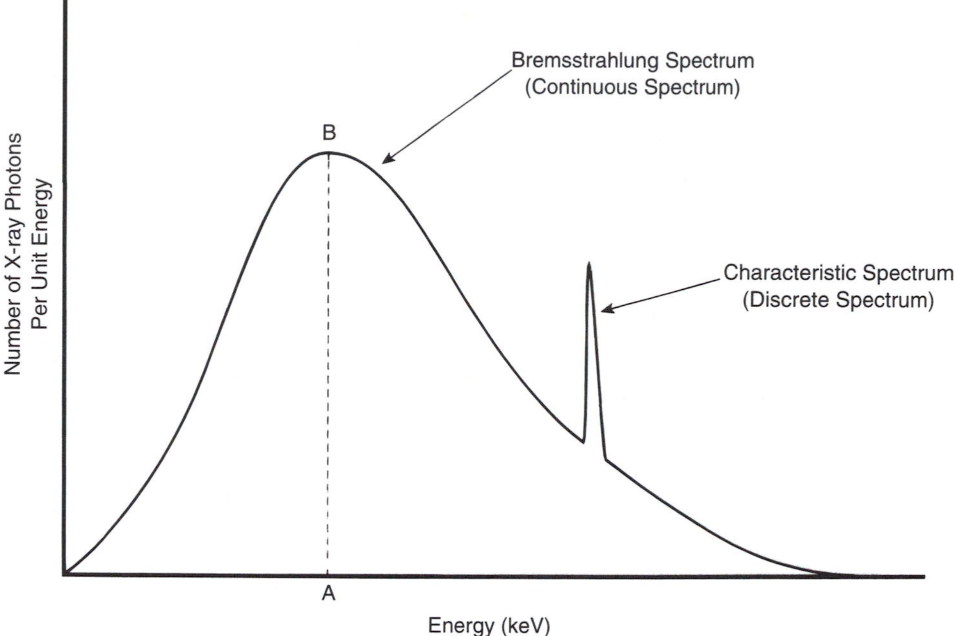

FIGURE 2-12. The general form and shape of both the discrete and continuous x-ray spectra. The line AB represents the amplitude of the continuous spectrum.

Factors Affecting X-Ray Quantity and Quality

The factors affecting the quantity and quality of x-rays were introduced earlier. This subsection is devoted to examining how these factors affect the size and relative position of both the continuous and discrete x-ray spectra.

kVp

The higher the kVp, the greater the beam quality. High kVp will also affect beam intensity (I) through the following expression:

$$I \propto (kVp)^2 \qquad (2\text{-}4)$$

This implies that as the kVp is doubled, the intensity will increase by a factor of four. Intensity problems can be solved using the following equation:

$$\frac{I_1}{I_2} = \left(\frac{kVp_1}{kVp_2}\right)^2 \qquad (2\text{-}5)$$

where I_1 and I_2 are the intensities at kVp_1 and kVp_2, respectively.

An increase in kVp will alter the spectrum by increasing the amplitude, or height of the wave, of the continuous spectrum (the area under the curve is increased), as shown in Figure 2-13. Note that the amplitude is increased and the position of the spectrum is shifted toward higher energies. The discrete spectrum remains the same because it is not influenced by kVp.

mA

The tube current (mA) determines the quantity of photons because it affects the quantity of electrons flowing from the filament to the target of the x-ray tube. The greater the mA, the greater the number of electrons and the greater the quantity of x-rays. The quantity of x-rays is directly proportional to the mA, that is:

$$I \propto mA \qquad (2\text{-}6)$$

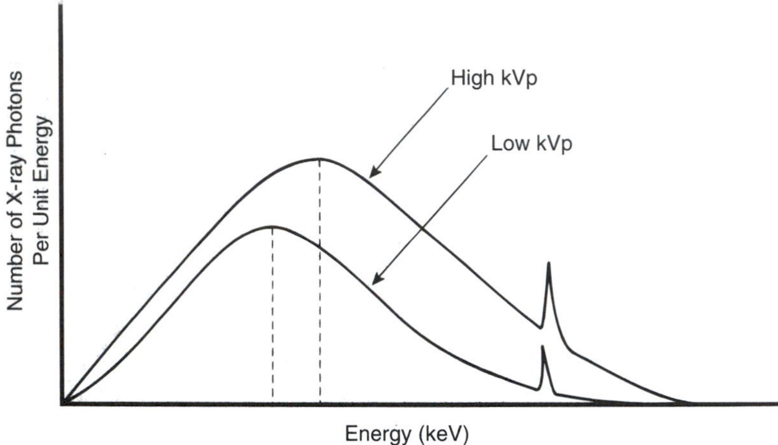

FIGURE 2-13. The effect of kVp on the intensity and quality of x-rays. Note that the discrete spectrum remains at the same position on the energy axis while the amplitude of the continuous spectrum shifts to the higher energy region. The continuous spectrum increases in amplitude for high kVp techniques.

If the mA is doubled, the quantity of x-rays doubles, as illustrated in Figure 2-14. Note that while the amplitude changes proportionately, the position of the continuous spectrum does not shift toward higher energies. The discrete spectrum is not influenced by mA. The same holds true for changes in mAs (milliamperage-seconds).

TARGET MATERIAL

The atomic number (Z) of the target material of the x-ray tube affects both the intensity and the quality of the beam. The higher the atomic number of the target material, the more efficient the production of Brems radiation. This means that the amplitude of the continuous spectrum is increased (increase in intensity) as the Z of the tar-

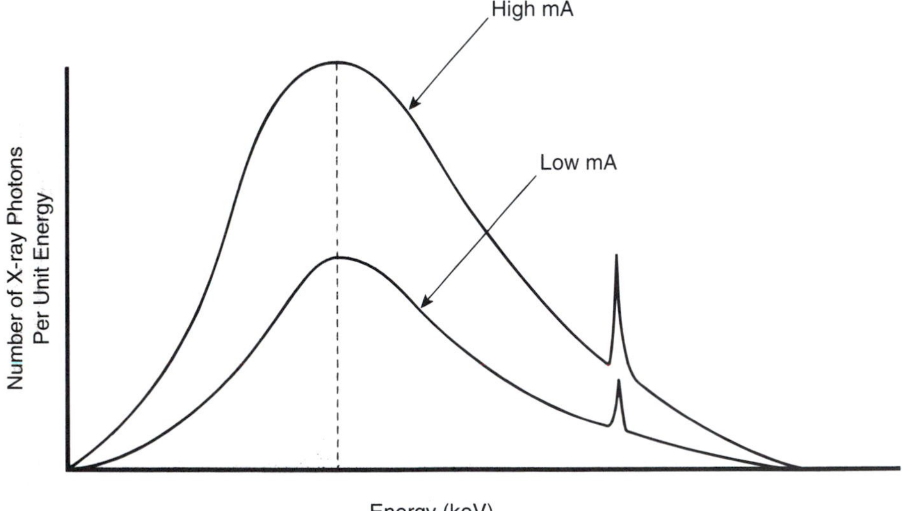

FIGURE 2-14. The effect of mA on x-ray spectra. The area under the curve increases proportionately as the mA increases. There is no shift of the amplitude on the photon energy axis, indicating that mA does not affect the beam energy.

get material increases (Fig. 2-15). Note now that there is a change in the position of the discrete spectrum. The Z of the target material influences the quality of the characteristic radiation.

REVIEW BOX:
Low energy photons have long wavelengths, whereas high energy photons have short wavelengths.

FILTRATION

The x-ray beam from the x-ray tube is a heterogeneous radiation beam comprised of low energy and high energy photons. A filter placed in the x-ray beam preferentially absorbs the low energy photons, which are less likely to reach the image receptor. These photons only increase the dose to the patient. With the removal of the low energy photons, the beam becomes harder, or more penetrating, that is, the mean energy of the beam is increased. Filtration, therefore, is intended to protect the patient.

An increase in filtration will change the shape and position of the continuous spectrum but leave the discrete spectrum unaffected. Figure 2-16 shows that for a constant kVp and mA, an increase in filtration will result in a decrease in x-ray intensity and an increase in the effective energy of the x-ray beam.

VOLTAGE WAVEFORM

The voltage waveform for the generation of x-rays depends on the type of x-ray generator. The type of generator affects the continuous x-ray spectrum but not the discrete spectrum, as illustrated in Figure 2-17. This will be discussed further in Chapter 8.

A GENERAL RELATIONSHIP

The general relationship between intensity (I) and kVp, mA, and atomic number is:

$$I \; \alpha \; kVp^2 \times mA \times Z \qquad (2\text{-}7)$$

This relationship is one of *direct proportionality*, which means that: (1) intensity increases proportionately as the mA increases; (2) intensity increases approximately as the square of the kVp; and (3) intensity increases proportionately as the atomic number of the target material increases.

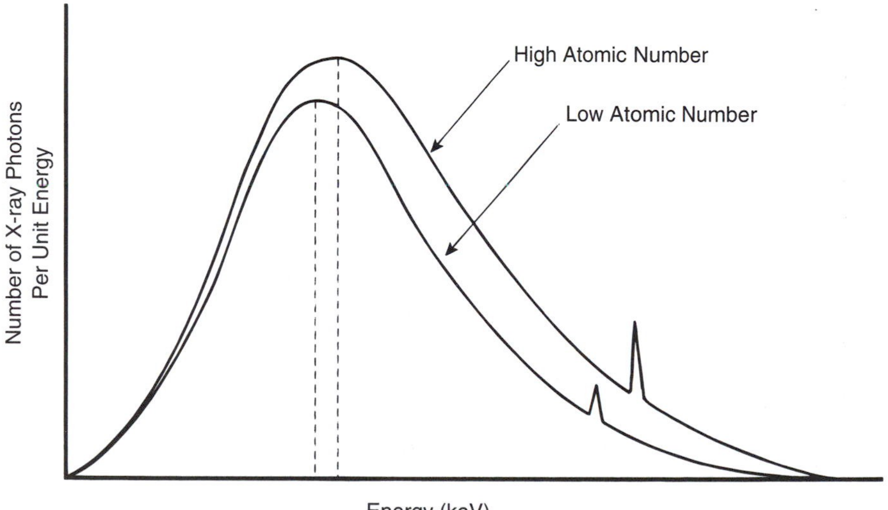

FIGURE 2-15. For higher atomic number target materials, there is an increase in quantity as well as quality of the beam compared with target materials of lower atomic number. Note that there is a change in the position of the discrete spectrum.

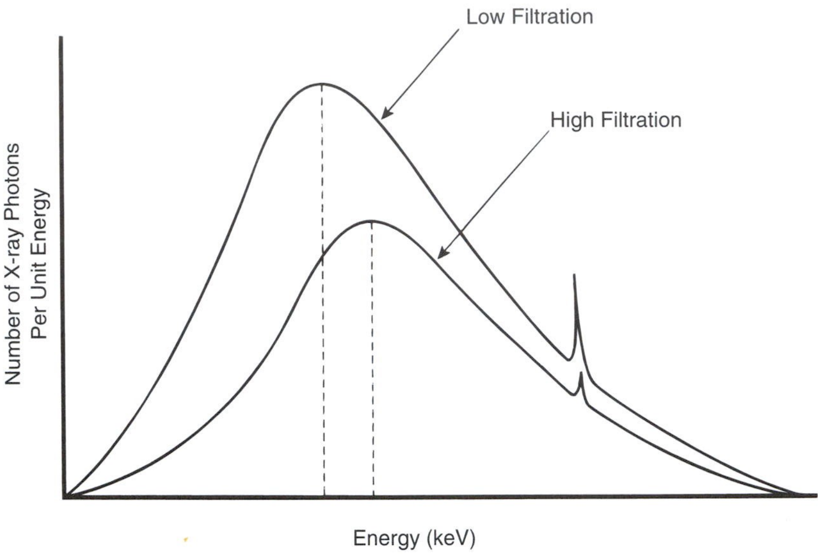

FIGURE 2-16. The effect of filtration on the x-ray spectra. For high filtration, there is a reduction in the intensity of the beam and an increase in the beam energy (the amplitude of the continuous spectrum shifts to the right on the energy axis). The position of the discrete spectrum remains the same.

If the distance from the x-ray tube target to the image receptor is introduced as another factor, then the expression (Eq. 2-7) becomes:

$$I \propto \frac{kVp^2 \times mA \times Z}{d^2} \tag{2-8}$$

The intensity is inversely proportional to the square of the distance. High kVp and low mA techniques result in a decreased dose to the patient for film-screen systems. This will be discussed further in Chapter 8.

Interaction of X-Rays with Matter

When radiation interacts with matter, some of the photons in the beam will be absorbed, some will be scattered, and others will penetrate the material. These processes (absorption, scattering, and penetration) depend on the energy of the photons as well as on the composition of the absorbing material, and contribute to the reduction of the number of photons (intensity) in the beam. This reduction is referred to as *attenuation*. Because we explore the intricacies of this phenomenon, it is important to consider the different mechanisms by which x-rays interact with matter. Because of the range of energies (low, moderate, and high) of x-rays, there are five different mechanisms: (1) classical, or Rayleigh, scattering, (2) Compton scattering, (3) photoelectric absorption (photoelectric effect), (4) pair production, and (5) photodisintegration. In this section, only the first three will be reviewed because they occur in diagnostic radiology. Because photodisintegration and pair production occur at very high energies beyond those used in diagnostic imaging, they will not be discussed in this book.

Mechanisms of Interaction in X-Ray Imaging

When the absorbing material has many atoms in a small volume, then the chance of an interaction is greater than when there are few

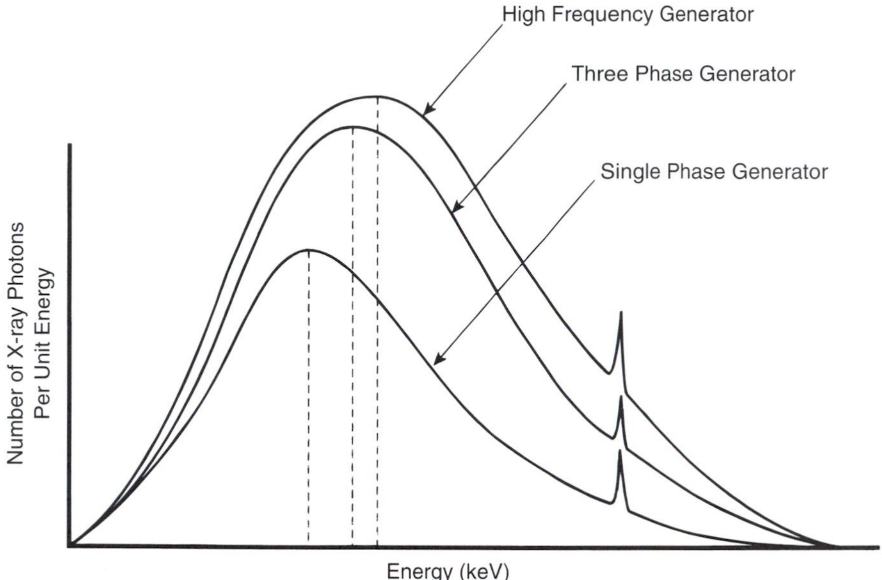

FIGURE 2-17. The effect of rectification on the x-ray spectra. For three phase and high frequency generators both the intensity and the effective energy of the beam increase.

atoms encompassed within the same volume. The chance that an interaction will occur is referred to as its *probability*. The probability that a given interaction will occur depends upon a number of factors, including the atomic number (Z) of the absorbing material and the energy of the photons.

CLASSICAL SCATTERING

When a low-energy photon (~10 keV) interacts with an atom, it is absorbed by the entire atom. There is no ionization, but the atom becomes excited and very quickly releases a photon with energy equal to that of the incident photon. The released photon is scattered in a different direction, as is illustrated in Figure 2-18. For energies used in radiography, <5% of x-ray interactions are due to classical scattering. This percentage contributes little to image formation and results in some degree of film fogging. Classical scattering is also referred to as elastic, or Rayleigh, scattering.

COMPTON SCATTERING

Another photon–electron interaction of vital importance to the technologist is *Compton scattering* (also referred to as inelastic or nonclassical scattering) because it is the predominant interaction in x-ray imaging. In Compton scattering (Fig. 2-19), an incident photon interacts with electrons in the outer shell of the atom. The incident photon has enough energy to eject the electron from its shell, resulting in ionization of the atom. The incident photon is scattered in a different direction, which is defined by the angle of deflection. The following points should be noted: The energy of the scattered photon is less than the energy of the incident photon. After the collision, the energy of the incident photon (E_i) is distributed between the energy of the scattered photon (E_s) and that of the ejected electron (E_{e^-}). The mathematical expression is:

$$E_s = \frac{E_i}{1 + \frac{E_i}{0.511\ M_{eV}}(1 - \cos\theta)} \quad (2\text{-}9)$$

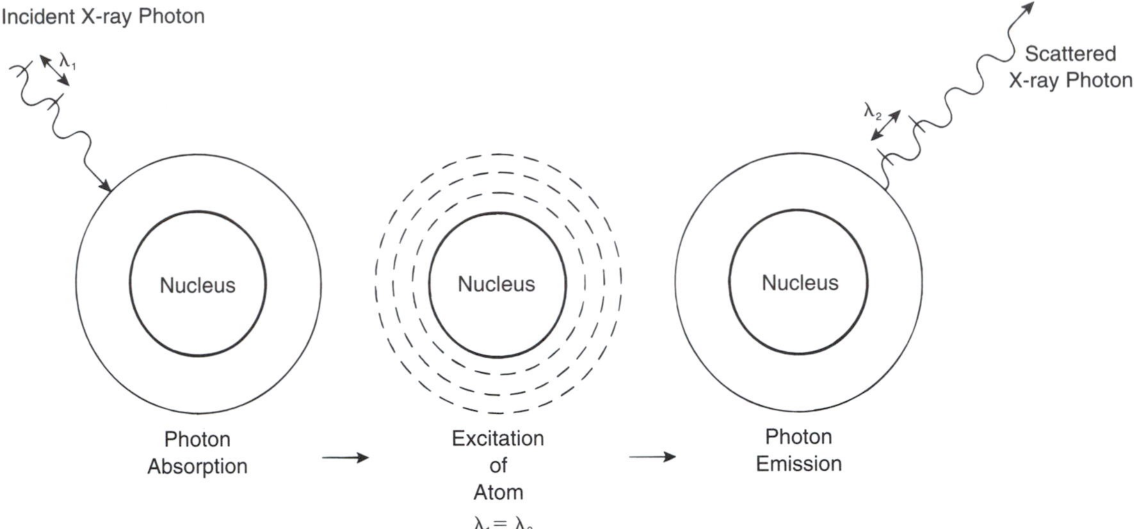

FIGURE 2-18. Classical scattering. A low energy photon is absorbed by the atom resulting in excitation. The excited atom quickly releases a photon with energy equal to that of the incident photon.

As shown in Figure 2-20, for a 70-keV incident photon, the energy of the scattered photon is large when the scattering angle is small. For a 100-keV incident photon energy, the energies of the scattered photon for 10°, 30°, 60°, 90°, and 180° are 99.6, 97.5, 91.2, 83.8, and 72.1 keV, respectively (Thompson et al, 1994).

The probability that Compton scattering will occur depends on the energy of the incident photon, and the electron density (number of electrons per gram of absorber × density). As the energy of the incident photon and the density of the absorber increase, the probability of Compton scattering increases (Bushong, 1993). The probability of Compton scattering does not depend on the atomic number of the absorber.

PHOTOELECTRIC ABSORPTION

Another mechanism of x-ray interaction with matter is that of photoelectric absorption, otherwise known as the photoelectric effect. This is schematically shown in Figure 2-21. The incident photon interacts with inner shell electrons (K or L) and transfers all of its energy to these electrons. The electron absorbs this energy (Fig. 2-21) and is ejected from the atom. The ejected electron is referred to as a photoelectron. The vacancy now left in the inner shell is filled by an electron in the neighboring outer shell, resulting in characteristic x-ray emission.

The energy of the photoelectron (E_{pe-}) is equal to the energy of the incident photon (E_i) minus the binding energy of the ejected electron (E_b). This can be expressed mathematically as:

$$E_{pe-} = E_i - E_b \tag{2-10}$$

Photoelectric absorption results in the following: (1) photoelectron, (2) ionization of the atom (what remains after the electron is ejected is a positive ion), and (3) characteristic x-rays. The probability of photoelectric absorption (P_{PE}) depends on the atomic number (Z) of the absorber and the energy of the incident photon (E), and is governed by the following relationship:

$$P_{PE} = \frac{Z^3}{E^3} \tag{2-11}$$

This means that the photoelectric absorption is greatest with high atomic number elements

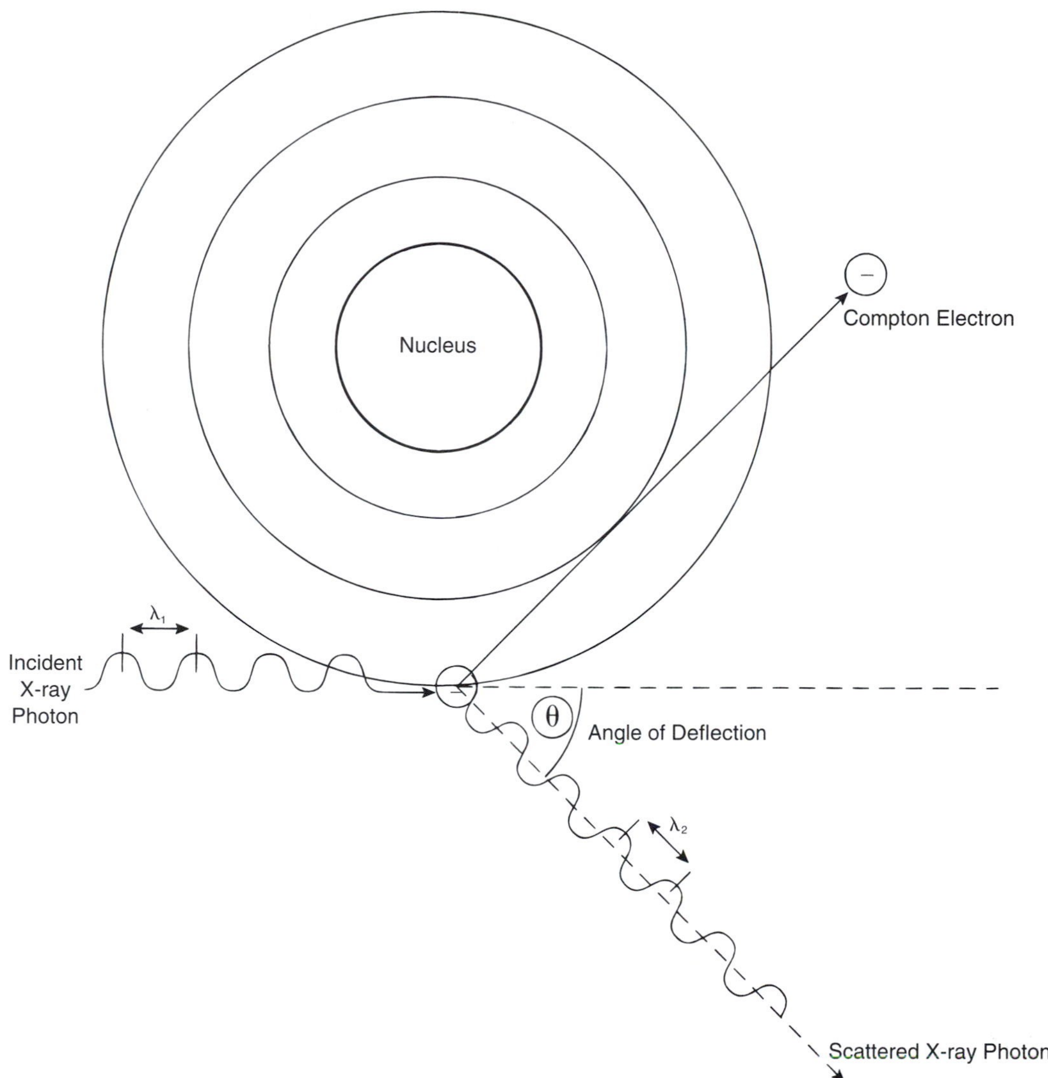

FIGURE 2-19. Compton scattering is a photon-electron interaction in which the incident photon interacts with electrons in the outer shell of the atom, resulting in a high-speed electron and scattered x-rays.

and low energy radiation. Thus, because bone has an effective Z of 13.8, it will absorb more radiation than soft tissue, which has an effective Z of 7.4. In addition, because the probability of photoelectric absorption is inversely proportional to the energy of the incident radiation, if this energy is increased by a factor of 2, photoelectric absorption decreases by a factor of 8.

The photoelectric absorption process is responsible for much of the high contrast in x-ray imaging; because it results in complete absorption of the photon, it contributes significantly to the radiation dose to the patient.

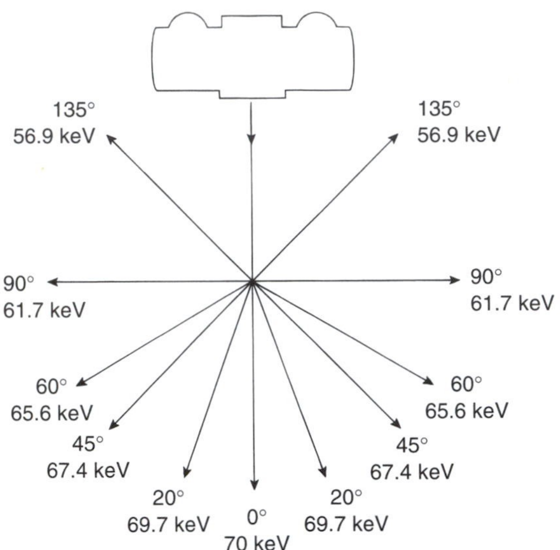

FIGURE 2-20. The energy of scattered photons in a Compton interaction. As the angle of deflection increases, the energy of the scattered photons decreases. At 20°, the energy of the scattered photon is about the same as that of the incident photon. [From Thompson, M.A., Hattaway, M.P., Hall, J.D., & Dowd, S.B. (1994). *Principles of imaging science and protection*. Philadelphia: W.B. Saunders. Reproduced by permission.]

Radiation Attenuation

Attenuation is the reduction of radiation as it passes through matter. The interactions or mechanisms just described are all examples of how radiation is attenuated.

LINEAR ATTENUATION COEFFICIENT

Consider Figure 2-22, which shows a beam of radiation passing through a block of material with thickness X. The attenuation of the beam is given by the following expression, known as the Lambert-Beer law, or the law of exponential attenuation:

$$I = I_o e^{-\mu x} \qquad (2\text{-}12)$$

where I is the transmitted intensity, I_o is the intensity of the incident or primary photons, e is the base of the natural logarithm, x is the thickness of material, and μ is the *linear attenuation coefficient.* μ represents the probability that a photon will be attenuated per centimeter (cm^{-1}) of the absorbing material. The unit of μ is cm^{-1}.

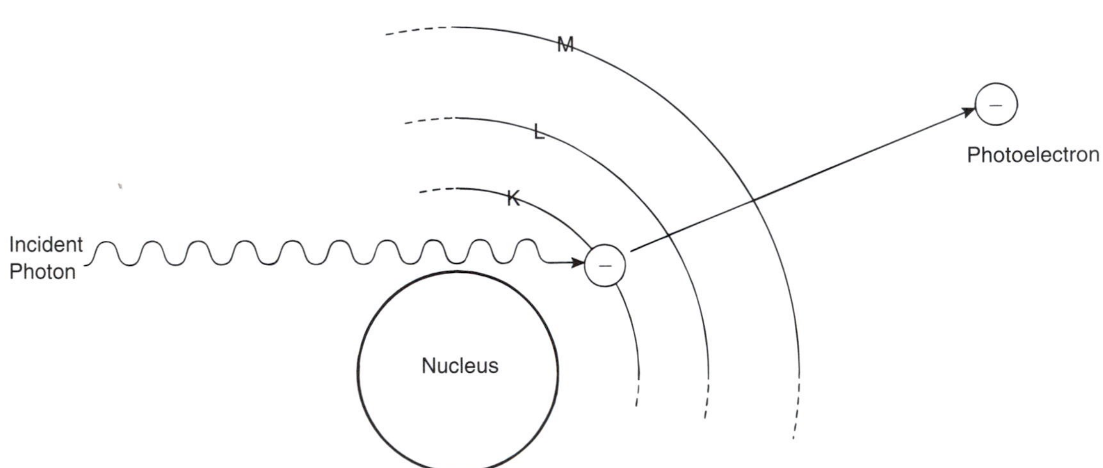

FIGURE 2-21. Photoelectric absorption is a mechanism of x-ray interaction with matter in which an incident photon interacts with inner shell electrons of the atom. The electron ejected from the atom is referred to as the photoelectron. The vacancy left in the inner shell is filled by an electron in a neighboring outer shell resulting in the production of characteristic x-rays.

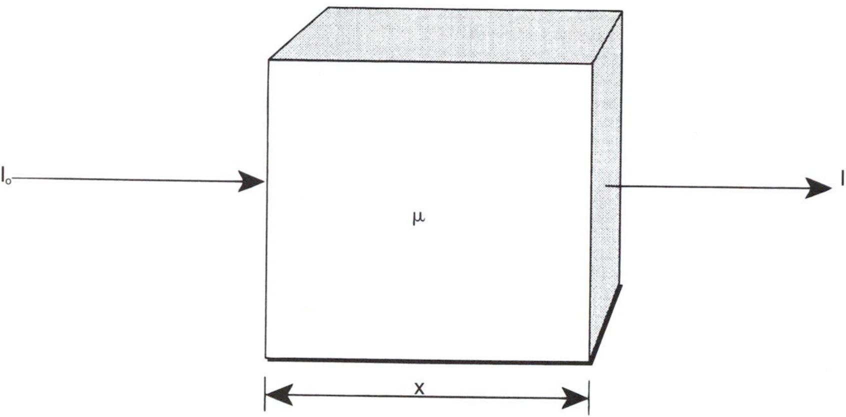

FIGURE 2-22. Radiation attenuation. As a beam of radiation of intensity I_o passes through an object of thickness X, it is reduced in intensity according to the law of exponential attenuation, governed by the equation $I = I_o e^{-\mu x}$.

The factors affecting the linear attenuation coefficient of a radiation beam include the following: (1) the energy of the beam, (2) the atomic number and density of the absorbing material, and (3) the electrons per gram of the absorber. Increasing the energy of the beam (going from 90 to 120 kV) increases the number of transmitted photons and hence decreases attenuation. Increasing the density, atomic number, and electrons per gram of the absorber leads to a decrease in the number of transmitted photons, thus leading to an increase in attenuation. For example, lead ($Z = 82$) will attenuate more radiation than gold ($Z = 79$).

In general, and with respect to radiation attenuation and dose in particular, the technologist should consider the following when imaging patients:

1. High kVp techniques decrease attenuation.
2. Low kVp techniques increase attenuation.
3. Bone attenuates more radiation than soft tissues because of its higher atomic number.
4. The probability of photoelectric absorption is seven times greater in bone than in soft tissues regardless of energy (Bushong, 1993).
5. As the density (mass per unit volume) of the tissue increases, attenuation increases.
6. Contrast media (containing iodine or barium) will attenuate more radiation than soft tissues because of their higher atomic number and densities, particularly with low kVp techniques.

MASS ATTENUATION COEFFICIENT

Another measure of radiation attenuation is the *mass attenuation coefficient* (μ_m), given by the algebraic expression:

$$\mu_m\,(\mathrm{cm^2/g}) = \frac{\mu(\mathrm{cm^{-1}})}{\text{density of absorber}\ (\mathrm{g/cm^3})} \qquad (2\text{-}13)$$

Whereas μ depends on the density (P) of the absorber (for example, $\mu_{water} > \mu_{ice} > \mu_{water\ vapor}$), μ_m does not depend on density ($\mu/P_{water} = \mu/P_{ice} = \mu/P_{water\ vapor}$).

μ_m would be used in radiology when weight is important. For example, "tin" attenuates more x-rays than lead because of K-edge absorption considerations, even though 1 mm of lead attenuates significantly more photons than does the same thickness of tin. In this case, a well-designed "tin" apron of a given weight would actually outperform a lead apron of the same weight in attenuating x-rays (Bushberg, 1994).

HALF VALUE LAYER

A practical measure of attenuation is the *half value layer* (HVL), which is defined as that thickness of material needed to reduce the intensity of a beam of radiation by 50%. The HVL expresses the quality, or penetrating power, of the beam.

For a homogeneous beam of radiation, in which all photons have the same energy, equal thicknesses of material will remove the same percentage of photons from the beam. The energy of the transmitted beam remains the same but there is a decrease in the quantity of photons. This is not the case with a heterogeneous beam, in which photons have different energies. The beam emanating from the x-ray tube is heterogeneous, and it is important to consider what happens to such a beam as it passes through matter. For a heterogeneous beam, equal thicknesses of material remove different amounts of photons from the beam. The transmitted beam has a higher effective energy than the incident beam because the low energy photons have been absorbed or filtered by the material (Fig. 2-23).

The radiation from the x-ray tube is filtered before it reaches the patient. This filtration protects the patient by removing some of the low energy photons that are destined to be absorbed by the patient rather than transferred to the film.

Interaction of Radiation with Tissue: Physical and Chemical Factors

The electrons ejected from atoms as a result of ionization such as those from Compton scattering (Compton recoil) and photoelectric absorption (photoelectron) travel through the patient's tissues and cause further ionizations along their path. In addition, these fast electrons transfer energy to the neighboring tissue, which subsequently leads to some sort of biological response caused by physical and chemical damage. For further insight into the events relating to radiation-induced injury, it is necessary to review the following: direct and indirect action of radiation, radiolysis of water, linear energy transfer, and the relative biological effectiveness.

Direct and Indirect Action

Direct and indirect action are two classes of radiation interaction that lead to biological responses in living things. Both of these are clearly illustrated in Figure 2-24. In *direct action* an ionizing particle or photon directly ionizes or excites a biological macromolecule, such as DNA, leaving it in a chemically unstable state. Alternatively, *indirect action* implies that an ionizing particle or photon ionizes or excites water, to form free radicals (highly reactive chemical species), which in turn attack biological macromolecules (DNA, RNA, proteins), thus leading to biological responses.

Radiolysis of Water

Because living systems contain ~70–85% water, most of the interaction of radiation with tissues is between radiation and water, particularly in diagnostic radiology. When a water molecule (H_2O) is irradiated, it absorbs energy and dissociates into a positive water ion (H_2O^+) and an electron (e^-) represented as:

$$_{\text{radiation}} + H_2O \rightarrow H_2O^+ + e^- \qquad (2\text{-}14)$$

The free electron will combine with another water molecule to produce a negative water ion (H_2O^-), represented as:

$$e^- + H_2O \rightarrow H_2O^- \qquad (2\text{-}15)$$

Since the two ions, H_2O^+ and H_2O^- are chemically unstable, each will dissociate to produce a hydrogen ion (H^+), a hydroxyl ion (OH^-), a hydrogen free radical ($H^{\cdot}$), and a hydroxyl free radical ($OH^{\cdot}$), represented as:

$$H_2O^+ \rightarrow H^+ + OH^{\cdot} \qquad (2\text{-}16)$$

and

$$H_2O^- \rightarrow H^{\cdot} + OH^- \qquad (2\text{-}17)$$

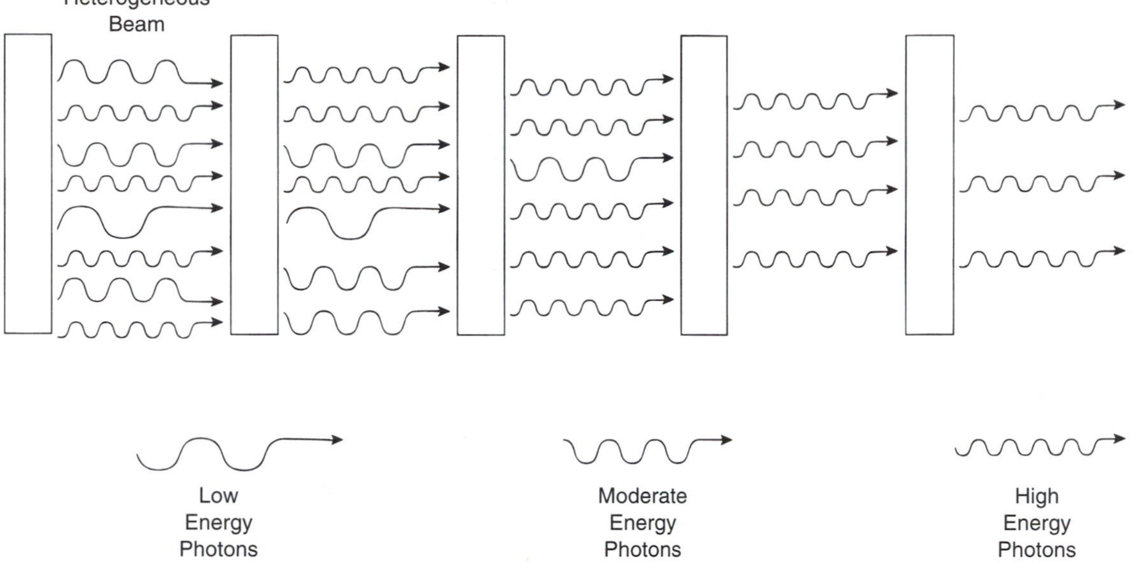

FIGURE 2-23. When a beam of heterogeneous radiation passes through several half value layers, the low energy photons are removed from the beam, thus increasing the effective beam energy. The beam becomes harder, or more penetrating.

The final products of the dissociation of water by radiation are two ions (H^+) and (OH^-) and two free radicals ($H^{\cdot} + OH^{\cdot}$)

Free radicals, symbolized by a dot (·) next to the chemical symbol, are atoms or molecules with an unpaired electron in the outermost shell. They are unstable and highly reactive chemical species. While the two ions (H^+ and OH^-) will recombine to form water, free radicals can combine with other free radicals to form water as well, in which case there is no damage to the cell. These reactions can be represented as follows:

$$H^+ + OH^- \rightarrow H_2O \qquad (2\text{-}18)$$

$$H^{\cdot} + OH^{\cdot} \rightarrow H_2O \qquad (2\text{-}19)$$

Free radicals can also combine with other free radicals to form other potentially cytoxic molecules, such as hydrogen peroxide (H_2O_2). This process is represented as:

$$OH^{\cdot} + OH^{\cdot} \rightarrow H_2O_2 \qquad (2\text{-}20)$$

Free radicals ($H^{\cdot}$) can, for example, combine with oxygen to form the highly reactive hydroperoxyl radical ($HO_2^{\cdot}$), represented as:

$$H^{\cdot} + O_2 \rightarrow HO_2^{\cdot} \qquad (2\text{-}21)$$

Free radicals react with cell components giving rise to chemical products that lead to biological damage. In diagnostic radiology most of the biological damage is attributed to the indirect action on water.

Linear Energy Transfer

The ability of ionizing radiation to cause biological damage can be determined by a physical factor referred to as the *linear energy transfer* (LET). Recall that the electrons ejected as a result of photoelectric absorption and Compton scattering move through tissue and deposit or transfer energy through ionizations. The rate at which an electron (or an x-ray photon that ejected it) transfers energy (as it moves through some length of tissue) to the surrounding tissue

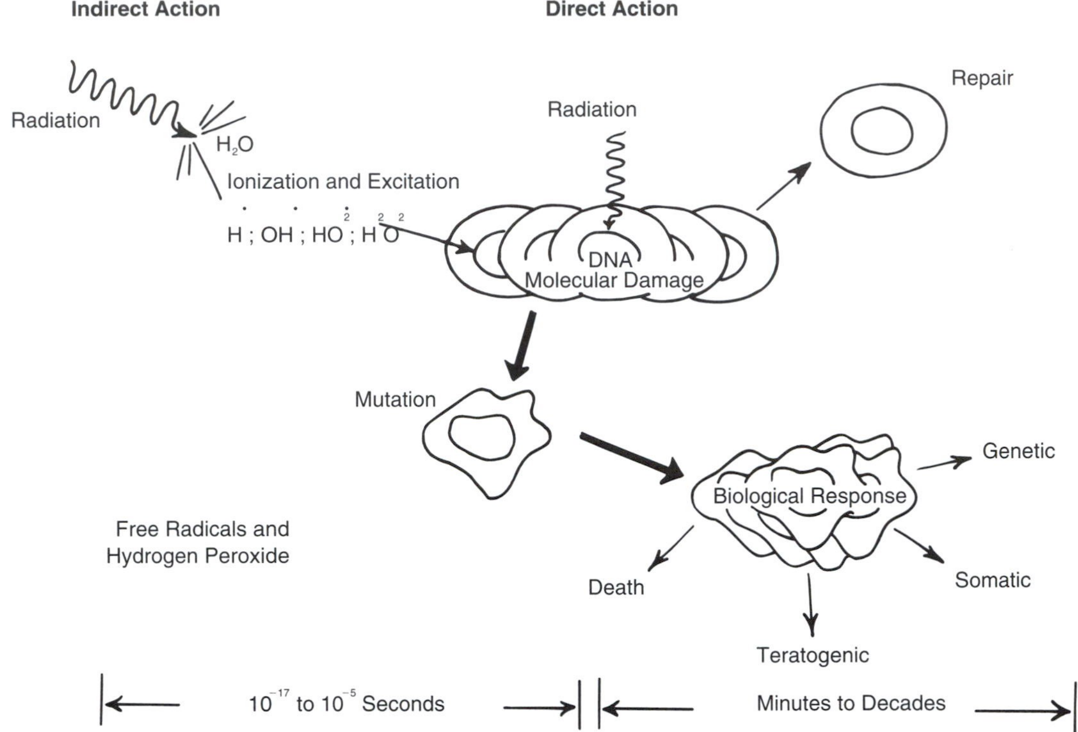

FIGURE 2-24. Direct and indirect action of radiation. [From Bushberg, J.T., Seibert, J.A., Leidholdt Jr, E.M., & Boone, J.M. (1994). *The essential physics of medical imaging*. Baltimore: Williams & Wilkins. Reproduced by permission.]

is referred to as LET. LET is expressed in units of keV per micrometer (μm) of path length (keV/μm). As the LET of the radiation increases, the biological response increases because more ionizations are produced along the path of travel of the electron, as shown in Figure 2-25.

The LET for diagnostic x-rays is 3.0 keV/μm, whereas it is 50 keV/μm for fast neutrons and 100 keV/μm for 5-MeV alpha particles. Therefore, 5-MeV alpha particles (high LET) are more damaging per unit of absorbed dose (gray) than fast neutrons and diagnostic rays (Bushberg, 1994).

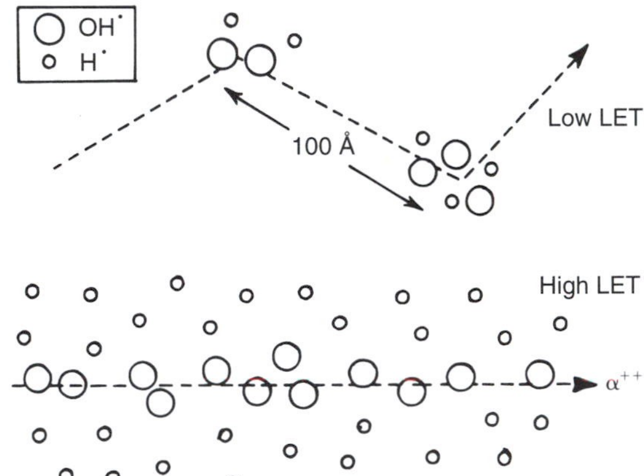

FIGURE 2-25. As the LET of the radiation increases (high LET), more ionizations are produced along the path through which the ionizing particle moves. [From Wolbarst, A.B. (1993). *Physics of radiology*. Norwalk, CT: Appleton & Lange. Reproduced by permission.]

Relative Biological Effectiveness

As mentioned in the preceding paragraph, different radiations (e.g., x-rays, neutrons, alpha particles) have different LET values. The higher the

LET, the greater the biological response. Even though different types of radiation produce the same kinds of biological response, the size of the effect varies per unit dose depending on the LETs. The effectiveness of different types of radiations and their associated LETs can be evaluated in experiments that compare a dose of the test radiation to a particular dose of a reference radiation in terms of how much of each is needed to generate the same specific biological response (typically 250 keV x-rays) (Bushberg, 1994, p. 658).

The effectiveness of the dose of test radiation (D_{test}) to the dose of the reference radiation ($D_{reference}$) is referred to as the *relative biological effectiveness* (RBE), which is expressed mathematically as:

$$RBE = \frac{D_{reference}}{D_{test}} \qquad (2\text{-}22)$$

If the test radiation is more effective than the reference radiation, the smaller the dose needed to produce the same biological effect and the greater will be the RBE.

The relationship between LET and RBE is a complex one that varies over the course of radiation. Initially, RBE is proportional to LET. That is to say, an increase in LET is mirrored by an increase in RBE (Fig. 2-26). This is so be-

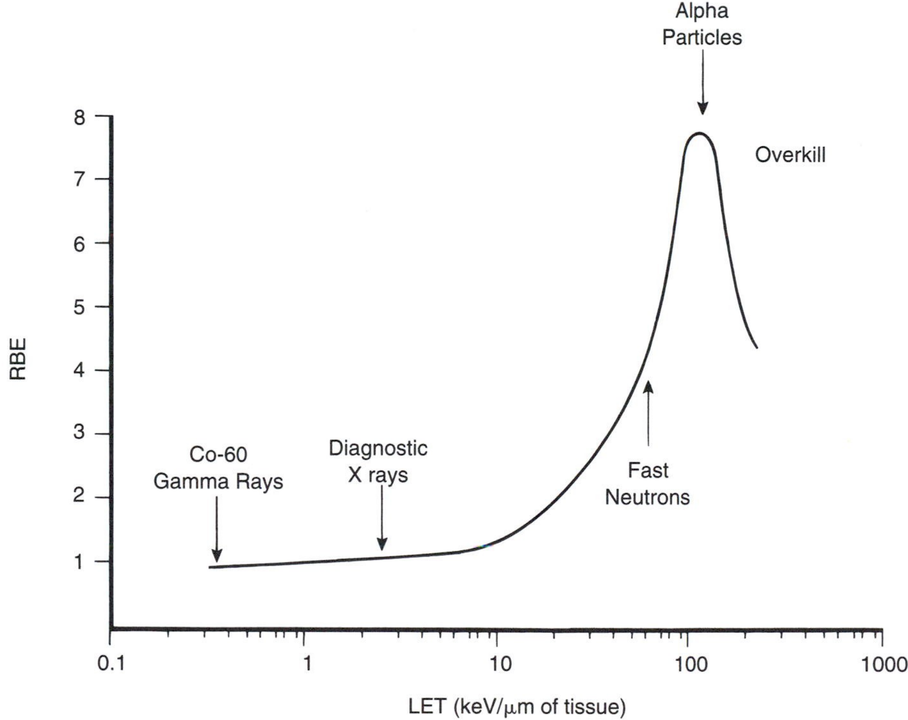

FIGURE 2-26. The relative biological effectiveness (RBE) of a given radiation is an empirically derived term that, in general, all other factors held constant, increases with the LET of the radiation. Note, however, that the radiation becomes less efficient beyond ~100 keV/μm. This is the result of overkill, in which the maximum potential damage has already been reached and the increases in LET beyond this point result in wasted dose. For example, at 500 keV/μm, many of the cells may have three or more ionizing events when only two are required to kill the cell. [From Bushberg, J.T., Seibert, J.A., Leidholdt Jr, E.M., & Boone, J.M. (1994). *The essential physics of medical imaging*. Baltimore: Williams & Wilkins. Reproduced by permission.]

cause high LET radiation produces higher specific ionization than does lower LET radiation, and high LET radiation is more heavily implicated in cellular damage. Once the tissue level of radiation goes beyond 100 keV/μm, the RBE decreases with increasing LET because of the *overkill effect*. The overkill effect comes into play when the amount of radiation in the tissue exceeds that which is necessary to kill the cells in that tissue.

In general the RBE ranges from <1 to >20. The specific RBE for a given type of radiation depends on the biological end point being used—"chromosomal mutation, cataract formation, or acute lethality" in test animals can all be used as end points—and the total dose and dose rate. Even given these limitations, the RBE is a useful tool for characterizing the potential damaging effects of different types of radiation (Bushberg, 1994).

REVIEW QUESTIONS

1. Which of the following represents Bohr's model of the atom?
   A. Electrons revolving about a small, dense, positively charged, central nucleus in prescribed orbits or energy levels.
   B. A dense nucleus revolving about a central group of electrons.
   C. A plum pudding in which the plums represent the electrons.
   D. Atoms have hooks and eyes which connect to form chemical compounds.

2. Which of the following is a positively charged particle?
   A. An electron.
   B. A neutron.
   C. A proton.
   D. All of the above.

3. The number of positively charged particles in the nucleus is called the:
   A. Atomic number.
   B. Atomic mass number.
   C. Nuclear coefficient.
   D. Elemental mass or atomic mass unit.

4. Which of the following electron orbit, or shell, is closest to the nucleus?
   A. K
   B. L
   C. M
   D. N

5. Which of the following expressions is used to find out the number of electrons contained in each of the electron shells, or orbits?
   A. $2n \times (n)^2$
   B. $n^3 + 2n$
   C. $2 + (n)^2$
   D. $2(n)^2$

6. The M shell of the atom can have ______ electrons.
   A. 18
   B. 9
   C. 15
   D. 36

7. Which of the following electrons has the greatest binding energy?
   A. Electrons in the L shell.
   B. Electrons in the K shell.
   C. Electrons in the M shell.
   D. Electrons in the O shell.

8. In excitation:
   A. Electrons are removed from the atom.
   B. Electrons absorb energy from the radiation beam and move into orbits farther away from the nucleus.
   C. The nucleus gains energy.
   D. Protons are ejected from the nucleus.

9. Ionization is:
   A. The removal of an electron from the K shell to the outermost shell of the atom.
   B. The removal of protons from the nucleus.
   C. The removal of neutrons from the nucleus.
   D. The removal of electrons from the atom.

10. Electromagnetic radiation consists of:
    A. An electric field moving through space.
    B. A magnetic field moving through space.
    C. Both electric and magnetic fields moving through space, perpendicular to each other.
    D. Particles such as alpha, beta, and protons.

11. All of the following belong to the electromagnetic spectrum except:
    A. Alpha particles.
    B. X-rays.
    C. Gamma rays.
    D. Radiowaves.

12. Which of the following is more penetrating?
    A. X-rays.
    B. Gamma rays.
    C. Alpha particles.
    D. Beta particles.

13. Which of the following is an example of nonionizing radiation?
    A. Ultrasound.
    B. X-rays.
    C. Gamma radiation.
    D. Beta particles.

14. The fundamental tenet of the wave-particle theory of electromagnetic radiation holds that:
    A. Radiation can behave both as a wave and as a particle.
    B. Radiation can behave only as waves.
    C. Radiation can behave only as particles.
    D. Radiation causes biological effects.

15. The wave equation implies that the:
    A. Velocity of a wave is inversely proportional to the wavelength.
    B. Velocity of a wave is inversely proportional to the frequency.
    C. Velocity of a wave is directly proportional to the wavelength and inversely proportional to the frequency.
    D. Velocity of a wave is directly proportional to the wavelength and frequency of the radiation.

16. Which equation would be used to find the wavelength (λ) of a proton (energy = E)?
    A. $\lambda = 12.4/E$
    B. $\lambda = E/12.4$
    C. $\lambda = E \times 12.4$
    D. $\lambda = 1.24/E$

17. The unit of energy in the above equation is the:
    A. Angstrom.
    B. Kiloelectron volt.
    C. Rad.
    D. Roentgen.

18. X-rays are produced in an x-ray tube when:
    A. High-speed electrons from the filament strike the target of the anode.
    B. Electrons are "boiled off" the filament.
    C. The target is heated to 2000°C.
    D. The filament is heated by 6 amperes.

19. The flow of electrons from cathode to anode of an x-ray tube is referred to as the:
    A. mA.
    B. kVp.
    C. Filament current.
    D. All of the above.

20. Characteristic x-rays are produced when:
    A. High-speed electrons collide with inner shell target electrons and cause ionization.
    B. Electrons interact with the nucleus of the atom.

C. Electrons are "boiled off" the filament.
D. None of the above is correct.

21. Bremsstrahlung radiation is produced when:
A. High-speed electrons collide with the inner shell target atoms and cause ionization.
B. High-speed electrons are decelerated by the force field of the nucleus, thus losing their kinetic energy and changing their direction of travel.
C. Electrons are raised to higher orbits.
D. The nucleus loses protons.

22. A plot of the number of x-ray photons emanating from the x-ray tube as a function of the energy of the photons is called the:
A. X-ray emission spectrum.
B. mA spectrum.
C. kVp spectrum.
D. Exposure technique factors.

23. The major controlling factor for beam quality that is under the direct control of the technologist is the:
A. Voltage waveform.
B. Filtration.
C. X-ray tube target material.
D. kVp.

24. Which of the following is the major controlling factor for beam quantity?
A. kVp.
B. Exposure time.
C. mA.
D. Filtration.

25. Filtration of the x-ray beam will result in:
A. A harder beam.
B. A more penetrating beam.
C. A decrease in x-ray quantity and an increase in beam quality.
D. All of the above.

26. Which of the following results in an increase in scattered radiation production?
A. Photoelectric absorption.
B. Classical scattering.
C. Pair production.
D. Compton effect.

27. Which of the following interactions will result in an increase in radiation dose to the patient?
A. Classical scattering.
B. Photoelectric absorption.
C. Compton effect.
D. Pair production.

28. Which of the following will attenuate more radiation?
A. Bone.
B. Muscle.
C. Fat.
D. Lung.

29. Which of the following affects radiation attenuation?
A. The energy of the beam.
B. The atomic number and the electrons per gram of tissue.
C. The density of the absorbing material.
D. All of the above.

30. The half value layer (HVL) of a radiation beam expresses the:
A. Beam quantity.
B. Voltage waveform.
C. Beam quality.
D. Attenuation.

31. Which of the following results in ionization of water to form free radicals?
A. Indirect action.
B. Direct action.
C. Filtration.
D. All of the above.

32. Which of the following are the final products of the dissociation of water by radiation?
    A. Hydrogen ion.
    B. Hydroxyl ion.
    C. Hydrogen and hydroxyl free radicals.
    D. All of the above.

33. The rate of energy transfer by an electron as it moves through tissue is referred to as:
    A. The relative biological effectiveness (RBE).
    B. The linear energy transfer (LET).
    C. Ionization.
    D. Excitation.

34. As the LET of the radiation increases, RBE:
    A. Increases.
    B. Decreases.
    C. Remains unchanged.
    D. There is no relationship between RBE and LET.

35. Which of the following has the highest LET?
    A. Alpha^{++} particles.
    B. X-ray photons.
    C. Neutrons.
    D. Protons.

REFERENCES

Bushberg, J.T., Seibert, J.A., Leidholdt Jr, E.M., & Boone, J.M. (1994). *The Essential physics of medical imaging.* Baltimore: Williams & Wilkins.

Bushong, S. (1993). *Radiologic science for technologists.* (5th ed.). St Louis: Mosby-Year Book.

Hall, E.J. (1988). *Radiobiology for the radiologist.* (3d ed.). Philadelphia: J.B. Lippincott.

Thompson, M.A., Hattaway, M.P., Hall, J.D., & Dowd, S.B. (1993). *Principles of imaging science and protection.* Philadelphia: W.B. Saunders.

Wolbarst, A.B. (1993). *Physics of radiology.* Norwalk, CT: Appleton and Lange.

Wootton, R. (Ed.). (1993). *Radiation protection of patients.* Cambridge, England: Cambridge University Press, 1993.

CHAPTER THREE

RADIATION EXPOSURE

LEARNING OBJECTIVES

Upon completion of this chapter, the reader should be able to:

1 ■ Identify two main sources of radiation exposure.

2 ■ Describe the contribution of radiation exposure from cosmic rays, earth sources, and internal sources.

3 ■ List several man-made sources of radiation exposure and state the reasons why medical radiation is of importance to the technologist.

4 ■ List two classes of medical radiation exposure.

5 ■ Describe each of the following types of exposure: occupational exposure, medical exposure, and public exposure.

6 ■ Explain what is meant by each of the following: radiation field, radiation concentration, and the international system of units.

7 ■ Define each of the following radiation quantities and their associated units:

(continued)

exposure, kerma, absorbed dose, dose equivalent, equivalent dose, and effective dose.

8 ■ Explain what is meant by each of the following terms: radiation weighting factor and tissue weighting factor.

9 ■ Define each of the following terms: skin dose, average organ dose, depth dose, average dose to the patient, and integral dose.

Introduction

In this chapter, we set the stage for the rest of this book by exploring the sources of radiation exposure, the types of exposure, and fundamental dosimetric quantities and their units.

Both natural and man-made sources of radiation exposure are important to the technologist. Of the man-made sources, medical radiation exposure is the most important. Because annual dose limits for individuals are established based on the types of exposure, it is mandatory that we have a clear understanding of the meaning of medical exposure and how it compares to both occupational and public exposure.

To understand dose limits, we define and explain the fundamental radiation quantities and their units. First, we introduce the International System of Units (SI units); this topic is followed by a discussion of radiation quantities such as exposure, kerma, absorbed dose, and dose equivalent, as well as their respective units, including their conversion to SI units.

Finally, the chapter concludes with a brief introduction to patient dose distributions and methods of reporting patient doses in diagnostic radiology.

Sources of Exposure

Radiation is all around us. Every day we are exposed to some form of radiation emanating from two main types of sources: those that are natural and those that are man-made. The contributions of each of these sources are shown in Figure 3-1.

Natural Radiation Sources

Natural radiation sources include cosmic radiation, earth sources, and internal sources.

Cosmic radiation consists of several types of radiation having different energies and includes solar and galactic radiation. Whereas solar radiation consists of protons and helium, for example, galactic radiation includes photons, gamma rays, high energy protons, neutrons, and several subatomic particles such as mesons and pions. In addition, galactic particles include protons and alpha particles, for example; exposure to these particles represents a particular hazard to those engaged in prolonged space flights (Luckey, 1991).

Exposure to cosmic radiation varies directly with altitude. In other words, as altitude increases, the rate of cosmic radiation exposure also increases. For each 2 km above sea level, cosmic radiation exposure doubles. This means that people living in New York City receive about half the exposure to cosmic radiation that people living in Denver receive. However, people who climb mountains are subjected to about three times more cosmic radiation exposure (at 3000 m) than people living on the coast. Luckey (1991) also pointed out that the crews of commercial aircraft and diplomatic carriers, who spend 500 hr/yr traveling at 11,000 m, are exposed to about 1.5 mGy/yr from cosmic radiation. Pilots and attendants traveling in supersonic aircraft at 13 km receive no more cosmic radiation than do other pilots. In fact, they may receive less as a result of decreased exposure time (Luckey, 1991).

Another natural source of radiation exposure is that of *earth radiation*, which includes

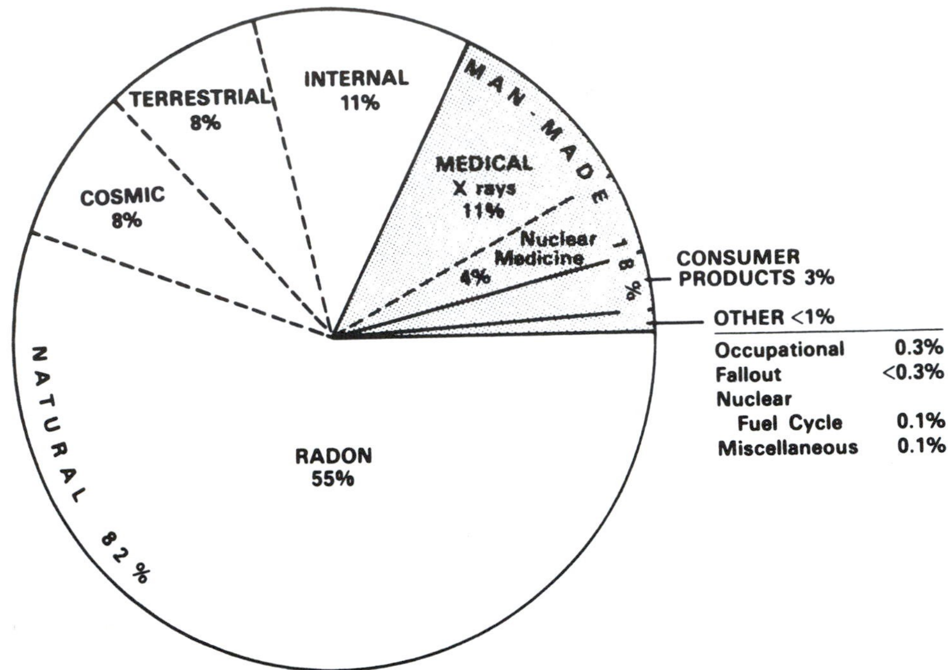

FIGURE 3-1. The percentage contribution of each of the sources of radiation to the U.S. population. [From Hall, E.J. (1994). *Radiobiology for the radiobiologist*. Philadelphia: J.B. Lippincott.]

radiation from the air, terrestrial radiation, radiation from buildings, radionuclides in food and drink, and endogenous radiation, which emanates from the human body.

Radiation from the air includes products from nuclear reactors, nuclear explosions, soil, coal, and cosmogenic reactions (these range from protons, electrons, tritium, and beryllium to thorium-232, uranium-238, potassium-40, and rubidium-87). Terrestrial radiation arises, however, from two categories of radionuclides: (1) the three families of uranium-238, uranium-235, and thorium-232 and (2) potassium-40 (Luckey, 1991).

Of particular concern is radiation exposure to *radon gas*, which is the major source of exposure of the general public (See Figure 3-1 for the percentage contribution of radon and various other sources of radiation exposure). Radon is of concern because its decay products, alpha emitters, when inhaled find their way to the bronchial epithelium and result in an increase in the incidence of lung cancer (Hart et al., 1990; Hendee and Doege, 1987).

Radon-222 (Rn-222) arises from the decay of uranium-238. It is a radioactive gas that is invisible, colorless, odorless, and chemically nonreactive. As shown in Figure 3-2, radon enters a building from the underlying soil as well as from water, building materials, and natural gas. As illustrated in the figure, the radon gas can be removed by proper ventilation.

Radiation from buildings arises from the concentrations of radionuclides in granite, stone, sandstone, limestone, and wood; granite contributes twice as much radiation as stone, which itself contributes twice the amount of radiation as sandstone and wood (Luckey, 1991).

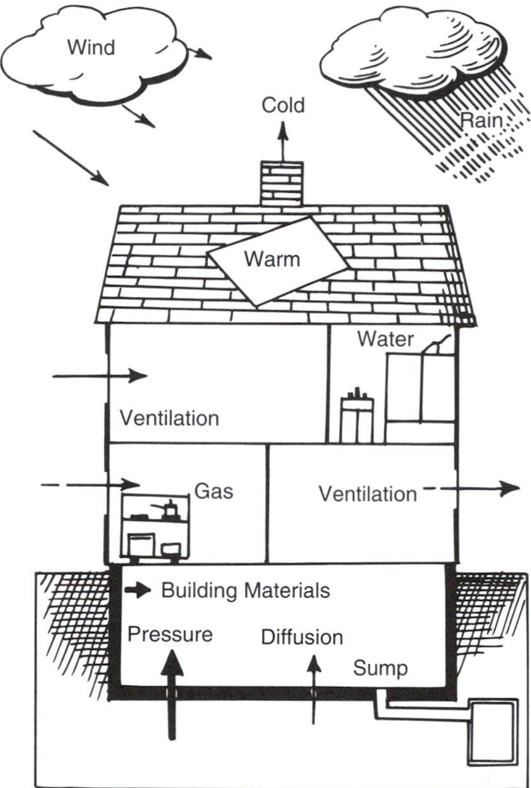

FIGURE 3-2. Sources of indoor radon gas and processes for its removal. [From Hart, B.L., Mettler, F.A., & Harley, N.H. (1989). Radon: Is it a problem? *Radiology, 172*, 593–599. Reproduced by permission.]

Luckey (1991), however, pointed out that a wooden house blocks as much cosmic and earth radiation as it contributes.

Radionuclides that normally occur in food and drink (dairy, eggs, meat, vegetables, fruit, seafood, cereals, etc.) are potassium-40, strontium-89, strontium-90, cesium-137, and several others.

But what about food that is irradiated for the purposes of sterilization? Do the foods themselves become radioactive as a result? The answer to this question is provided by Luckey (1991), who stated that cobalt-60, the 1.3-MeV gamma ray source of ionizing radiation used in food sterilization, is powerful enough to kill microbes but not powerful enough to induce radioactivity in the exposed foodstuffs.

Finally, *endogenous radiation* refers to radiation produced within or caused by factors within the body. This radiation arises from several radionuclides, including carbon-14, potassium-40, rubidium-87, strontium-90, radon-222, and thorium-232.

Various organs of the body are exposed to different amounts of radiation from different radionuclides. The liver, for example, receives most radiation exposure from plutonium, which is also found in lymph nodes and bone, as well as in the lungs, gonads, spleen, and the kidneys.

Internal radionuclides make each and every one of us a source of radiation. In this regard, Luckey (1991) indicated that:

> An adult emits about 100 gamma rays per second. Sleeping with an adult adds about 0.04 mGy/year to one's exposure. Family, friends and coworkers may add another 0.02 mGy/year. You may receive more if the persons close to you smoke or have been given radionuclides for medical purposes. Endogenous radiation begins at conception, is continuous through death, and becomes more intense with cremation; radionuclides in the ashes are about ten times more concentrated than in the body (p. 19–20).

Man-Made Radiation Sources

It was the Curies who discovered man-made sources of radiation toward the end of the 19th century. Man-made sources include those arising from industry, nuclear fallout, and medicine.

Industrial radiation sources include those from mining, nuclear power plants, and consumer products. In mining, it was the radioactivity in uranium mines (in which uranium ores were mined for radium) that caused exposure to miners in Arizona, Colorado, New Mexico, Nevada, and Utah. The natural decay of uranium-238 into radon-222 (a noble gas that itself decays through the emission of alpha, beta, and gamma radiation), represents a means of radiation exposure.

Do you recall Three Mile Island and Chernobyl? These names were made infamous by their association with nuclear power plant accidents. In 1979, a major meltdown occurred at Three Mile Island in Pennsylvania, during which radioactive materials were released into the atmosphere. On Saturday, April 25, 1987, at 1:23 AM, a reactor at the nuclear power station at Chernobyl exploded, releasing a plume of radioactive materials and gases, such as iodine-131, cesium-137, and strontium-90, into the environment.

In addition, nuclear power plants emit, as a matter of course, airborne wastes in the form of radioactive gases such as krypton and xenon, as well as other radioactive materials (e.g., strontium-89 and barium-140).

A wide variety of consumer products utilize radioactive materials. These include smoke alarms, which contain americium; watches and clocks that feature luminous dials and numbers, which contain tritium, strontium-90, radium-226, and promethium-147; and cardiac pacemakers, which contain plutonium-238.

Other consumer products such as televisions and video display terminals (VDTs) are of concern as well because they use cathode ray tubes (CRTs), which are known to be sources of radiation. Because the average operating hours for these devices are about 7 hr/day, exposures have been reported at an annual dose of up to 0.3 mGy (Pomroy and Noel, 1984). "For children who sit too close, the dose to the eye may become more important than the gonadal dose" (Luckey, 1991, p. 28).

Fallout refers to radiation produced as a result of nuclear testing and chemical explosions in nuclear facilities. While atomic testing can release tritium, atmospheric bomb tests can release iodine-131 in addition to cerium-144, cesium-137, and strontium-90, the latter two of which emit beta radiation. The amount of cesium-134 released during the explosion at Chernobyl was greater than that associated with the detonation of atomic bombs (Luckey, 1991).

Finally, *medical radiation* constitutes the last category of man-made radiation to be discussed in this book. Medical radiation is important to technologists for several reasons:

1. It represents the greatest source of exposure to the population.
2. It is this radiation to which our patients are exposed.
3. The radiation protection recommendations with which we are concerned in this text have been established for medical radiation.
4. It represents low-level radiation, which has received much attention in terms of both stochastic and deterministic biological effects.
5. Medical radiation exposure of the patient should always result in some benefit.
6. Medical radiation exposure of the patient is determined by a set of technical factors that are under the direct control of the technologist. These factors include technique factors (kVp and mAs), collimation, shielding, positioning, and patient instructions.

For these reasons, we explore medical radiation in more detail in the next section.

Medical Radiation Exposure

Medical radiation exposure arises from two classes of radiation: ionizing and nonionizing. Whereas medical radiation technologies that utilize ionizing radiation include diagnostic radiology, nuclear medicine, and radiation therapy, technologies based on nonionizing radiation include diagnostic medical sonography (ultrasound) and magnetic resonance imaging. These technologies were described briefly in Chapter 1 and will not be treated here; however, it is important to review the major sources of radiation used, particularly in diagnostic radiology.

The main source of radiation in diagnostic radiology is the x-ray tube (Fig. 3-3). The essential features of the tube are two electrodes, an anode and a cathode, positioned opposite each other and sealed in a vacuum by a surrounding glass envelope. X-rays are produced when electrons from the filament of the cathode are accelerated at high speeds across the vacuum to strike the target region of the anode.

The radiation beam emanating from the x-ray tube is a heterogeneous beam consisting of x-rays of both long and short wavelengths. Whereas the high-energy short wavelength x-ray photons penetrate the patient's body to form an image on the film, the long, less penetrating wavelength photons are usually absorbed by the patient, thus increasing patient dose. These x-rays are unwanted, and in radiography every effort is made to remove these low energy photons.

In nuclear medicine, several different radionuclides are used. These range from I-123, I-131, and Tc-99 to Fe-59, Ga-67, In-111, Xe-133, Hg-197, and Au-199, to mention only a few.

In radiation therapy, x-rays, neutrons, protons, heavy ions, and pions are used to irradiate tumor cells in patients.

Finally, in MRI the radiation used is a burst of radiowaves, which are part of the electromagnetic spectrum as described in Chapter 2.

Types of Exposure

Now that we have identified the various sources of radiation exposure, it is essential

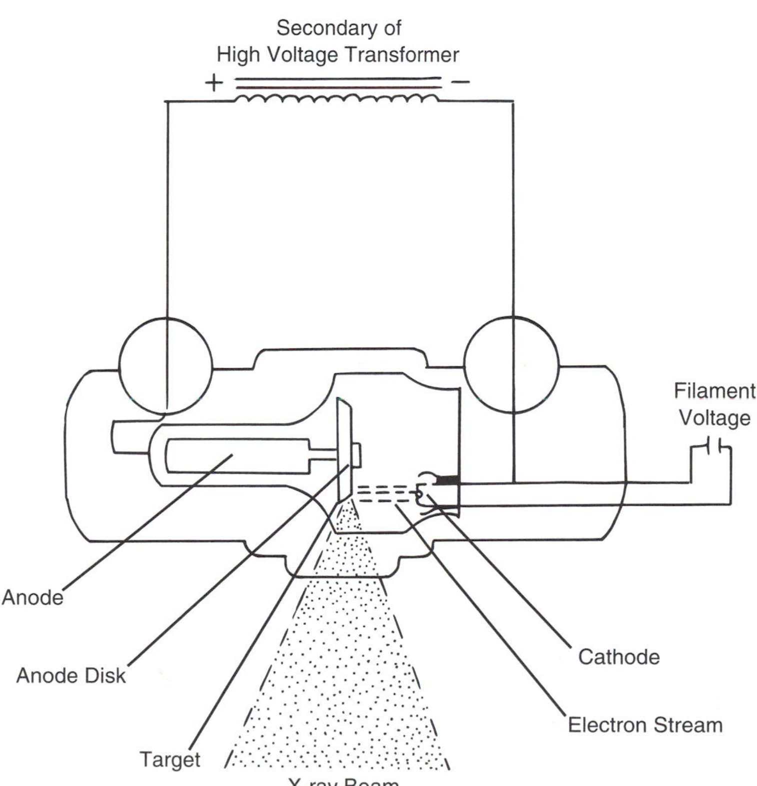

FIGURE 3-3. The essential features of a rotating anode x-ray tube used in diagnostic radiology. [From Seeram, E. (1985). *X-ray imaging equipment: An introduction*. Springfield, IL: Charles C. Thomas.]

that we consider the types of radiation exposure, that is, the situations in which individuals are exposed to the various sources, because dose limits depend on them. These situations include exposure at work (occupational exposure), exposure due to medical diagnosis or radiation therapy (medical exposure), and all other exposures (public exposure). Each of these will now be described briefly. In doing so, we quote the ICRP (1991) with respect to the various types of exposure.

Occupational Exposure

Occupational exposure refers to exposures received at work. A more elaborate definition of this is given by the ICRP (1991) as "... exposures incurred at work as a result of situations that can reasonably be regarded as being the responsibility of the operating management" (p. 33).

For radiologic technologists, this refers to work in the radiology department and includes activities in general radiography and fluoroscopy, special procedures such as angiography and CT, mobile radiography and fluoroscopy, and operating room radiography. In addition, the ICRP (1991) pointed out that "any exposure at work (excluding any medical exposure at work) as a result of artificial sources in, or associated with, the workplace should be included in occupational exposure, unless the sources have formally been excluded from regulatory control or exempted from the relevant aspects of regulatory control by the regulatory agency" (p. 34).

The previous statement would appear to indicate that if a diagnostic radiologic technologist is exposed to a patient who is radioactive while in the radiology department, this would constitute occupational exposure. Also, if the radiologic technologist is exposed to radionuclides while in the nuclear medicine department, this would be included in the occupational exposure category.

Medical Exposure

The ICRP provides us with the following definition of *medical exposure*:

> Medical exposure is confined to exposure incurred by individuals as part of their own medical diagnosis or treatment and to exposures (other than occupational) incurred knowingly and willingly by individuals helping in the support and comfort of patients undergoing diagnosis or treatment. Exposure of an individual to other sources, such as stray radiation from the diagnosis or treatment of other persons, is not included in medical exposure. Nor is any occupational exposure of staff (p. 34).

Should a technologist receive a chest x-ray for the purpose of managing his or her own illness, the dose resulting from this exposure is considered medical exposure and is therefore not included in his or her occupational exposure.

Public Exposure

What is meant by public exposure? Once again, the ICRP (1991) provided us with a serviceable definition:

> Public exposure encompasses all exposures other than occupational and medical exposures. The component of public exposure due to natural sources is by far the largest, but this provides no justification for reducing the attention paid to smaller but more readily controlled exposures to artificial sources (p. 34).

This statement indicates that even though the public receives exposure from natural sources, such exposures should not interfere with the decision to expose the individual to medical radiation in order to restore health.

Fundamental Dosimetric Quantities and Units

Radiation Field

Now that we have a general idea of the types of exposure, it is essential that we understand exposure quantities and their respective units.

The radiation beam emanating from the x-ray tube describes an area consisting of an average number of rays referred to as the *radiation field.* The field can be shaped or collimated to cover any size appropriate to the anatomy of interest.

The patient is exposed to the radiation field, which is characterized by several quantities, as shown in Figure 3-4. Two of these, the *integral exposure* and the *integral dose,* relate to the total amount of radiation falling on the patient. In addition, the radiation beam is concentrated on a particular point on the patient (the square in the middle of the beam in Fig. 3-4). This *radiation concentration* (number of photons passing through the area on the patient) can be described by three fundamental dosimetric quantities, exposure, absorbed dose, and dose equivalent (Sprawls, 1990), each of which is described in subsequent sections of this text.

These radiation quantities, as they are often referred to, have special units. While the conventional units were specified in the centimeter-gram-second (cgs) system, there has been a strong movement to specify these same units in the International System (SI) of units. Because the SI system is now common in science and technology, and radiation protection in particular, we examine its essential elements in the next subsection.

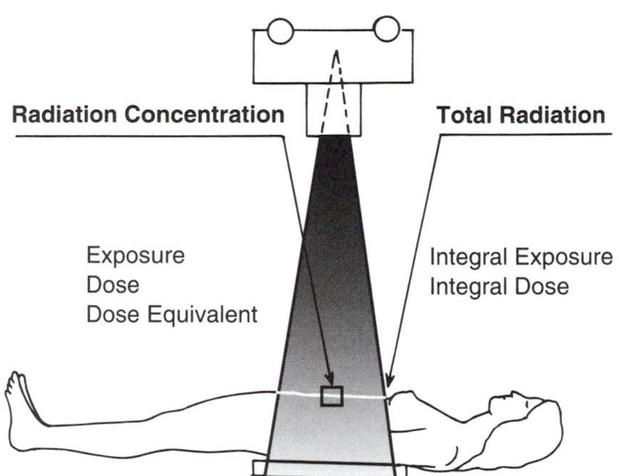

FIGURE 3-4. In diagnostic radiology, the patient is exposed to the radiation field emanating from the x-ray tube. The field is characterized by several quantities that describe both the radiation concentration and the total radiation incident on the patient. [From Sprawls, P. (1990). *Principles of radiography for technologists.* Rockville, MD: Aspen. Reproduced by permission.]

International System of Units

In 1960, an extension of the metric system, referred to as *Le Système International d'Unités* (SI), translated as the *International System of Units,* was adopted by the General Conference of Weights and Measures for all branches of science. These include radiation sciences (radiation physics, radiation chemistry, and radiation biology), radiation protection, diagnostic radiology, nuclear medicine, and radiation therapy.

In 1977, the ICRP began using SI units in their reports and for a period of time, SI units slowly preceded the former or conventional units, which were enclosed in parentheses. In addition, the International Commission on Radiological Units and Measurements (ICRU) recommended that SI units be adopted by 1985.

SI units are now commonplace in the literature and have been adopted by several countries, including Canada. In the United States, the NCRP (1990) made the following statement with respect to SI units in radiation protection and measurements:

> After 1989, it is recommended that SI units be used exclusively. In tables, graphs, and radiation records, one system of units would be used with a footnote containing conversion factors to the other system (p. 2).

Throughout this book, SI units will be used. For studies that have reported doses in the old units, these will be cited and it is left up to the reader to make the conversion to SI units.

There are two classes of units in the SI system: *base units* and *supplementary units.* The base units are the meter (m), kilogram (kg), and the second (s) for the physical quantities of length, mass, and time, respectively; the supplementary units are the radian (rad) and the steradian (S), which are used, respectively, to denote the plane angle and the solid angle. From these units, other units can be derived using basic mathematics (products or quotients).

The NCRP (1990) indicated that "a major argument in favor of the SI is the simplicity and coherence of the system" (p. 21). Coherence implies that 1 (and no other factor) is used to convert from the base and supplementary units. The example cited by the NCRP in the coherent SI for "absorbed dose" (p. 50), is as follows:

$$1 \text{ Gray (Gy)} = \frac{1 \text{ joule (J)}}{1 \text{ kilogram (kg)}}$$

$$= 1 \cdot \text{Jkg}^{-1} \text{ or } 1 \text{ J/kg}$$

Finally, the SI system uses prefixes to generate multiples and submultiples of these units. These prefixes are listed in Table 3-1.

Exposure and Its Unit

Technologists think of *exposure* as the quantity of radiation falling on the patient. Actually, exposure is more narrowly defined as "a quantity that expresses the concentration of radiation delivered to a specific point, rather than the total radiation delivered to the patient's body or other object" (Sprawls, 1990, p. 32).

In Figure 3-4, the concentration of radiation in the region of the small square is not the same as the concentration covering the total area of the beam falling on the patient. If the technologist changes the area of the beam by collimating it to cover a larger region of the patient, for example, the entire abdomen, it would do nothing to alter the center of the area, although it would obviously change the total amount of radiation entering the body (Sprawls, 1990, p. 33).

TABLE 3-1. SI PREFIXES USED TO GENERATE MULTIPLES AND SUBMULTIPLES OF RADIATION UNITS

Prefix	Symbol	Factor	Unit	Symbol
centi	c	10^{-2}	centigray	cGy
milli	m	10^{-3}	milligray	mGy
			millisievert	mSv
micro	μ	10^{-6}	microgray	μGy
			microsievert	μSv
nano	n	10^{-9}	nanosievert	nSv
pico	p	10^{-12}	picocoulombs	pC

If we place an ionization chamber in the region of the small square, we can measure the exposure. The radiation beam will ionize the air in the chamber and the exposure can then be defined. Exposure is the radiation quantity used as a measure of the amount of ionization produced in a specific mass of air by x or gamma radiation. The ionization tells us something about the amount of radiation to which an individual is exposed.

The conventional unit of exposure is the *roentgen* (R), which was proposed in 1928 by the ICRU. The roentgen is defined as "the amount of x or gamma rays that produces a given amount of ionization in a unit of air, 0.000258 coulomb per kilogram (c/kg) or 1.0 electrostatic unit (esu) in 0.0001293 g of air" (NCRP, 1989, p. 4). The roentgen produces 2.58×10^{-4} *coulombs per kilogram* of air at standard temperature and pressure, or 2.1×10^{9} ion pairs per cubic centimeter of air at 0°C.

The student may notice that while older studies in the literature report exposure in milliroentgens (mR), a much smaller unit (1 R = 1000 mR), more recent studies report exposure in SI units. The SI unit of exposure is the coulomb per kilogram (C/kg or $C \cdot kg^{-1}$).

$$1 \text{ R} = 2.58 \times 10^{-4} \text{ C} \cdot \text{kg}^{-1}$$

or

$$3876 \text{ R} = 1 \text{ C} \cdot \text{kg}^{-1}$$

Submultiples of the roentgen are as follows:

$$1 \text{ R} = 258 \text{ microcoulombs/kilogram } (\mu\text{C} \cdot \text{kg}^{-1})$$

$$1 \text{ mR} = 258 \text{ nanocoulombs/kilogram } (\text{nC} \cdot \text{kg}^{-1})$$

$$1 \text{ μR} = 258 \text{ picocoulombs/kilogram } (\text{pC} \cdot \text{kg}^{-1})$$

A concept related to exposure is *exposure rate.* If a technologist delivers a certain amount of exposure to the patient per unit time at a given point, the exposure rate can be calculated as follows:

$$\text{Exposure} = \text{Exposure rate} \times \text{Time} \quad (3\text{-}1)$$

Another concept related to exposure is the *surface integral exposure* (SIE), and it is extremely important in terms of reducing the amount of radiation delivered to the patient. The SIE takes into account both the exposure and the area of the beam falling on the patient (Sprawls, 1990), and it can be expressed as follows (for uniform exposure):

$$\text{SIE} = \text{Exposure} \times \text{area of the radiation beam} \quad (3\text{-}2)$$

Equation 3-2 has implications for the importance of collimation (i.e., limiting the radiation beam to the anatomy of interest) during an examination. If the beam size is small, then the total radiation to the patient is also small. Therefore, the technologist must always collimate the beam only to the area of interest and to the size of the image receptor (film cassette) or smaller.

Kerma and Its Unit

When the patient is exposed to a beam of radiation, two events occur:

1. The photons from the beam interact with the atoms in the patient and may eject an electron from its orbit. In this event, energy transfer occurs. Specifically, kinetic energy is transferred from the beam (photons) to the patient (electrons). This energy transfer is called *kerma*, that is, the kinetic energy released in the material. While the old unit of kerma is the erg per gram ($\text{erg}\cdot\text{g}^{-1}$), the SI unit is the joule per kilogram ($\text{J}\cdot\text{kg}^{-1}$).
2. Kinetic energy from the ejected electron, which takes place by ionization and excitation (Chapter 2), is absorbed. This event leads to the quantity referred to as the absorbed dose.

Whereas kerma deals with the transfer of energy at a point, absorbed dose refers to the absorption of energy along the path that the ejected electron travels in the patient's tissue.

Absorbed Dose and Its Unit

The roentgen (R) is a unit of measure whose use is restricted to photons, but other kinds of ionizing radiation transfer energy to the absorbing medium as well. The amount of energy absorbed per unit mass is referred to as the *absorbed dose.*

The original unit of absorbed dose, the *rad*, was defined in terms of an energy deposition of 100 erg/g of absorber. In SI units, the unit of absorbed dose is called the *Gray* (Gy) in honor of Louis Harold Gray, an English radiobiologist who played a major role in setting up procedures to measure radiation absorbed dose.

The Gray is defined as 1 joule (J) of energy deposition in 1 kg of material. This can be expressed as:

$$1\ \text{Gy} = 1\ \text{J/kg} = 1\ \text{J}\cdot\text{kg}^{-1}$$
$$\text{or } 1\ \text{rad} = 10^{-2}\ \text{Gy}$$
$$\text{or } 100\ \text{rad} = 1\ \text{Gy}$$

Submultiples of the Gray are:

1 centigray (cGy) = 1 rad

1 milligray (mGy) = 100 millirad (mrad)

1 microgray (μGy) = 100 microrad (μrad)

1 nanogray (nGy) = 100 nanorad (nrad)

It should be noted that 1 rad (1 R) is approximately equal to an absorbed dose of 0.01 Gy. We can also calculate the tissue or organ absorbed dose through the following relationship:

$$\text{Tissue or organ dose} = \frac{\text{Total energy delivered to tissue or organ}}{\text{Mass of tissue or organ}} \quad (3\text{-}3)$$

Dose Equivalent and Its Unit

Earlier in this chapter, we described several types of natural and man-made radiation that differ in terms of their energy (quality). For example, cosmic and gamma rays have more energy than x-rays. Biological effects are attributed not only to the absorbed dose but also depend on the type and energy of the radiation. Radiation with a high linear energy transfer (LET) is, in general, more destructive to biological material than low LET radiation. For example, Martin and Harbison (1979) pointed out that 0.01 Gy of fast neutrons produce about the same biodamage as 0.1 Gy of gamma radiation. Because of this, a special quantity and unit are needed to address these differences in biological effectiveness. This quantity is the *dose equivalent*, H, and its conventional unit is the *rem* (rad equivalent man).

The dose equivalent can be calculated using the absorbed dose, D, as follows:

$$H = DQ \tag{3-4}$$

where Q is a quality factor of the particular radiation. Other modifying factors can be included, but they are not routinely used (Turner, 1986). The *quality factor* reflects the effectiveness of a particular type of radiation resulting in the same biological effect as another type of radiation.

The radiation badges worn by technologists record occupational exposures and are evaluated in terms of the unit of dose equivalent. The SI unit of dose equivalent is the *Sievert* (Sv), named after the Swedish physicist Rolf Maximilian Sievert, who played a major role in the application of radiation physics to clinical problems.

The Sievert is related to the Gray as follows:

$$\text{Sievert} = \text{Gray} \times W_R \tag{3-5}$$

where W_R is a *radiation weighting factor* (to be discussed subsequently).

Submultiples of the Sievert are as follows:

$$1 \text{ Sv} = 100 \text{ rem}$$
$$1 \text{ mSv} = 100 \text{ mrem}$$
$$1 \text{ µSv} = 100 \text{ µrem}$$
$$1 \text{ nSv} = 100 \text{ nrem}$$

In diagnostic radiology, because we are concerned only with x-rays, for the sake of simplicity, we could write:

$$1 \text{ roentgen} = 1 \text{ rad} = 1 \text{ rem}$$

or in SI units:

$$2.58 \times 10^{-4} \text{ C}\cdot\text{kg}^{-1} = 0.01 \text{ Gy} = 0.01 \text{ Sv}$$

To convert conventional units (for the radiation quantities just discussed, i.e., exposure, absorbed dose, dose equivalent) to SI units, the following can be used:

$$1 \text{ roentgen} \times 2.58 \times 10^{-4} = \text{C}\cdot\text{kg}^{-1}$$
$$1 \text{ rad} \times 0.01 = 1 \text{ Gy}$$
$$1 \text{ rem} \times 0.01 = 1 \text{ Sv}$$

RADIATION WEIGHTING FACTOR

From Eq. 3-4, the absorbed dose, D, is weighted at a point and the weighting factor has been referred to as the quality factor (Bushong, 1993). The ICRP (1991) stated that "in radiological protection, it is the absorbed dose over a tissue or organ (rather than a point) and weighted for the radiation quality that is of interest. The weighting factor for this purpose is now called the radiation weighting factor, W_R, and is selected for the type and energy of the radiation incident on the body . . ." (p. 5).

The W_R for photons of all energies is 1, while for neutrons it can range from 5 to 20 depending on the energy. The W_R for alpha particles is 20. (W_R is dimensionless.)

Equivalent Dose

In the 1990 recommendations of the ICRP (ICRP, 1991), the term dose equivalent (the weighted absorbed dose at a point) has been superseded by the term *equivalent dose* (H_T). This is a weighted absorbed dose in a tissue or organ, and it is obtained by weighting the absorbed dose by the radiation weighting factor, W_R. Mathematically, this can be expressed as follows:

$$H_T = \sum_R W_R \cdot D_{T,R} \quad (3\text{-}6)$$

This is read as follows: the equivalent dose is equal to the sum of the weighted absorbed doses, where H_T is the equivalent dose, W_R is the radiation weighting factor, and $D_{T,R}$ is the absorbed dose averaged over the tissue or organ, T, for the radiation R (ICRP, 1991). $\sum_R$ (sigma) is read as summing over the radiation.

TISSUE WEIGHTING FACTOR

Radiation biological effects depend not only on the type and energy of the radiation but also on the type of tissue or organ that has been exposed. Because of this, the ICRP (1991) introduced another factor, the *tissue weighting factor*, W_T, "which represents the relative contribution of that organ or tissue to the total detriment due to those effects resulting from uniform irradiation of the whole body" (p. 7). These tissue weighting factors were recently revised by the ICRP based on current knowledge of radiobiological effects. A comparison of the old (1977) weighting factors with the new (1991) is given in Table 3-2.

TABLE 3-2. A COMPARISON OF OLD AND NEW TISSUE WEIGHTING FACTORS USED IN QUANTIFYING THE RISK OF RADIATION EXPOSURE

	Tissue Weighting Factors	
Organ	**New (1991)**	**Old (1977)**
Gonads	0.20	0.25
Bone marrow	0.12	0.12
Lung	0.12	0.12
Breast	0.05	0.15
Thyroid	0.05	0.03
Bone surface	0.01	0.03
Remainder	0.05	0.30

SOURCE: International Commission on Radiological Protection. (1991). *1990 Recommendations of the ICRP* (ICRP Publication No. 60). Elmsford, NY: Pergamon Press; and International Commission on Radiobiological Protection. (1977). *Recommendations of the ICRP*. (ICRP Publication No. 26). Elmsford, NY: Pergamon Press.

Effective Dose

If the equivalent dose, H_T, is weighted by the tissue weighting factor, W_T, we arrive at another quantity, which the ICRP (1991) refers to as the *effective dose*, E. (This was previously referred to as the effective dose equivalent, H_E.) E is a quantity designed to quantify the risk from partial body exposure to that from an equivalent whole body dose. It is defined as the "sum of the weighted equivalent doses in all tissues and organs of the body" (ICRP, 1991, p. 7). Mathematically, this can be expressed as:

$$E = \sum_T W_T \cdot H_T \quad (3\text{-}7)$$

where E, T, H_T, and W_T function as previously defined.

The average annual effective dose equivalent to the United States population is shown in Table 3-3. It should be noted that radon contributes the largest effective dose equivalent (2 mSv) compared with other sources. The effective dose equivalent from x-ray diagnosis is 0.39 mSv. In addition, the effective dose equivalent for various diagnostic x-ray examinations such as those of the chest, lumbar spine, upper gastrointestinal tract, and abdomen, as well as the barium enema and the intravenous pyelogram, are 0.06, 1.3, 2.45, 0.55, 4.05, and 1.6 mSv, respectively (NCRP, 1987).

What do these numbers mean? An effective dose equivalent of 4.05 mSv for a barium enema implies that the risk from a barium enema is equivalent to the risk of an x-ray exposure of 4.05 mSv to the whole body.

Patient Dose Distributions in Diagnostic Radiology

When a beam of radiation falls upon a patient, the dose is distributed spatially as shown in Figure 3-5. The distribution gives rise to the skin dose, the average organ dose, the depth dose, the average dose in the beam, and the integral dose.

TABLE 3-3. AVERAGE ANNUAL EFFECTIVE DOSE EQUIVALENT OF IONIZING RADIATION TO A MEMBER OF THE U.S. POPULATION

	Dose Equivalent[a]		Effective Dose Equivalent	
Source	mSv	mrem	mSv	%
Natural				
Radon[b]	24	2,400	2.0	55
Cosmic	0.27	27	0.27	8.0
Terrestrial	0.28	28	0.28	8.0
Internal	0.39	39	0.39	11
Total natural	—	—	3.0	82
Artificial				
Medical				
X-ray diagnosis	0.39	39	0.39	11
Nuclear medicine	0.14	14	0.14	4.0
Consumer products	0.10	10	0.10	3.0
Other				
Occupational	0.009	0.9	<0.01	<0.3
Nuclear fuel cycle	<0.01	<1.0	<0.01	<0.03
Fallout	<0.01	<1.0	<0.01	<0.03
Miscellaneous[c]	<0.01	<1.0	<0.01	<0.03
Total artificial	—	—	0.63	18
Total natural and artificial	—	—	3.6	100

[a] To soft tissues.

[b] Dose equivalent to bronchi from radon daughter products. The assumed weighting factor for the effective dose equivalent relative to whole-body exposure is 0.08.

[c] Department of Energy facilities, smelters, transportation, etc.

SOURCE: National Council on Radiation Protection and Measurements. (1987). *Radiation exposure of the US population from consumer products and miscellaneous sources* (Report No. 95). Bethesda, MD: NCRP.

While the *skin dose* is the exposure to the entrance surface of the skin (also referred to as the *entrance skin dose*), the *average organ dose* refers to the average radiation energy absorbed by the particular organ. On the other hand, the *depth dose* is an absorbed dose at some point below the skin surface. The *average dose to the patient* is "an average of the dose received by each bit of tissue contained within the geometrically defined x-ray beam" (Whalen and Balter, 1984, p. 11).

Finally, the *integral dose* is the total amount of energy absorbed by a particular mass of tissue. The radiation risk to a patient is directly proportional to the integral dose; hence, technologists must make every effort to reduce this dose by using techniques such as collimation (Whalen and Balter, 1984).

Reporting Patient Dose in Diagnostic Radiology

The literature is replete with articles reporting patient dose in radiography, fluoroscopy, computed tomography, digital radiography, angiography, and mammography. In general, most of the studies have reported patient doses in terms

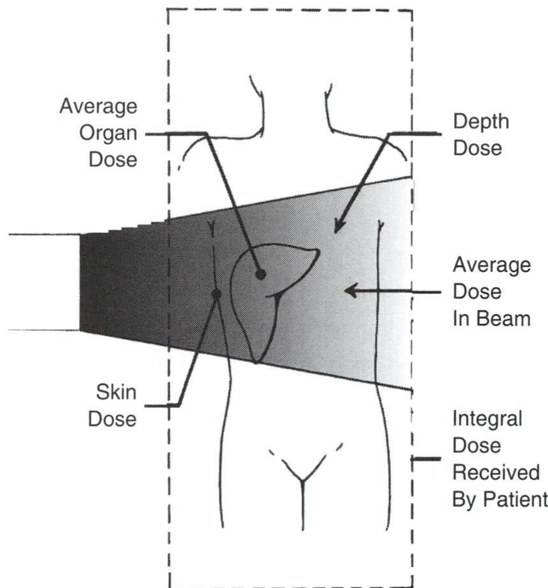

FIGURE 3-5. The spatial distribution of dose as the radiation beam falls on the patient. [From Whalen, J.P., & Balter, S. (1984). *Radiation risks in medical imaging.* Chicago: Year Book Medical. Reproduced by permission.]

of gonadal dose, bone marrow dose, and the genetically significant dose. These dose studies are the subject of Chapter 11.

REVIEW QUESTIONS

1. Which of the following belong to the class of natural radiation?
   A. X-rays.
   B. Fallout from nuclear testing.
   C. Radiation from cardiac pacemakers.
   D. Cosmic rays.

2. Which of the following has the highest percentage contribution to radiation exposure of the population?
   A. Radon gas.
   B. Cosmic rays.
   C. X-rays.
   D. Fallout.

3. Natural radiation sources include all of the following except:
   A. Cosmic rays.
   B. Radon gas.
   C. Endogenous radiation.
   D. X-rays.

4. Man-made radiation includes all of the following except:
   A. Industrial radiation.
   B. Cosmic rays.
   C. Radiation from nuclear power plants.
   D. X-rays used in radiology.

5. The highest percentage contribution of radiation exposure to the population from man-made sources is from:
   A. Nuclear medicine procedures.
   B. Diagnostic x-ray procedures.
   C. Consumer products.
   D. Nuclear fallout.

6. The reason(s) why medical radiation exposure is of importance to the technologist is (are):
   A. It contributes the highest percentage of exposure to the population.
   B. It represents low-level radiation for which biological effects are of concern.
   C. Exposure of the patient in radiology is under the direct control of the technologist.
   D. All of the above.

7. The following are classified as ionizing radiation except:
   A. X-rays.
   B. Gamma rays.
   C. Beta particles.
   D. Ultrasound.

8. The main source of x-rays from an x-ray tube is the:
   A. Target.
   B. Filament.

C. Glass envelope.
D. Focusing cup.

9. Which of the following techniques uses nonionizing radiation?
   A. Diagnostic x-ray procedures.
   B. Magnetic resonance imaging.
   C. Nuclear medicine.
   D. Radiation treatment planning.

10. Which of the following refers to exposures received during the course of work?
   A. Occupational exposure.
   B. Medical exposure.
   C. Public exposure.
   D. All of the above.

11. When an individual is exposed to radiation as part of the clinical diagnosis or therapy, it is referred to as:
   A. Occupational exposure.
   B. Medical exposure.
   C. Public exposure.
   D. All of the above.

12. The exposure of a patient waiting in the hallway just outside the x-ray room is classified as:
   A. Medical exposure.
   B. Occupational exposure.
   C. Public exposure.
   D. All of the above.

13. When a technologist is exposed to a chest x-ray during the course of his or her work, the dose resulting from such exposure is considered:
   A. Medical exposure.
   B. Occupational exposure.
   C. Public exposure.
   D. All of the above.

14. The following are radiation quantities except:
   A. The radiation field.
   B. Exposure.
   C. Absorbed dose.
   D. Dose equivalent.

15. The NCRP indicated that in the U.S., SI units be used exclusively after the year:
   A. 1989.
   B. 1990.
   C. 1995.
   D. 1996.

16. Which of the following refers to the quantity of radiation falling upon the patient?
   A. Absorbed dose.
   B. Exposure.
   C. Dose equivalent.
   D. Equivalent dose.

17. Each of the following refers to kerma except:
   A. The SI unit of kerma is joules per kilogram (J/kg).
   B. The kinetic energy released in the material.
   C. The quantity of radiation falling on the patient.
   D. The kerma deals with the transfer of energy at a point.

18. The energy absorbed per unit mass is referred to as the:
   A. Absorbed dose.
   B. Exposure.
   C. Dose equivalent.
   D. Effective dose.

19. The radiation quantity that deals with differences in biological effectiveness is the:
   A. Exposure.
   B. Absorbed dose.
   C. Dose equivalent.
   D. All of the above.

20. The SI unit of exposure is the:
   A. Sievert.
   B. Gray.

C. Coulombs per kilogram.
D. Roentgen.

21. The traditional or conventional unit of exposure is the:
 A. Sievert.
 B. Gray.
 C. Coulombs per kilogram.
 D. Roentgen.

22. The SI unit of absorbed dose is the:
 A. Coulombs per kilogram.
 B. Gray.
 C. Sievert.
 D. Rad.

23. The SI unit of dose equivalent is the:
 A. Coulombs per kilogram.
 B. Gray.
 C. Sievert.
 D. Rad.

24. The term dose equivalent has been superseded by the term:
 A. Equivalent dose.
 B. Radiation weighting factor.
 C. Tissue weighting factor.
 D. Effective dose equivalent.

25. The term used to quantify the risk from partial body exposure to that from an equivalent whole body dose is the:
 A. Exposure.
 B. Absorbed dose.
 C. Equivalent dose.
 D. Effective dose.

26. The skin dose is the:
 A. Entrance skin dose.
 B. Exposure to the entrance surface of the skin.
 C. Absorbed dose below the skin surface.
 D. A and B are correct.

27. Which of the following refers to the average dose absorbed by a particular organ?
 A. Skin dose.
 B. Average organ dose.
 C. Depth dose.
 D. Integral dose.

28. The total amount of energy absorbed by a particular mass of tissue is the:
 A. Entrance skin dose.
 B. Average dose to the patient.
 C. Depth dose.
 D. Integral dose.

29. Which of the following refers to the absorbed dose at some point below the skin surface?
 A. Entrance skin dose.
 B. Depth dose.
 C. Integral dose.
 D. Average organ dose.

30. Most studies in radiology have reported patient doses in terms of:
 A. Gonadal dose.
 B. Bone marrow dose.
 C. Genetically significant dose.
 D. All of the above.

REFERENCES

Bushong, S. (1993). *Radiologic science for technologists* (5th ed.). St. Louis: Mosby-Year Book.

Hart, B.L., Mettler, F.A., & Harley, N.H. (1989). Radon: Is it a problem? *Radiology, 172*, 593.

Hendee, W.R., & Edwards, M. (1986). ALARA and an integrated approach to radiation protection. *Seminars in Nuclear Medicine, 16*, 142.

International Commission on Radiological Protection (1977). Recommendations of the ICRP (ICRP Publication No. 26). Elmsford, NY: Pergamon Press.

International Commission on Radiological Protection (1991). 1990 recommendations of the ICRP (ICRP Publication No. 60). Elmsford, NY: Pergamon Press.

Luckey, TD. (1991). *Radiation hormesis*. Boca Raton, FL: CRC Press.

Martin, A., & Harbison, S.A. (1979). *An introduction to radiation protection* (2nd ed.). London: Chapman and Hall.

National Council on Radiation Protection and Measurements. (1987). *Recommendations on limits from ionizing radiation* (Report No. 91). Bethesda, MD: NCRP.

National Council on Radiation Protection and Measurements. (1990). *SI units in radiation protection and measurements* (Report No. 82). Bethesda, MD: NCRP.

Pomroy, C., & Noel, L. (1984). Low background radiation measurements on video display terminals. *Health Physics, 46*, 413.

Sprawls, P. (1990). *Principles of radiography for technologists.* Rockville, MD: Aspen.

Turner, JE. (1986). *Atoms, radiation and radiation protection.* Elmsford, NY: Pergamon Press.

Whalen, J.P., & Balter, S. (1984). *Radiation risks in medical imaging.* Chicago: Year Book Medical.

Part II
Bioeffects of Radiation

CHAPTER FOUR

BIOEFFECTS OF RADIATION

ELIZABETH TRAVIS

LEARNING OBJECTIVES

Upon completion of this chapter, you should be able to:

1 ■ Define the term radiobiology.
2 ■ State five generalizations about the effects of radiation on living organisms.
3 ■ Describe the direct and indirect action of radiation interaction in matter.
4 ■ Describe the types of damage to DNA produced by radiation.
5 ■ Describe the types of radiation damage to chromosomes.

(continued)

6 ■ State the role of oncogenes and suppressor genes in the transformation of a normal cell into a malignant cell.
7 ■ Describe how irradiated cells die.
8 ■ Explain what is meant by cell survival.
9 ■ Discuss how the following factors modify cell survival: LET, RBE, and cell cycle.
10 ■ Describe the effects of radiation on the total body with respect to each of the following: sources of high dose exposure of humans, radiation syndromes, total body radiation in humans, and lethal dose for the hematopoietic syndrome.
11 ■ Describe the effects of radiation on the embryo and fetus.
12 ■ List the data sources regarding the carcinogenic effect of radiation in humans.
13 ■ Explain the concept of risk estimates.
14 ■ Outline radiation-induced cancers in humans.
15 ■ List the three potential mechanisms by which radiation may induce cancer.
16 ■ Discuss the hereditary effects of radiation.

Introduction

Definition of Radiobiology

The discovery of x-rays by Roentgen over 100 years ago heralded a new age in biology and medicine. Although these rays were initially hailed as wholly beneficial, they were soon observed to have damaging effects as well. In the past 100 years, the discovery of x-rays has changed the practice of medicine dramatically, and we have learned a great deal about their effects on biological systems. In addition, our basic understanding of biology and biological processes has been enhanced by using x-rays as a tool to study cells and tissues in animal models.

The goal of this chapter is to serve as a small window into the now vast fund of knowledge of the effects of radiation on biological systems, the study of which is referred to as *radiobiology*.

Basic Concepts of Radiobiology

Generalizations About Radiation Effects on Living Organisms

When considering the effects of radiation on living organisms, it is important to keep the following generalizations in mind:

1. The interaction of radiation in cells is a probability function or a matter of chance, i.e., an interaction may or may not occur. Furthermore, the occurrence of an interaction does not necessarily mean that damage will result. In fact, damage is frequently repaired.
2. The initial deposition of energy occurs very rapidly, within 10^{-18} seconds.
3. Radiation deposits energy in a cell in a random fashion.
4. Radiation produces no unique changes in cells, tissues, or organs. The changes induced by radiation are indistinguishable from damage produced by other types of trauma.
5. The biological changes in cells, tissues, and organs do not appear immediately. They occur only after a period of time (latent period), ranging from hours (e.g., after accidental overexposures to the total body resulting in failure of organ systems and death) to as long as years (e.g., in the case of radiation-induced cancer) or even generations (such as is the case if the damage occurs in a germ cell leading to heritable changes). The length of the latency period depends on factors related to the radiation, e.g., the dose given, as well as to biological characteristics of the cells irradiated, e.g., how often they divide.

Radiation Interactions in Matter: Direct vs. Indirect Action

Strong circumstantial evidence indicates that the biological effects of radiation, including cell killing, mutagenesis, and carcinogenesis, are due to damage primarily to one molecule, DNA, the critical target. Radiation may deposit energy directly within the *critical target* or, conversely, may interact with other molecules in the cell, one of the most important of which is water. The site of this initial interaction determines whether the initial interaction is direct or indirect.

REVIEW BOX:
Direct action occurs when radiation is absorbed by a molecule known to be critical to maintaining the life of the cell (e.g., DNA), thus initiating a series of events that lead to changes that may be lethal to the cell. *Indirect action*, on the other hand, occurs when radiation interacts with other molecules in the cell, most importantly water.

Because the cell is more than 70% water, the majority of radiation interactions occur via indirect action. Although there are a number of free radicals that may be produced as a result of indirect action, the oxidizing agent OH is considered the most damaging. It is estimated to account for approximately two thirds of all x-ray damage to DNA in mammalian cells. Although both direct action and indirect action initiate a series of molecular, biochemical, and biological events that lead to the overt expression of damage over a course of months to years later, these interactions remain poorly understood. (The time scale for these events is shown in Fig. 4-1.)

Radiation Damage to DNA

As stated previously, it is generally accepted that DNA is a critical target for radiation. Indeed, experiments show that lower doses of radiation are needed to induce cell death when only the nucleus is irradiated than when the cytoplasm is

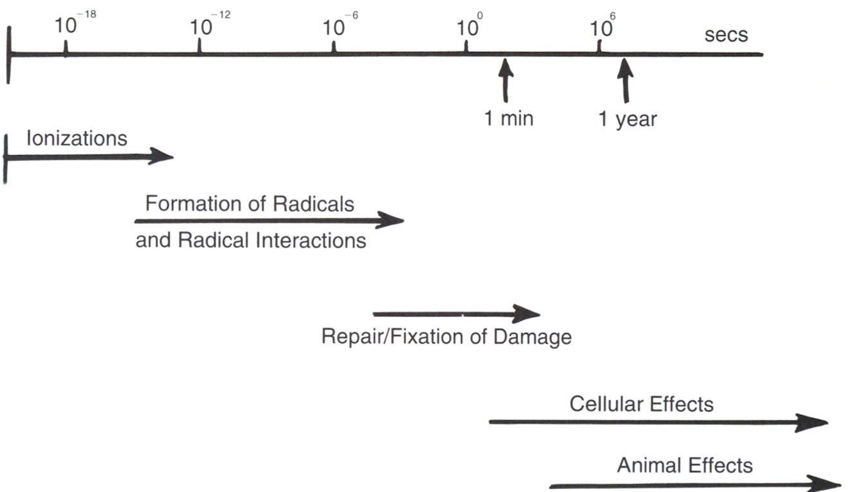

FIGURE 4-1. Schematic of time course of events occurring after irradiation of biological systems.

irradiated. Also, studies in a number of different organisms in which DNA content was correlated with radiosensitivity provide substantial evidence that the critical site for cell killing is in the nucleus and not the cytoplasm of the cell. It is the nuclear DNA that is the most likely target.

DNA consists of two strands that form a double helix. The backbone of each strand is made up of sugar moieties and phosphate groups, which serve as the framework for the four bases—adenine, guanine, cytosine, and thymine (Fig. 4-2). The bases are attached to a sugar on opposite sides of the strand and are complementary; adenine pairs with thymine and guanine pairs with cytosine. The order of these bases on the sugar-phosphate backbone spells out the genetic code.

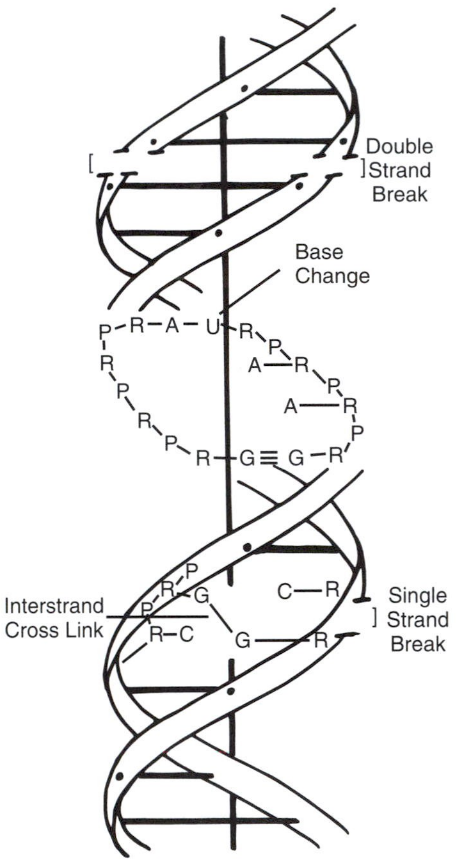

FIGURE 4-2. Lesions produced in DNA by irradiation. (Courtesy of Drs. Raymond Meyn and Ron Humphrey, M. D. Anderson Cancer Center.)

Radiation can damage either the backbone of DNA, producing strand breaks, or it can produce alterations or loss of bases (Fig. 4-2). Strand breaks may occur in only one of the strands (a single strand break, SSB), or in both strands (a double strand break, DSB). The critical question is as follows: which of these lesions is most likely to result in cell death? Studies that use new techniques to quantitate specific types of DNA damage, specifically SSBs and DSBs, show a high degree of correlation between DSBs and cell killing. SSBs, however, do not show a correlation with cell death. Both SSBs and DSBs can be and often are repaired after radiation. SSBs are more readily repaired, most likely because they can use the opposite unbroken strand as a template. DSBs, particularly if they are opposite each other or separated by only a few base pairs, are repaired less efficiently and at a slower rate than SSBs. This is presumably because the opposite strand is not intact, which may account for the correlation between this DNA lesion and cell death. These studies indicate that the ability of DNA to repair damage may be related to cellular sensitivity to radiation. Support for the relationship between DNA repair capability and cellular radiosensitivity comes from studies on fibroblasts isolated from patients with ataxia telangiectasia, a rare genetic disorder associated with a deficiency in DNA repair capacity. When irradiated, these fibroblasts are exquisitely sensitive compared with fibroblasts from normal individuals. However, whether DSBs are the lesion responsible for cell death remains to be proven.

Chromosomal Effects

Cell division in somatic cells is the process by which one "parent" cell replicates an exact copy of its DNA, packages it, condenses it into chromosomes, and finally divides into two "daughter" cells, each of which contains an exact copy of the DNA from the original parent cell. The cell cycle can be divided into the period in which actual division occurs, termed *mitosis*, and the remainder of the cycle, termed *interphase*, in which the quantity of DNA is doubled and each chromosome lays down an exact copy of itself next to itself. By far the greatest part of the life of the cell is spent in interphase.

Mitosis consists of four distinct phases: prophase, metaphase, anaphase, and telophase, all of which can be visualized using a conventional light microscope. The processes occurring during interphase, however, cannot be seen under the light microscope. *Prophase* begins when the chromatin condenses into coiled strands distributed throughout the nucleus, which can be stained and observed with a conventional light microscope. It ends with the formation of chromosomes, each complete with a centromere, a constriction in the chromosome from which the arms extend. At this point, the nuclear membrane also has disappeared, allowing free movement of the chromosomes within the cell. The next phase, *metaphase*, is characterized by lining up of the chromosomes at the center of the cell, at the cell's equator. The spindle is composed of fibers that stretch across the cell, connecting the two poles. Metaphase is completed when the centromere of each chromosome divides and attaches to the spindle. During *anaphase*, the chromosomes, attached by their centromeres, move along the spindle to the poles of the cell. At the end of anaphase, one copy of each chromosome is located at each pole of the cell. During the last phase of mitosis, *telophase*, the chromosomes uncoil, lose their distinctive appearance, and take on the appearance of an interphase nucleus. The nuclear membrane reappears and the cell divides into two cells, each of which now contains an exact replica of DNA and chromosomes.

Radiation produces breaks in chromosomes, termed *aberrations*, which can be observed during the next division after exposure, during metaphase, when the chromosomes are formed. Aberrations are further specified as either *chromosomes* or *chromatid* aberrations depending on whether they occur before or after DNA synthesis. Chromosome aberrations are those that occur early in interphase, before the genetic material is duplicated. In this situation, the break occurs in only one strand of the DNA and is then duplicated during DNA synthesis. Aberrations occurring after the DNA has been duplicated, when the chromatin consists of two strands, are termed chromatid aberrations.

Because the broken ends of chromosomes are "sticky," they can join easily with other broken ends. The general consequences of these breaks are as follows:

1. The ends of the same chromosome may rejoin, a process called *restitution*. This causes no changes.
2. The sticky end of one chromosome may join with that of another, leading to reassortment of the genetic material and an aberration visible at the next metaphase.
3. The broken ends may not rejoin and will appear as an acentric fragment at the next mitosis. The genetic material contained in the acentric fragment will be lost from the cell and will be scored as a deletion.

Many of these changes are visible at the next mitosis as a range of gross structural changes, including (1) acentric fragments, (2) dicentric chromosomes (single chromosomes that have two centromeres), (3) ring chromosomes (the result of breaks in and subsequent joining of the sticky ends in each arm of the same chromosome before replication), and (4) anaphase bridges (the result of breaks occurring late in interphase, after the chromosomes have been replicated, in which breaking and subsequent joining of the sticky ends may lead to attachment of each centromere to opposite poles, thus stretching the chromosome between them at anaphase, and ultimately producing a break in the stretched portion). Figure 4-3 shows examples of these aberrations in irradiated human cells.

Although it is easy to see why the loss of a significant amount of genetic material results in cell death, it is not only the amount of genetic material that is important to the cell but also the arrangement of the bases on the sugar phosphate backbone of DNA, the sequence of which contains the genetic code. Thus, chromosomal aberrations that result in a rearrangement of the sequence of the genetic code carried by the chromosome can have profound effects on the cell. Such aberrations include an exchange of the same amount of genetic material between two different chromosomes (i.e., symmetrical translocations, inversions of genetic material on the same chromosome, and small deletions of genetic material). Symmetrical translocations must be visualized by techniques other than conventional microscopy, such as fluorescence *in situ* hybridization, or chromosome painting, as it is commonly called. This technique uses fluorescent probes that are specific for a given chromosome, making it possible to visualize when an exchange of material has occurred between two different chromosomes. It is now known that all of these types of chromosomal aberrations are associated with malignancies. Burkitt's lymphoma was the first tumor shown to involve a translocation of a specific gene. Other tumors now known to be associated with translocations include acute promyelocytic

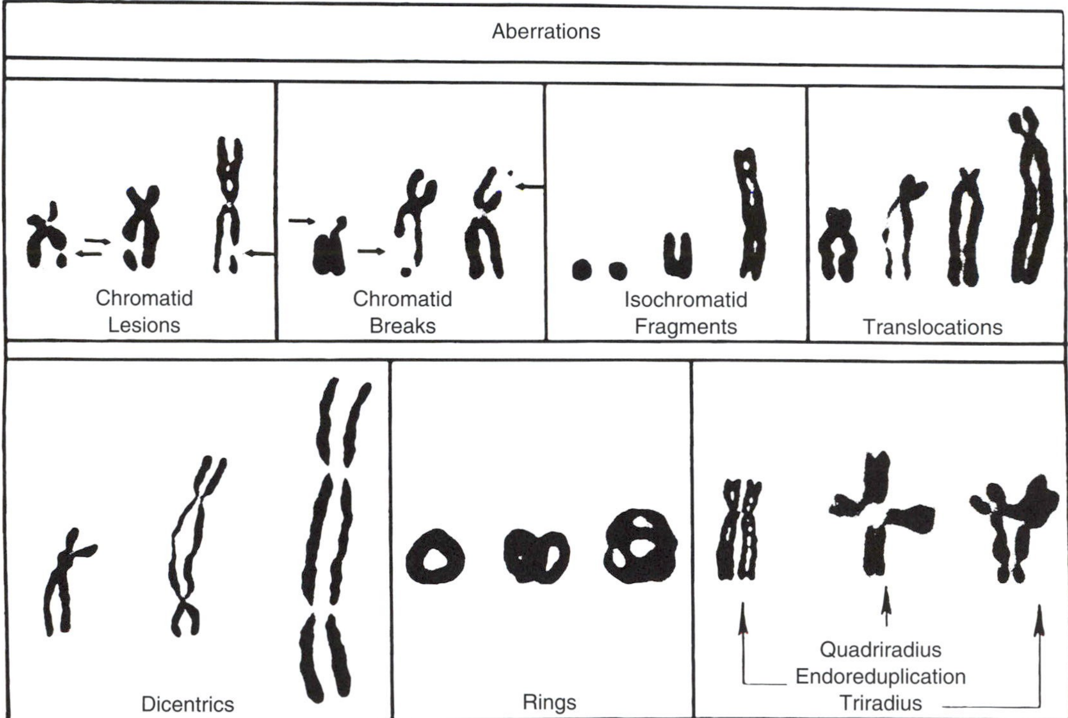

FIGURE 4-3. Chromosomes from a patient undergoing radiation therapy, illustrating many types of aberrations. [From Amarose, A.P., Plotz, E.J. & Stein, A.A. (1967). Residual chromosomal aberrations in female cancer patients after irradiation therapy. *Journal of Experimental and Molecular Pathology, 7*, 58. Reproduced by permission.]

leukemia and ovarian cancer. Tumors associated with deletions include small cell lung cancer, neuroblastoma, retinoblastoma, and Wilms' tumor.

Oncogenes, Suppressor Genes, and Radiation

Oncogenes are mutated genes that are thought to be involved in the transformation of a normal cell to a malignant phenotype. The normal counterparts of oncogenes, proto-oncogenes, are present in mammalian cells, and many have been shown to function in regulating cell growth. Radiation can activate oncogenes through a number of mechanisms including point mutations, chromosomal rearrangement, or chromosomal translocations. Table 4-1 shows a list of known oncogenes, the human cancers associated with them, and the accompanying chromosomal changes. *Suppressor genes* may also be involved in the change to a malignant phenotype via a chromosomal aberration. It has been suggested that all normal cells contain genes that suppress the induction of tumors. If a radiation-induced break in a chromosome results in loss of that part of the chromosome that contains the suppressor gene, it could be conducive to the expression of the malignant phenotype.

Cell Death and Cell Survival

How Irradiated Cells Die

Irradiated cells die either by mitotic death, also called reproductive failure, or by apoptosis, formerly termed interphase death. *Mitotic death* occurs when an irradiated cell attempts to undergo mitosis. Death does not occur necessarily at

TABLE 4-1. CHROMOSOMAL CHANGES LEADING TO ONCOGENE ACTIVATION AND THE HUMAN MALIGNANCIES ASSOCIATED WITH THEM

Oncogene	Chromosomal Changes	Human Cancers
N-*ras*	Deletion (1)	Neuroblastoma
Blym	Deletion (1)	Neuroblastoma
fms	Deletion (5)	Acute nonlymphocytic leukemia
H-*ras*	Deletion (11)	Sarcoma
c-*abl*	Translocation (9–12)	Chronic myelogenous leukemia
c-*myc*	Translocation (8–14)	B-cell lymphoma
	Translocation (2–8)	Burkitt's lymphoma
N-*myc*	Translocation (2–8)	Burkitt's lymphoma
raf	Translocation (3–8)	Parotid gland tumor
myb	Translocation (6–14)	Carcinoma
mas	Translocation (3–8)	Acute myelocytic leukemia
abl	Translocation (9–22)	Chronic myelogenous leukemia
sis	Translocation (9–22)	Chronic myelogenous leukemia
	Translocation (8–22)	Burkitt's lymphoma
N-*myc*	Gene amplification	Neuroblastoma
neu	Gene amplification	Breast carcinoma

SOURCE: Hall, E.J. (Ed.). (1994). *Radiobiology for the radiologist* (4th ed.) (p. 60). Philadelphia: J.B. Lippincott. Reproduced by permission.

the first postirradiation mitosis. A cell may go through one, two, or even three divisions before finally dying. Mitotic death occurs after relatively small doses and is the type of cell death assayed in clonogenic assays *in vivo* and *in vitro*.

A second, nonmitotic form of cell death also has been recognized for many years. As the term implies, cells die before attempting mitosis, during the interphase portion of the cell cycle. With the exception of the small lymphocyte, which has long been known to die by interphase death, this form of cell death was thought to be rare in other cells. It is now known that this form of cell death is *apoptosis*, or programmed cell death. Apoptosis is a natural form of cell death that occurs spontaneously without a cytotoxic insult. For example, apoptosis frequently occurs during embryonic development and is the process by which tadpoles lose their tails. Apoptosis is characterized by a well-defined and recognizable sequence of events that can be divided into two phases. In the first phase, the cell condenses and forms small membrane-enclosed buds. These bodies are then phagocytosed and digested by neighboring cells. Because apoptosis is a discrete event, apoptotic bodies tend to be found scattered throughout an irradiated tissue rather than in clumps. Apoptosis does not elicit an inflammatory response, a common feature of other forms of cell death in tissues. Apoptosis occurs in tumors and in normal tissues, although its contribution to tumor control and normal tissue damage after doses in the therapeutic range is unclear.

Radiation Survival Curves for Mammalian Cells

Cell survival curves show the relationship between radiation dose and the proportion of cells surviving. In the sense used here, *cell survival* refers to the ability of the cell to sustain unlimited proliferation, i.e., it measures the reproductive integrity of a cell. Cells that retain all other functions, including the ability to synthesize DNA, or those that divide once or twice after irradiation, are considered "dead." A cell survival curve represents the sum total of cells that survive both mitotic death and apoptosis, the two forms of radiation-induced cell death discussed above. The reproductive integrity of a cell can be measured *in vitro* or *in vivo* for specific tissues and organs, and represents the ability of a single cell to divide repeatedly, forming a colony of cells known as a clone. The cell forming the colony is termed a "clonogenic" cell.

Shape of Survival Curves

The techniques outlined above have been used to obtain cell survival curves for a wide variety of normal tissues and tumors. Based on these data, survival curves for irradiation of mammalian cells with sparsely ionizing radiations, i.e., low linear energy transfer (LET), e.g., x-rays, fall into two basic categories as shown in Figure 4-4. In these figures cell survival is plotted on a logarithmic scale as a function of dose on a linear scale. In general, these curves can be defined by their shape. In the low-dose region of the curve in Figure 4-4A, there is evidence of a shoulder. As the dose increases, the survival curve becomes steeper and straight; in this portion of the curve, survival is an exponential function of dose. The continuously bending curve in Figure 4-4B is characteristic of some types of cells and is represented by the lack of a terminal exponential slope. For densely ionizing radiations (high LET) such as alpha particles, the survival curve is a straight line from the origin. Survival is thus shown to be an exponential function of dose over the entire dose range.

Factors Modifying Cell Survival

LET AND RBE

The quality of the radiation has an effect not only on cell survival but on all biological responses.

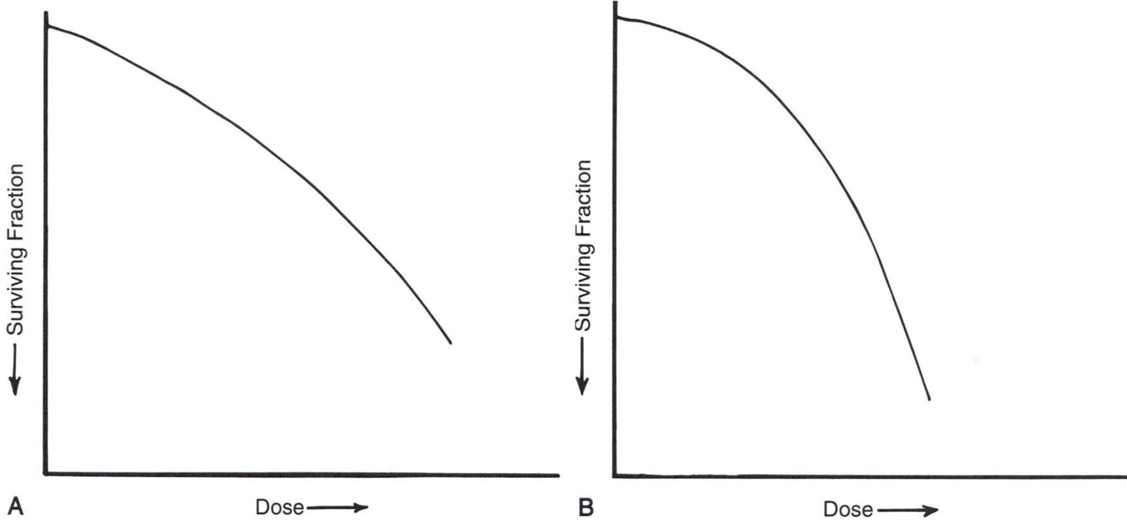

FIGURE 4-4. Two different shapes of survival curves in mammalian cells. A: Straight survival curve with small shoulder and terminal exponential slope. B: Continuously bending "curvy" survival curve that does not exhibit a final exponential slope.

REVIEW BOX:
The rate at which an electron (or an x-ray photon that ejected it) transfers energy (as it moves through some length of tissue) to the surrounding tissue is referred to as linear energy transfer (LET).

The ionizations produced by x-rays are spaced far apart; thus, x-rays are sparsely ionizing and have a low LET. The ionizations from radiations such as alpha particles, however, are spaced close together and are densely ionizing; thus, alpha particles and some neutrons are high LET radiations. In general, both the shoulder and the slope of the survival curve for mammalian cells are reduced when irradiated with high LET radiations compared with low LET radiations (Fig. 4-5). The term relating the biological effectiveness of radiations with different LETs is relative biological effect (RBE).

REVIEW BOX:
The RBE is the ratio of the dose of a standard type of radiation, usually 250 kVp x-rays, to the dose of the test radiation to produce the same biological effect: $RBE = \frac{D_{reference}}{D_{test}}$

RBE has no units; it is simply a ratio of two doses. Because the shoulder of the survival curve is reduced with high LET radiations, the RBE is not a constant over the entire dose range but increases as the dose is reduced (Fig. 4-5). Although the change in RBE with dose is well established, the relationship between RBE and dose is critically dependent on the shape of the initial portion of the cell survival curve and thus will vary between cells and tissues.

CELL CYCLE

The cell cycle consists of the four phases G1, S, and G2 (the three phases that make up inter-

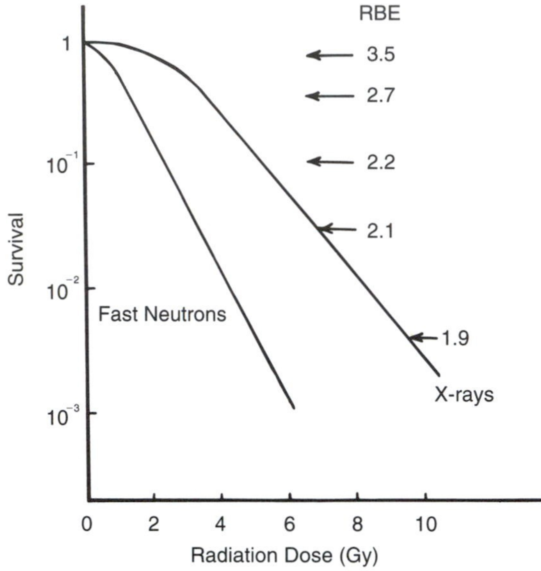

FIGURE 4-5. Comparison of survival curves after x-rays and fast neutrons showing that the relative biological effectiveness (RBE) is not constant over the dose range but increases as the dose decreases.

phase) and mitosis. The order of these phases is G1, S, G2, M. The sensitivity of cells in different phases of the cell cycle is not uniform, as shown in Figure 4-6. In general, the variation in radiosensitivity through the cell cycle can be summarized as follows:

1. Mitosis is the most sensitive phase of the cell cycle.
2. The G2 phase is similarly sensitive.
3. The S phase is the most resistant phase of the cycle.

Radiation causes a delay of the progression of cells through the cell cycle, which is largely due to a block of cells in the G2 phase. This phenomenon is termed *division delay*. Because cells in mitosis are the most sensitive, radiation induces a decrease in the mitotic index of a population of cells. This is so for two reasons: (1) mitotic cells are preferentially killed and (2) surviving cells do not enter division, due to the G2 block. Cells in mitosis, however, continue to progress through the cell cycle. This has the effect of partially synchronizing the irradiated population. However, after a period of time that is dependent on the dose and the type of cell, delayed cells will begin to progress through mitosis and the population again will become asynchronous.

The field of molecular biology has greatly increased our ability to study the regulation of the cell cycle, thus increasing our understanding of the effects of radiation. It is now known that the cell cycle is regulated by genes called *molecular checkpoint genes*, which ensure that the correct sequence of events occurs. The genes involved with radiation halt the progression of cells in G2 so that the damage can be surveyed and repaired before the cell continues into mitosis. If this damage is not repaired, cells continue into mitosis with chromosomal aberrations, making them more susceptible to any DNA-damaging agent, including radiation. One checkpoint gene controls the formation of the spindle during prophase, such that if spindle formation is blocked, the cells are halted from progressing through mitosis. The mechanism of action of checkpoint genes involves p34 protein kinase, the levels of which control progression through mitosis. If these checkpoint genes are damaged or lacking in a cell, it is likely that these cells would be more sensitive to radiation. In addition, the lack or malfunction of checkpoint genes could permit damaged chromosomes to complete mitosis, resulting in aberrations such as translocations and other chromosome changes known to be associated with the malignant phenotype.

Effects of Radiation on the Total Body

Although much of what we know about the effects of total body radiation is based on animal experiments, sufficient numbers of humans have been irradiated to the whole body such that these acute effects in humans also are well

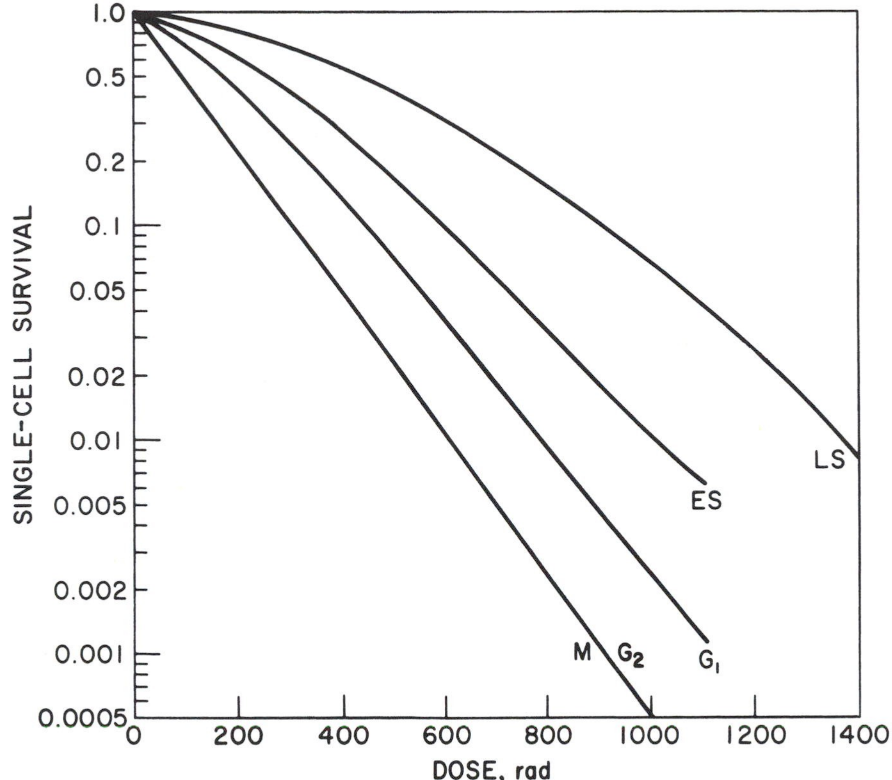

FIGURE 4-6. The relationship of position in the cell cycle to radiosensitivity. [From Sinclair, W.K. (1968). Cyclic responses in mammalian cells in vitro. *Radiation Research, 33*, 620. Reproduced by permission.]

documented. Data on humans have been obtained from studies on individuals exposed at Hiroshima and Nagasaki, the Marshall Islanders exposed to fallout radiation, the victims of the few accidents at nuclear installations, including that at Chernobyl, and patients in radiation therapy.

The primary effect of a high acute exposure to the whole body is lethality occurring within days to weeks after exposure. The time of death is dependent on the dose given and is preceded by a specific set of signs and symptoms that is directly related to damage and cell death in a particular organ system. The term *total body syndrome*, or radiation syndrome, is used to describe this condition. Three distinct syndromes have been defined after whole-body irradiation resulting from damage to three specific organ systems—the cerebrovascular syndrome, the gastrointestinal syndrome, and the hematopoietic, or bone marrow, syndrome. Figure 4-7 shows the relationship between dose and survival time for each of these three syndromes.

In the first part of the curve, after doses between 2 and 10 Gy, the time of death is dependent on the magnitude of the dose. The higher the dose, the earlier death occurs. Within this dose range, death occurs within weeks after exposure and is characterized by a decrease in the number of circulating blood cells. The major

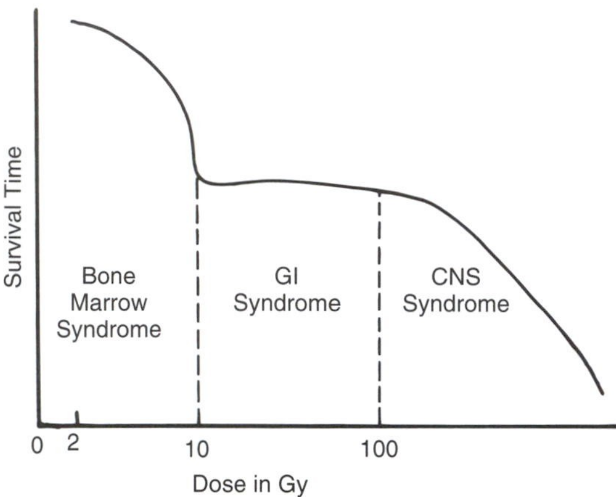

FIGURE 4-7. Schematic of dose dependence of total body radiation, showing three defined syndromes: bone marrow, gastrointestinal (GI), and central nervous system (CNS). Although the dose range over which each syndrome occurs is different for different species, each syndrome occurs within the dose ranges shown. Each syndrome is named for the specific organ that fails. [From Pizzarello D.J., & Witcofski R.L. (1967). *Basic radiation biology.* Philadelphia: Lea & Febiger. Reproduced by permission.]

organ system that ultimately fails and causes death is the bone marrow and other blood-forming organs; thus, this syndrome is known as the hematopoietic, or bone marrow, syndrome. The mechanism of death is well established and is a result of killing and depleting the stem cells in the bone marrow.

In the second part of the curve, between the doses of 10 and 100 Gy, the time of death appears to be unrelated to dose. However, in a recent study in mice that were checked hourly after exposure to these high doses to the total body, the time of death was determined to be related to dose. In this dose range, death occurs within 1 to 2 weeks after irradiation and is due to damage and depletion of stem cells of the gastrointestinal mucosa. This mode of death is therefore termed the gastrointestinal syndrome. Death occurs more quickly in the gastrointestinal syndrome than in the bone marrow syndrome because the cells of the gastrointestinal tract, particularly the crypt cells, have a high cell replacement and a shorter life expectancy than the cells in the circulating blood.

The third part of the curve again shows a marked time-dependent relationship between time of death and dose. The doses that induce this syndrome are considered supralethal, >100 Gy (10,000 rads). Death after this supralethal dose reflects failure of the central nervous system and cardiovascular system and is termed the cerebrovascular syndrome. The cause of death in the cerebrovascular syndrome is poorly understood, but one possibility is that blood vessels in the brain are damaged by the radiation and become leaky, causing edema, vasculitis (inflammatory changes in the vessels), and meningitis (inflammation of the meninges). Death results from a buildup of pressure inside the skull, resulting from the edema.

These dose ranges are not specific for humans but represent a compilation of data from many different mammals, exposed either accidentally or intentionally (for medical purposes) to total body irradiation. Humans are the most sensitive of the mammals studied; thus, in humans each syndrome occurs at the lower end of these dose ranges.

Total Body Radiation in Humans

The least understood of the three syndromes is the cerebrovascular, which occurs after doses of 50 Gy (5000 rads) and higher to the whole body, although doses of 20 Gy may induce this syndrome. Death occurs in 100% of the exposed population, and in the few reported cases of humans exposed to doses in the range of the cerebrovascular syndrome, death has occurred within 2 days.

An acute total body dose >10 Gy will result in signs and symptoms of the gastrointestinal syndrome in most mammals studied, although in humans signs of this syndrome appear after a dose of 6 Gy. In humans without medical intervention, death usually occurs within 3 to 10 days after exposure. To date, no human has survived a dose of 10 Gy even with medical support. Until the nuclear accident at Chernobyl in the Ukraine, there was only one victim of the gastrointestinal syndrome resulting from an accidental overexposure. However, both workers and firefighters at Chernobyl died of the gastrointestinal syndrome.

Total body doses between 2 and 8 Gy may cause death as a result of killing of the radiosensitive precursor cells in the bone marrow that supply mature functional cells to the circulating blood. In most mammals the first deaths are seen as soon as 10 days after exposure, peak at 2 weeks, and are complete by 30 days. In humans, however, deaths from the hematopoietic syndrome begin later and peak later (at 30 days) and continue for a prolonged period (up to 60 days) when they are complete.

Mean Lethal Dose or LD_{50} for the Hematopoietic Syndrome

The lethal dose 50 (LD_{50}) is a term borrowed from the field of pharmacology and is defined as the dose of an agent that causes mortality in 50% of a given population in a given period of time. The $LD_{50/30}$ can be measured in experimental animals providing a precise estimate of its value. In humans the $LD_{50/60}$ can only be estimated from data from the atomic bomb explosions at Hiroshima and Nagasaki and from accidental exposures. Based on these data and the observation that, with medical support, humans have survived a total body dose of 4 Gy, estimates of the LD_{50} for humans range from 3 to 4 Gy. The threshold dose for this syndrome in humans is <1 Gy. At Chernobyl, ~200 employees, firefighters, and emergency personnel were exposed to doses >1 Gy and exhibited overt signs of the hematopoietic syndrome. Thirty-five of these individuals had severe bone marrow failure and 13 of these died. The remainder survived with medical support. Table 4-2 shows a comparison of LD_{50} for hematopoietic syndromes in humans and other species.

TABLE 4-2. $LD_{50/30}$ VALUES FOR DIFFERENT SPECIES

Species	$LD_{50/30}$ (Gy)[a]
Human	3.0–4.0
Monkey	4.0
Dog	3.0
Rabbit	8.0
Rat	9.0
Mouse	9.0
Chicken	6.0
Frog	7.0
Goldfish	20.0

[a] In humans the expression $LD_{50/60}$ may be more useful (for explanation, see the text). In addition, this expression is an estimate based on the small number of accidental overexposures; more data may change these estimates.

Effects of Radiation on the Embryo and Fetus

Most of our information and knowledge concerning the effects of radiation on the developing fetus and embryo has been obtained from studies in mice and rats because these animals have large litters and the gestational times are short. Based on the characteristics of fetal development and the fact that radiosensitivity is related to mitotic activity and differentiation, the fetus can be expected to be highly vulnerable to the lethal effects of radiation as well as to the induction of gross abnormalities recognizable at birth.

The classic effects of radiation on the developing embryo and fetus can be divided into three categories, known as the "classic triad" of radiation embryologic syndromes:

Classic Triad of Radiologic Embryologic Syndromes

1. *Lethal effects.* These are induced before or immediately after implantation of the fertilized ovum in the uterine wall or at any time during intrauterine development. Death can

occur before birth (prenatal death) or at about the time of birth (neonatal death).

2. *Congenital malformations.* These are expressed after birth and are induced by radiation exposure during the time of major organogenesis. Specific malformations reflect the organ system developing at the time of *in utero* irradiation.
3. *Growth disturbances.* These can occur before birth, at which time they would be intrauterine, or after birth, when they would be considered extrauterine. In general, disturbances in growth occur without the presence of other malformations.

The probability of finding one or more of these effects in an embryo is dependent on a number of factors, principally the dose and the time of gestation during which exposure occurred. The dose rate is also important because it is known that reducing the dose rate reduces the effects on the embryo and fetus.

These radiation-induced effects must be viewed relative to the spontaneous incidence of each of the effects in the general population. In the human, the incidence of malformations at birth is ~6%, but because some malformations are expressed with growth, the incidence of malformations in humans roughly doubles to 12% if grown children are included in the estimate.

Fetal Development and Radiation Effects

Radiation-induced lethality and specific gross abnormalities in the embryo and fetus are dependent on the day of gestation, in fact the *part of the day* of gestation in which exposure occurs. Russell and Russell have divided fetal development into three gestational stages:

- Preimplantation, the time between fertilization and attachment of the embryo onto the uterine wall;
- Organogenesis, the period during which all major organs develop;
- Fetal stage, primarily a period of growth of the newly formed organs.

The times postconception of the three phases of development for mice and humans are shown in Figure 4-8. In the rodent, the three stages are equal in time, whereas in the human the fetal, or growth, stage occupies the majority of fetal development.

The *preimplantation stage* is characterized by repeated divisions of the fertilized ovum, such that it forms a ball of cells that are highly undifferentiated. Exposure during this stage results in a high incidence of prenatal deaths. This phase of fetal development is exquisitely sensitive to radiation; doses as low as 0.1 Gy (10 rads) are fatal to the mouse embryo during this time. Those embryos that do survive exhibit few congenital abnormalities at birth, with the exception of one specific abnormality, exencephaly, i.e., brain hernia, or protrusion of the brain through the top of the skull.

Implantation of the embryo in the uterine wall signals the onset of the second stage, *major organogenesis*, which extends through the seventh week postconception in humans. During this time the cells of the embryo begin differentiating into the various stem cells that eventually will form all the organs of the body. The incidence of congenital abnormalities in mouse embryos increases dramatically when exposure occurs during major organogenesis. Gross abnormalities have been observed in the mouse embryo exposed to 0.25 Gy (25 rads) during this stage. Because differentiation of cells to form various organs begins on specific days, irradiation on certain gestational days produces specific abnormalities. The greatest variety of congenital abnormalities is produced when radiation is given during the 8th to the 12th day in the mouse, corresponding to the 23rd to 37th day in humans.

The majority of the effects of radiation on the fetus during this period of development are manifested in the central nervous system and in

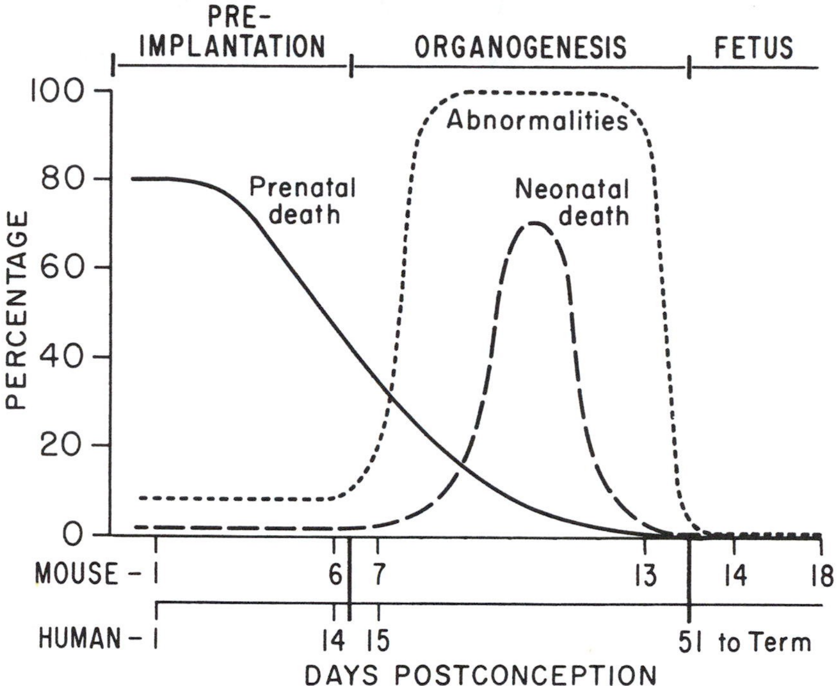

FIGURE 4-8. The effects of 2.0 Gy *in utero* exposure on mouse embryos. The upper scale is mouse gestational time; the lower scale is the equivalent in humans. [From Russell, L.B., & Russell, W.L. (1954). An analysis of the changing radiation response of the developing mouse embryo. *Journal of Cell Physiology, 1* (Suppl 43), 103. Reproduced by permission.]

related sense organs, such as the eye. The most common abnormalities include brain abnormalities, behavioral abnormalities, and skeletal abnormalities, as listed in Table 4-3.

The incidence of prenatal death decreases when exposure occurs during major organogenesis; however, there is an increase in the incidence of neonatal death (death at birth). This may be partially due to the presence of abnormalities in the fetus that are fatal at term.

At the end of this time, the embryo is termed a fetus and enters the *fetal stage*, primarily a period of growth. The fetus at this time contains most organ systems and many types of cells, ranging from undifferentiated stem cells to more differentiated cells. Irradiation during the fetal period results in fewer obvious abnormalities and a decreased incidence in both prenatal and neonatal deaths. Higher doses are necessary during this time to produce lethality and gross abnormalities. Irradiation during this period of gestation may result in effects that occur later in life (e.g., cancer) or in functional disorders after birth.

Data from Humans

The 1600 survivors irradiated *in utero* when the atomic bombs were dropped on Hiroshima and Nagasaki provide dramatic data on the effects of irradiation at various stages of human gestation. The two main effects observed and reported in the survivors irradiated *in utero* are microcephaly (small head circumference) and mental retardation. Significant harmful effects of radiation on the developing brains of children ex-

TABLE 4-3. SOME MAJOR ABNORMALITIES FOUND IN MAMMALS (HUMANS, RABBITS, MICE) AFTER FETAL IRRADIATION

Central Nervous System	Skeletal	Ocular	Others
Exencephaly	Stunting	Absence of eye(s)	Leukemia
Microcephaly	Abnormal limbs	Microphthalmia (small eyes)	Genital deformities with sterility
Mental retardation	Small head		
	Cleft palate	Strabismus	
Skull malformations	Club feet	Cataract	
Hydrocephaly	Deformed arms	Absence of lens	
	Spina bifida		

SOURCE: Rugh, R. (1963). The impact of ionizing radiation on the embryo and fetus. *American Journal of Roetgenology, Radium Therapy and Nuclear Medicine, 89*; 182. Reproduced by permission.

posed *in utero* were observed only for those exposed during the periods 8 to 15 weeks and 16 to 25 weeks after conception.

Small head size was noted more than 50 years ago in children who had been irradiated *in utero* at Hiroshima and Nagasaki. This abnormality was maintained into adulthood. Although it is impossible to estimate with any accuracy the amount of radiation to which those persons were exposed, it has been shown that doses as low as 0.09 Gy (9 rad) caused a detectable increase in the number of microcephalic individuals, regardless of the gestational age at exposure. This is particularly important, as it is generally believed that microcephaly is the most common sequelae of *in utero* exposure after the first trimester. A dose–response relationship was found with a clear increase observed after doses as low as 0.1 to 0.19 Gy (10 to 19 rad).

Thirty of these 1600 children also have been diagnosed as clinically severely retarded with IQs below 68. Although five of these cases were not radiation related, the remaining incidence is still well above normal. This effect is dependent on dose and the gestational age at the time of irradiation. Assuming a linear dose–response, the probability of induction of mental retardation is estimated to range from 0.4 per Gy to 0.1 per Gy. It has been estimated also that a dose of 1 Gy (100 rads) causes a 30-point decrease in the IQ score. To put this in the context of diagnostic radiology, where doses are on the order of 0.5 Gy (5 rads), the decrease in IQ would not be detected.

Carcinogenesis: Stochastic Effects

The previous two sections dealt with the consequences of radiation-induced cell killing on tissues and organisms. Although these effects are important, of equal importance to the individual are the consequences of cells that survived the irradiation with subsequent modification. Two consequences of these viable but modified cells are carcinogenesis and hereditary effects. Both radiation-induced cancers and hereditary effects are *stochastic effects*, i.e., they are random events that probably do not have a threshold. In addition, the severity of the effect is not dose dependent. For example, in somatic cells, the probability of cancer induction increases with dose, but the severity of the cancer is not dose related.

Data Sources

The first case of radiation-induced cancer was reported 6 years after Roentgen's discovery; within 15 years 100 cases of skin cancer were reported in occupationally exposed persons. Since these early reports, a large body of data has been collected in humans, indicating that radiation does cause cancer. The most compelling data regarding the carcinogenic effect of radiation in humans are derived from the following:

1. Increased incidence of many types of cancer, including leukemia and solid tumors, in survivors of the atomic bombings in Hiroshima and Nagasaki;
2. Increased incidence of leukemia in irradiated patients with ankylosing spondylitis;
3. Increased incidence of leukemia in radiologists;
4. Increased incidence of thyroid cancer in children irradiated for ringworm or for enlarged thymus.

Risk Estimates

The question of most concern regarding radiation-induced cancers is as follows: What is the risk of developing cancer after irradiation? This is not an easy question to answer because of the long and variable latency period between exposure and the appearance of cancer. Another question is whether an individual is at risk for the whole of his life, or if, after a time, his risk returns to that of the "normal," unirradiated population. There is no single answer to this question, for the risk of developing some kinds of cancers is a discrete event, i.e., the risk increases for a period of time and then decreases, i.e., the risk is *absolute*. The incidence of radiation-induced leukemia follows this pattern. For other types of cancer, the individual is at risk throughout his life and the risk is increased by a constant factor for all ages, i.e., the risk is *relative*. With the exception of radiation-induced leukemia, whether the risk for other types of cancers is relative or absolute is not clear.

A second important issue is to estimate risk for occupationally exposed persons or for persons exposed to diagnostic procedures using radiation. Currently, the estimates for these low-dose exposures must be made from data obtained after higher doses. The two models used, the linear model and linear quadratic model, both fit the high-dose data reasonably well, but when extrapolated to low doses, the linear model overestimates the risk, whereas the linear quadratic model underestimates the risk. Experimental data do not permit a rejection of either model, although most radiobiologists favor the linear quadratic model because damage to many other cells and tissues is fitted well by this model.

Radiation-Induced Cancers in Humans

LEUKEMIA

The cancer most frequently associated with radiation exposure is leukemia. Studies on the survivors of the atomic bombs at Hiroshima and Nagasaki and patients treated for ankylosing spondylitis provide a large study population; thus, the best estimates of risk are available for this type of cancer. Only two types of adult leukemia are increased by radiation exposure, acute and chronic myeloid leukemia. Exposure during childhood, however, results in an increase in acute lymphatic leukemia. The increased risk of radiation-induced leukemia peaks between 7 and 12 years and then returns to that of the normal population. The incidence of leukemia in the survivors of the atomic bomb was 3 to 5 times higher than the expected incidence in an unexposed population. Estimates of risk in the low-dose Japanese survivors at Hiroshima are also higher than for the normal population, indicating that the risk of leukemia induction is dose dependent.

BREAST CANCER

The most compelling data indicating that breast cancer is induced by radiation comes from two primary sources: (1) female survivors of the atomic bombings in Japan, and (2) Canadian women administered multiple fluoroscopic examinations for tuberculosis in which the doses were estimated to range from 0.04 to 0.2 Gy, i.e., 4 to 20 rads.

Both of these data sets provide convincing evidence that breast cancer increases with radiation dose, although the Canadian study has the advantages of large sample size and reasonable estimates of dose. The data from the Canadian study, shown in Figure 4-9, can be fitted reasonably well by a straight line, suggesting that, at least for this one cancer, the relationship between incidence of breast cancer and radiation dose is a linear function of dose.

LUNG CANCER

Risk estimates for radiation-induced lung cancer come from two primary sources: (1) Japanese survivors of the atomic bombings, and (2) miners exposed to radon, a radioactive gas released in the decay of naturally occurring radioactive materials in the earth.

Although it is accepted that radiation does increase the incidence of lung cancer, estimates of risk are difficult to calculate with any certainty because radiation is only one of many agents known to cause lung cancer, including cigarettes and asbestos. Estimates of dose also are difficult to obtain in the exposed populations, particularly in the miners, because of inherent uncertainties in the exposure conditions.

OTHER TUMORS

Osteosarcoma and thyroid carcinoma are two other malignancies known to be associated with radiation. At this point it is safe to assume that radiation may be carcinogenic to any tissue and organ in the body, although tissues such as breast, lung, and thyroid seem to be particularly susceptible. Early follow-up of the Japanese survivors of the atomic bombs indicated that leukemia, with its short latency time, was the primary malignancy in the irradiated group. However, an increased incidence of a variety of solid tumors began to emerge with extended follow-up times and, in fact, these tumors now outnumber the earlier cases of leukemia. However, the total incidence of solid tumors in this population will not be known until all known survivors have died. It is estimated that the ratio of solid tumors to leukemias will be 2 to 3.

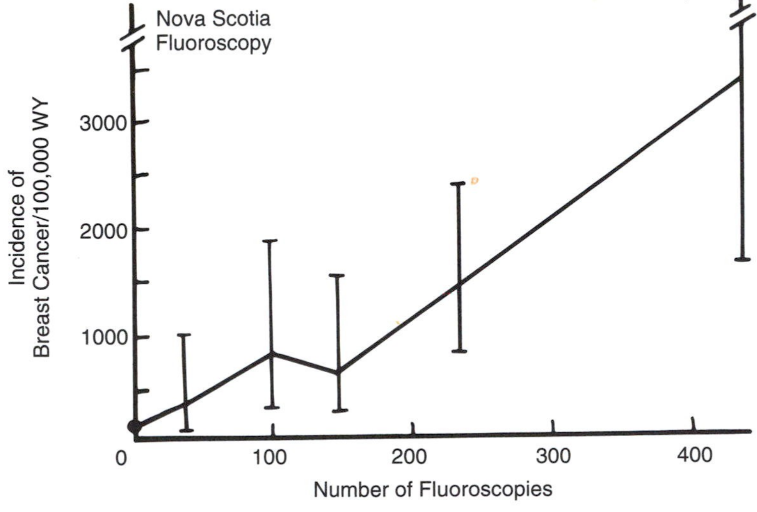

FIGURE 4-9. Incidence of breast cancer in a group of Canadian women exposed to multiple fluoroscopic examinations for tuberculosis. The incidence of breast cancer shows a linear dose–response. [From Boice, J.D., Land, C.E., Shore, R.E., Norman, J.E. & Tokunaga, M. (1979). Risk of breast cancer following low dose exposure. *Radiology, 131*, 589–597. Reproduced by permission.]

Mechanisms of Radiation-Induced Cancer

The development of the field of molecular biology has led to progress in our understanding of the molecular genetics of cancer. As discussed earlier, there are three potential mechanisms by which radiation may induce changes leading to cancer: checkpoint genes that control cellular proliferation and differentiation may be disrupted, or cells may be converted from normal to malignant by either the activation of oncogenes or the loss of suppressor genes. In some cancers, more than one of these mechanisms may be involved.

Hereditary Effects of Radiation: Stochastic Effects

The irradiation of the reproductive organs carries the risk of causing a mutation in the germ cells, i.e., the spermatozoa or the ova. Mutations can occur in the chromosome or in the genes that make up the chromosome. Chromosomal mutations have been associated with a number of diseases and include aberrations as discussed above or changes in chromosome distribution, a familiar example of which is Down's syndrome, in which there is an extra chromosome 23. Gene mutations can be a change in the composition or the sequence of bases, or both, on the DNA molecule. It might seem unlikely that small alterations in the DNA can cause significant changes in the individual, but this is not true. Sickle cell anemia, for example, results from the substitution of a single base on the DNA. Thus, radiation can cause profound changes in the genome, which can be passed on to future generations.

Animal Studies

The study of radiation-induced mutations is made difficult by the fact that radiation induces no new mutations; it only increases the incidence of spontaneous mutations in the general population. Because the data in humans are few, almost all of our knowledge of the hereditary effects of radiation is derived from animal data.

The majority of our information on genetic effects of radiation comes from one study, the "megamouse project" conducted at Oak Ridge National Laboratory by Russell and Russell. These investigators used an inbred strain of mice in which specific locus mutations occurred and produced a phenotype that could be observed with the eye, for example, coat color. The increase in the number of these specific phenotypes was scored after a range of radiation doses, dose rates, and dose fractionation schedules. A summary of the most important findings is listed below:

1. All mutations did not show the same sensitivity to radiation.
2. A substantial dose rate effect was found in the mouse, data that were in contrast to earlier studies in Drosophila (fruit flies) in which no dose rate effect was found.
3. The male was much more sensitive to radiation-induced mutations than the female such that, after low-dose rate irradiation, the burden of genetic effects in the population is carried by the male.
4. The genetic effects of a given dose can be reduced by allowing a period of time to elapse between radiation and conception.
5. The estimate of the doubling dose for humans, calculated from low-dose rate data in the mouse, is 1 Gy. The *doubling dose* is defined as the dose required to double the spontaneous mutation rate, or the dose that causes an increase in mutations equal to the number of spontaneous mutations.

Genetic Effects in Humans

Little data are available for humans with the exception of the Japanese survivors of Hiroshima and Nagasaki. Four genetic indicators have been studied in this population for 40 years; the data have been stratified by dose, low-dose exposures of 0.01 to 0.09 Gy, i.e., 1 to 9 rads, and high-dose exposures >1 Gy, i.e., 100 rads, and both parents of children from both cities were studied. The doubling dose calculated from these data is estimated at 156 rems.

Given the uncertainties in the data and the extrapolation of data on genetic effects in mice, the important points regarding the genetic effects of radiation in humans are:

1. Most mutations are harmful;
2. Any dose of radiation, no matter how small, can cause genetic changes;
3. There is a linear relationship between dose and number of mutations, thus information after low doses can be extrapolated from high-dose data;
4. Man is not more sensitive than mouse, and may, in fact, be less sensitive; and
5. Mouse data provide reasonable estimates of the risk of radiation-induced genetic effects in humans.

REVIEW QUESTIONS

1. Radiobiology is:
   A. A branch of cytogenetics.
   B. A branch of molecular biology.
   C. The study of the effects of radiowaves on living organisms.
   D. The study of the effects of radiation on biological systems.

2. When radiation interacts with living organisms:
   A. The interaction is a matter of chance.
   B. Certain parts of the cell are targeted for the interaction.
   C. The interaction produces unique changes in the cell.
   D. Cell changes occur immediately.

3. Which of the following has been labeled a critical target?
   A. Cytoplasm.
   B. Water.
   C. Lysosome.
   D. DNA.

4. Which of the following refers to direct action?
   A. Ions produced by the ionization of water react with other water molecules before they interact with a critical target.
   B. Radiation is absorbed by the critical target initiating a series of events leading to biological damage.
   C. Radiation interacts with water producing free radicals that reach critical targets.
   D. All of the above.

5. Free radicals are:
   A. Ions.
   B. Electrons.
   C. Molecules or atoms having an unpaired electron in their outer shell.
   D. Charged particles.

6. An ion is all of the following except:
   A. An electron.
   B. A water molecule that has lost an electron.
   C. H_2O^+.
   D. H_2O^-.

7. Which of the following accounts for about two thirds of all x-ray damage to DNA?
   A. The electron.
   B. The hydrogen free radical.
   C. The positive water ion.
   D. The hydroxyl free radical.

8. Radiation can damage DNA by producing:
   A. Single strand breaks.
   B. Double strand breaks.
   C. Loss of base pairs.
   D. All of the above.

9. Which of the following is most likely to produce cell death?
   A. DNA single strand break.
   B. DNA double strand break.

C. Ionization in the cytoplasm.
D. Loss of an electron from a water molecule.

10. Which of the following is not one of the phases of mitosis?

A. Anaphase.
B. Interphase.
C. Prophase.
D. Metaphase.

11. The term used to describe breaks in chromosomes due to radiation exposure is:

A. Aberrations.
B. Ionizations.
C. Excitations.
D. Fractures.

12. Chromosome breaks leading to deletions of genetic material can result in all of the following except:

A. Ovarian cancer.
B. Neuroblastoma.
C. Retinoblastoma.
D. Wilms' tumor.

13. Oncogenes can be activated by radiation through the following mechanisms:

A. Point mutations.
B. Chromosomal aberrations.
C. Chromosomal translocation.
D. All of the above.

14. Irradiated cells can die by which of the following:

1. Mitotic death.
2. Reproductive failure.
3. Interphase death.
4. Apoptosis.

A. 1, 2, and 3.
B. 2 and 3.
C. 3 and 4.
D. All are correct.

15. Which of the following shows a relationship between radiation dose and the proportion of cells that remain alive?

A. Cell-life curve.
B. Dead cell curve.
C. Cell survival curve.
D. Reproductive integrity curve.

16. A survival curve is a plot of cell survival as a function of:

A. kVp.
B. mAs.
C. Dose.
D. Cell death.

17. The transfer of energy from radiation per unit path length is called the:

A. Relative biological effectiveness.
B. Linear energy transfer.
C. Energy of the radiation.
D. Bragg peak.

18. The ratio of the dose of a standard type of radiation to the dose of a test radiation needed to produce the same biological response is called the:

A. Linear energy transfer.
B. Biological response.
C. Relative biological effectiveness.
D. Dose ratio.

19. Which of the following is not a part of interphase?

A. G1.
B. S.
C. G2.
D. Mitosis.

20. Which is the most radiosensitive portion of the cell cycle?

A. Mitosis.
B. G1.
C. S.
D. Interphase.

21. Which portion of the cell cycle is most radioresistant?

A. Mitosis.
B. G2.

C. G1.
D. S-phase.

22. Which of the following play(s) a role in regulating the cell cycle?
A. Checkpoint chromosomes.
B. Checkpoint genes.
C. Cytoplasm.
D. Time of day.

23. Data on total body irradiation of humans have been obtained from:
1. Survivors of the Hiroshima and Nagasaki bombings.
2. Marshall Islanders.
3. Chernobyl nuclear installation.
4. Patients in radiation therapy.
A. 1, 2, and 3.
B. 1 and 3.
C. 2 and 4.
D. All are correct.

24. The syndrome(s) that result due to a high acute exposure to the whole body is (are):
A. Hematopoietic syndrome.
B. Gastrointestinal syndrome.
C. Cerebrovascular syndrome.
D. All are correct.

25. Which of the following syndromes will occur due to a whole-body exposure of 2 to 10 Gy (200 to 1000 rads)?
A. Cerebrovascular syndrome.
B. Gastrointestinal syndrome.
C. Hematopoietic syndrome.
D. All of the above.

26. When death occurs (as a result of an acute high exposure to the whole body) as a result of killing and depletion of stem cells in the bone marrow, this is called the:
A. Cerebrovascular syndrome.
B. Gastrointestinal syndrome.
C. Hematopoietic syndrome.
D. a and b are correct.

27. At a whole-body exposure of 100 Gy (10,000 rads) or more, death is due to a failure of the:
A. Bone marrow.
B. Gastrointestinal system.
C. Central nervous system or cerebrovascular system.
D. a and b are correct.

28. The term $LD_{50/30}$ means that:
A. 50% of the population will die in 30 minutes.
B. 50% of the population will die in 30 days.
C. 30% of the population will die in 50 days.
D. 30% of the population will die in 50 minutes.

29. Most of the information on the effects of radiation exposure on the embryo and fetus are obtained from studies on:
A. Mice and rats.
B. Fruit flies.
C. Humans exposed in uranium mines.
D. Humans exposed in radiation therapy.

30. The "classic triad" of radiation embryologic syndromes include all of the following except:
A. Lethality.
B. Congenital abnormalities.
C. Growth disturbances.
D. Cerebrovascular syndrome.

31. Exposure at the preimplantation stage of fetal development results in a high incidence of:
A. Congenital abnormalities.
B. Neonatal deaths.
C. Prenatal deaths.
D. Cancer.

32. Exposure at the major organogenesis stage of fetal development results in a high incidence of:

A. Prenatal deaths.
B. Cancer.
C. Neonatal deaths.
D. Congenital abnormalities.

33. Exposure during the fetal stage of fetal development results in:

A. Neonatal death.
B. Congenital abnormalities.
C. Effects that occur later in life, such as cancer.
D. Exencephaly.

34. The two main effects observed and reported in the survivors of Hiroshima and Nagasaki who were irradiated *in utero* are:

1. Mental retardation.
2. Brain protrusion.
3. Skeletal abnormalities.
4. Microencephaly.

A. 1 and 2.
B. 2 and 3.
C. 2 and 4.
D. 1 and 4.

35. Which of the following are stochastic effects of radiation?

A. Carcinogenesis.
B. Hereditary effects.
C. Cataracts.
D. a and b are correct.

36. The data supporting the carcinogenic effect of radiation in humans are derived from:

1. Survivors of Hiroshima and Nagasaki bombings.
2. Patients irradiated for ankylosing spondylitis.
3. Children irradiated for enlarged thymus.
4. Radiologists.

A. 1, 2, and 3.
B. 2 and 3.
C. 3 and 4.
D. All are correct.

37. Which of the following dose–response models is most favored by radiobiologists in estimating the risk of exposure to diagnostic radiation?

A. Linear model.
B. Supralinear model.
C. Linear quadratic model.
D. All of the above.

38. Radiation-induced cancers in humans include:

A. Leukemia.
B. Breast cancer.
C. Lung cancer.
D. All of the above.

39. The mechanism(s) by which radiation may induce changes leading to cancer is (are):

A. Disruption of checkpoint genes that control cellular proliferation and differentiation.
B. Activation of oncogenes.
C. Loss of suppressor genes.
D. All of the above.

40. Which of the following can produce a hereditary effect?

A. A mutation in the germ cells.
B. A gene mutation.
C. A change in the sequence of bases on the DNA molecule.
D. All of the above.

41. Which of the following provides most of the information on the genetic effects of radiation?

A. The genome project.
B. Hiroshima and Nagasaki survivors.
C. Megamouse project at Oak Ridge National Laboratory.
D. Fruit fly experiments.

42. For humans, the following is (are) important regarding genetic effects:

1. Most mutations are harmful.
2. Any dose of radiation, no matter how small, can cause genetic effects.

3. There is a linear relationship between dose and the number of mutations.
4. The human is more sensitive than the mouse.

A. 1, 2, and 3.
B. 2 and 4.
C. 3 and 4.
D. All are correct.

REFERENCES

Bedford, J.S., & Mitchell, J.B. (1973). Dose-rate effects in asynchronous mammalian cells in culture. *Radiation Research, 54,* 316–327.

Bender, M. (1963). Induced aberrations in human chromosomes. *American Journal of Pathology, 43,* 26a.

Bronte, R.J. (1988). Chernobyl retrospective. *Seminars in Nuclear Medicine, 18,* 16–24.

Champlin, R. (1987). The role of bone marrow transplantation for nuclear accidents: Implication of the Chernobyl disaster. *Seminars in Hematology, 24,* 1–4.

Committee on the Biological Effects of Ionizing Radiation. (1980). *The effects on populations of exposure to low levels of ionizing radiation.* Washington, DC: National Academy of Sciences.

Committee on the Biological Effects of Ionizing Radiation. (1990). *Health effects of exposure of low levels of ionizing radiations.* Washington, DC: National Academy of Sciences/National Research Council.

Cornforth, M.N., & Bedford, J.S. (1983). X-ray-induced breakage and rejoining of human interphase chromosomes. *Science, 222,* 1141–1143.

Court-Brown, W.M., & Doll, R. (1958). Expectation of life and mortality from cancer among British radiologists. *British Medical Journal, 2,* 181.

Court-Brown, W.M., & Doll, R. (1958). Mortality from cancer and other causes after radiotherapy for ankylosing spondylitis. *British Medical Journal, 2,* 1327.

Dekaban, A.S. (1968). Abnormalities in children exposed to x-radiation during various stages of gestation: Tentative timetable of radiation injury to the human fetus. *Journal of Nuclear Medicine, 9,* 471.

Elkind, M.M. (1984). Repair processes in radiation biology. *Radiation Research, 100,* 425–449.

Evans, J.H. (1962). Chromosome aberrations induced by ionizing radiation. *International Review of Cytology, 13,* 221.

Frankenberg, D., Frankenberg-Schwager, M., & Harbich, R. (1984). Split-dose recovery is due to the repair of DNA double-strand breaks. *International Journal of Radiation Biology, 46,* 541–553.

Geard, C.R. (1982). Effects of radiation on chromosomes. In D. Pizzarello (Ed.), *Radiation Biology* (pp. 83–110). Boca Raton, FL: CRC Press.

Gould, M.N., & Clifton, K.H. (1977). The survival of mammary cells following irradiation in vivo: A directly generated single-dose survival curve. *Radiation Research, 72,* 343–352.

Hall, E.J. (1988). *Radiobiology for the radiologist* (3rd ed.). Philadelphia: J.B. Lippincott.

Hall, E.J., & Freyer, G.A. (1991). The molecular biology of radiation carcinogenesis. *Basic Life Sciences, 58,* 3–25.

Hartwell, L.H., & Weiner, T.A. (1989). Checkpoints: Controls that ensure the order of cell cycle events. *Science, 246,* 629–634.

Hempelmann, L.H. (1968). Risk of thyroid neoplasms after irradiation in childhood: Studies of populations exposed to radiation in childhood show a dose response over a wide dose range. *Science, 160,* 159–163.

Hewitt, H.B., & Wilson, C.W. (1959). A survival curve for mammalian cells irradiated in vivo. *Nature, 183,* 1060–1061.

Hollstein, M., Sidvansky, D., Vogelstein, B., & Harris, C.C. (1991). Mutations in human cancers. *Science, 253,* 49–53.

Howard, A., & Pelc, S.R. (1953). Synthesis of deoxyribonucleic acid in normal and irradiated cells and its relation to chromosome breakage. *Heredity, 6* (Suppl), 261–273.

Kellerer, A.M., & Rosso, H.H. (1972). The theory of dual radiation action. *Current Topics: Radiation Research Quarterly, 8,* 85–158.

Kerr, F.R., Jr., & Searle, J. (1980). Apoptosis: Its nature and kinetic role. In R.E. Meyn, & H.R. Withers (Eds.), *Radiation Biology in Cancer Research* (pp. 367–384). New York: Raven Press.

Krall, J.F. (1956). Estimation of spontaneous and radiation induced mutation rates in man. *Eugenics Quarterly, 3,* 201.

Lea, D. (1956). *Actions of radiations on living cells* (2nd ed.). Cambridge, England: Cambridge University Press.

Linnemann, R.E. (1987). Soviet medical response to the Chernobyl nuclear accident. *JAMA, 258,* 637–643.

Lushbaugh, C.C. (1969). Reflections on some recent progress in human radiobiology. In L.C. Augustein (Ed.), *Advances in Radiation Biology* (pp. 277–314). New York: Academic Press.

McKenzie, I. (1965). Breast cancer following multiple fluoroscopies. *British Journal of Cancer, 19,* 1.

Miller, R.W., & Blot, W.J. (1972). Small head size after in utero exposure to atomic radiation. *Lancet, 2,* 784.

Miller, R.W., & Mulvihill, J.J. (1986). Small head size after atomic irradiation. In J.L. Sever, & R.L. Brent (Eds.), *Teratogen Update, Environmentally Induced Birth Defect Risks* (pp. 141–143). New York: Alan R. Liss.

Munro, T.R. (1970). The relative radiosensitivity of the nucleus and cytoplasm of the Chinese hamster fibroblasts. *Radiation Research, 42,* 451–470.

Myrden, J.A., & Hiltz, J.E. (1969). Breast cancer following multiple fluoroscopies during artificial pneumothorax treatment of pulmonary tuberculosis. *Canadian Medical Association Journal, 100,* 1032–1034.

Otake, M., & Schull, W.J. (1984). In utero exposure to A-bomb radiation and mental retardation: A reassessment. *British Journal of Radiology, 57,* 409–414.

Puck, T.T., Marcus, T.I. (1956). Action of x-rays on mammalian cells. *Journal of Experimental Medicine, 103,* 653.

Rugh, R. (1963). The impact of ionizing radiation on the embryo and fetus. *American Journal of Roentgenology, Radium Therapy and Nuclear Medicine, 89,* 182.

Rugh, R. (1971a). *From conception to birth: The drama of life's beginnings.* New York: Harper & Row.

Rugh, R. (1971b). X-ray induced teratogenesis in the mouse and its possible significance to man. *Radiology, 99,* 433–443.

Russell, L.B. & Russell, W.L. (1954). An analysis of the changing radiation response of the developing mouse embryo. *Journal of Cellular Physiology, 43* (suppl 1), 103.

Russell, L.B., & Montgomery, C.S. (1966). Radiation sensitivity differences with cell-division cycles during mouse cleavage. *International Journal of Radiation Biology and Related Studies in Physics, Chemistry and Medicine, 10,* 151.

Russell, W.L. (1963). Genetic hazards of radiation. *Proceedings of the American Philosophical Society, 107,* 11.

Russell, W.L. (1965). Studies in mammalian radiation genetics. *Nucleonics, 23,* 53.

Schull, W.L., Otake, M., & Neal, J.V. (1981). Genetic effects of the atomic bomb: A reappraisal. *Science, 213,* 1220–1227.

Sinclair, W.K. (1969). *Dependence of radiosensitivity upon cell age.* Upton, NY: BNL Report 50203 (C-57).

Taylor, A.M.R., Harnden, D.G., Arlett, C.F., Harcourt, S.A., Lehmann, A.R., Stevens, S., & Bridges, B.A. (1975). Ataxia telangiectasia: A human mutation with abnormal radiation sensitivity. *Nature, 258,* 427–429.

Terasima, T., & Tolmach, L.J. (1961). Changes in the x-ray sensitivity of He-La cells during the division cycle. *Nature, 190,* 1210–1211.

Terasima, R., & Tolmach, L.J. (1963). X-ray sensitivity and DNA synthesis in synchronous populations of HeLa cells. *Science, 140,* 490.

Thames, H.D., Withers, H.R., Peters, L.J., & Fletcher, G.H. (1982). Changes in early and late radiation responses with altered dose fractionation: Implications for dose-survival relationships. *International Journal of Radiation, Oncology, Biology, Physics, 8,* 219–226.

Thoma, G.E., Jr., Wald, N. Acute radiation syndrome in man. In: *Fundamentals of Radiological Health, Training Manual of the National Center for Radiological Health, DHEW Training Publication No. 3n.* Washington, D.C.: U.S. Department of Health, Education and Welfare.

Travis, E.L. (in press 1996). *Primer of medical radiobiology* (3rd ed.). Chicago: Year Book Medical Publishers.

United Nations Scientific Committee on the Effects of Atomic Radiation. (1986). *Sources and effects of ionizing radiation.* New York: UNSCEAR.

Wanebo, C.K., Johnson, K.G., Sato, K., & Thorsland, T.W. (1968). Lung cancer following atomic radiation. *American Review of Respiratory Disease, 988,* 778–787.

Wanebo, C.K., Johnson, K.G., Sato, K., & Thorslund, T.W. (1968). Breast cancer after exposure to the atomic bombings of Hiroshima and Nagasaki. *New England Journal of Medicine, 279,* 667–671.

Wolff, S. (1963). *Radiation-induced chromosome aberrations.* New York: Columbia University Press.

Wood, J.W., Johnson, K.G., & Omori, Y. (1967a). In utero exposure to the Hiroshima atomic bomb: Follow-up at 20 years. *Pediatrics, 39,* 385–392.

Wood, J.W., Johnson, K.G., Omoro, Y., Kawamoto, S., & Keehn, R.J. (1967b). Mental retardation in children exposed in utero to the atomic bomb in Hiroshima and Nagasaki. *American Journal of Public Health, 57,* 1381–1390.

Zirkle, R.E. (1957). Partial cell irradiation. *Advances in Biology and Medical Physics, 5,* 103.

Part III
Principles of Radiation Protection

CHAPTER FIVE

Radiation Protection Concepts

Learning Objectives

Upon completion of this chapter, the reader should be able to:

1. Identify two types of radiation risks and list examples of each.
2. State the benefits of medical radiation exposure.
3. Discuss the benefit-risk concept of radiation exposure as applied to medicine.
4. State the objectives of radiation protection.
5. Discuss the following three principles of radiation protection: justification/net benefit; ALARA, and dose limitation.
6. Discuss the second triad of radiation safety, including time, shielding, and distance.
7. Compare and contrast radiation detection devices and radiation dosimeters.
8. Describe the characteristic features of the thermoluminescent dosimeter.
9. State the purpose of a personnel dosimeter and explain where it should be worn during radiography and fluoroscopy.
10. Explain the important elements of a dosimetry report.
11. State the purpose of radiation surveys.
12. Explain the basic requirements of the following five phases of a radiation protection survey: investigation, inspection, measurement, evaluation, and recommendations.
13. Describe each of the following major elements of a radiation protection program: administration, radiation safety committee, radiation safety officer, guidelines and recommendations, radiation protection records, and education and training.

Introduction

In this chapter, we explore the fundamental concepts of radiation protection, a few of which were introduced in Chapter 1. A firm understanding of these concepts and their underlying principles is mandatory for radiologic technologists.

We focus on analyzing the potential benefits and risks associated with radiation as well as describing specific radiation protection actions. In addition, we describe the detection and measurement of radiation, personnel dosimetry, and radiation protection surveys. The chapter concludes with a discussion of the essential elements of a radiation protection program.

Understanding the Potential Risks and Benefits of Medical Exposure

Risks

The risks of radiation exposure are well known. These risks were addressed in Chapter 4 by Elizabeth Travis, who described them in terms of stochastic and deterministic effects. Whereas stochastic effects are those for which the *probability* of occurrence increases with increasing radiation dose, deterministic effects are those for which the *severity* of the effect increases with increasing dose. Whereas no threshold dose exists for stochastic effects, deterministic effects have a threshold dose. In other words, any dose of radiation, no matter how small, has the potential to cause a stochastic effect, whereas for deterministic effects, there is a threshold dose that must be exceeded before the effect is observed. Cancer induction and genetic effects are examples of stochastic effects. Anyone exposed to even low doses of radiation, such as those delivered in radiology, is considered to be at risk for these health problems. Examples of deterministic effects are cataracts (opacification of the lens of the eye), blood changes, and impairment of fertility, such as a decrease in sperm count in males and sterilization in females.

Benefits

The idea that medical exposure to radiation should be of some benefit to the individual undergoing it is central to the decision-making process that always precedes diagnostic and therapeutic radiation.

The benefits of diagnostic exposure have been discussed by Dalrymple et al. (1984), who presented clinical examples in which radiation exposure is of great benefit, limited benefit, and no benefit to the patient. For example, they argued that although radiation is essential in screening programs such as mammography, it may, in fact, be of questionable value in other instances, such as diagnosing acute appendicitis, in repeated upper gastrointestinal series in patients with known peptic ulcers, and using repeated radiography of uncomplicated fractures. However, they suggested that radiation is usually not necessary in diagnosing or treating most psychiatric illnesses, ophthalmologic problems, and dermatologic conditions.

In a recent symposium of the Radiological Society of North America (RSNA) and the American Association of Physicists in Medicine (AAPM) on screening mammography, Tabar (1990) discussed the benefits of mammographic screening in terms of their social importance, and not simply in terms of their relevance to specific individuals. He reported that the collective findings of several major studies on mammography screening conducted in the United States and Sweden indicate that mass screening for breast cancer could significantly reduce mortality from the disease by detecting the cancer in its early stages, when it is treatable.

Benefit–Risk Analysis

Because radiation exposure is not without its hazards, no decision to expose an individual can be undertaken without weighing the benefits of exposure against the potential risks. The primary benefit of exposure to radiation is to help to restore the health of the sick or injured individual. The potential risks are, of course, the stochastic and deterministic effects we have already discussed.

One of the radiologic technologist's most important tasks is to explain these risks and benefits to the patient, for only then can the patient make an informed decision about whether to accept or reject the procedure. In equipping the patient to make an informed choice, the radiologic technologist transfers the responsibility for the outcome of the procedure to the patient. It must be made clear to the patient that along with the decision to accept any radiologic procedure comes the responsibility for accepting the possibility of an adverse outcome (Hendee, 1991, p. 110).

When the benefits of exposure clearly outweigh the risks, the decision to reject or, in many cases, to accept radiation is not difficult to make. Examinations that are considered to have a high benefit–risk ratio are coronary arteriogram in patients with cardiovascular problems and computed tomography (CT) of the brain in patients with cerebral hemorrhage. Decision making becomes more complicated in situations in which there is a low benefit–risk ratio. In these cases, the potential benefit of the procedure is small or negligible, and the potential risk, even though it too is small or negligible, is perceived to be greater than the benefit. Screening mammography of asymptomatic women younger than 35 years of age is considered to have a low benefit–risk ratio (Fabrikant, 1983).

These benefit–risk ratios are useful in helping to establish radiation protection guidelines. For example, the Radiation Protection Bureau (RPB) in Canada recommended the following with respect to screening mammography (Health and Welfare Canada, 1992):

1. Mammography *must not* be offered as a screening test to women of all ages.
2. Screening of women over 50 years can be accepted in the interim until the benefits and risks can be evaluated. Low dose techniques must be used for these purposes (p. 34).

In a symposium examining mammography screening, Feig and Ehrlich (1990) presented an update on the radiation risks for women exposed in screening mammography programs; they discussed recent epidemiologic studies, dose response models, age at exposure, risk models and risk estimates, radiation dose, lifetime risk, and a comparison of the risks and benefits from screening. These investigators came to the following conclusion:

> Although the risks and benefits from screening mammography are not precisely known, it is clear that the radiation risk is not only theoretical but negligible when compared with the proved benefits from earlier detection, fulfilling the American Cancer Society criteria for a screening test. Mammography screening cannot prevent breast cancer but can often prolong survival and prevent death from breast cancer. Though only an interim measure, mammography screening does represent a major step in the control of breast cancer (p. 646).

The benefit–risk analysis applies not only to patients but also to occupationally exposed individuals. An example of this is given in Appendix 5–1.

Current Radiation Protection Standards

In Chapter 1, we introduced the basic radiation protection framework of the ICRP. This framework addresses the overall objective of radiation protection as well as the principles that can be used to achieve that objective. In addition, these principles call for certain primary actions to be taken to protect not only patients but also personnel from the harmful effects of radiation exposure. We now address each of these ideas.

Objectives of Radiation Protection

Given the vast amount of data on the health risks of radiation, the ICRP (1991) stated that the overall objective of radiation protection is "to provide an appropriate standard of protection for man without unduly limiting the beneficial practices giving rise to radiation exposure" (p. 25). Furthermore, the ICRP (1991) suggested that current standards of protection are meant "to prevent the occurrence of deterministic effects, by keeping doses below relevant thresholds, and to ensure that all reasonable steps are taken to reduce the induction of stochastic effects" (p. 25).

The NCRP (1993), however, issued a similar statement in Report No. 116, *Limitation of exposure to ionizing radiation* (an update of Report No. 91): "the goal of radiation protection is to prevent the occurrence of serious radiation-induced conditions (acute and chronic deterministic effects) in exposed persons and to reduce stochastic effects in exposed persons to a degree that is acceptable in relation to the benefits to the individual and to society from the activities that generate such exposure" (p. 8).

The fundamental duty of the radiologic technologist is to meet this goal by adhering to the current standards of radiation protection. These standards are governed by three essential principles.

Principles of Radiation Protection

Current radiation protection standards advocated by the ICRP (1991) are based on three general principles. These principles have been used by various radiation protection organizations (NCRP and RPB-Canada) to provide guidelines for the safe use of radiation in medicine.

The ICRP (1991) states these principles as follows:

> (a) No practice involving exposures to radiation should be adopted unless it produces sufficient benefit to the exposed individuals or to society to offset the radiation detriment it causes (the *justification* of a practice).
> (b) In relation to any particular source within a practice, the magnitude of the individual doses, the number of people exposed and the likelihood of incurring exposures where these are not certain to be economic and

social factors being taken into account. This procedure should be constrained by restrictions on the doses to individuals (dose constraints), or risks to individuals in the case of potential exposures (risk constraints) so as to limit the inequity likely to result from the inherent economic and social judgments (the *optimization* of protection).

(c) The exposure of individuals resulting from the combination of all the relevant practices should be subject to dose limits, or to some control of risk in the case of potential exposures. These are aimed at ensuring that no individual is exposed to radiation risks that are judged to be unacceptable from these practices in any normal circumstances. Not all sources are susceptible to control by action at the source and it is necessary to specify the sources to be included as relevant before selecting a dose limit (*individual dose and risk limits*) (p. 28).

These three principles, namely justification, optimization, and dose and risk limits, have been referred to as one of the two triads of radiation safety (Wolbarst, 1993). The other triad, which incorporates the concepts of time, distance, and shielding, will be discussed subsequently.

Whereas *justification* refers to a positive net benefit of the activity involved in the radiation exposure of an individual, *optimization* refers to the ability to achieve that benefit by administering a dose that is *as low as reasonably achievable* (ALARA). *Dose limitation*, on the other hand, deals with the idea of establishing annual dose limits for occupational exposures, public exposures, and exposures to the embryo and fetus, a topic that is discussed in Chapter 7.

We now examine net benefit and ALARA, which are considered to be of "greater importance" than dose and risk limitation, at least from the point of view of radiation protection in medicine (Edwards, 1991).

JUSTIFICATION/NET BENEFIT

Any new technology that is introduced into the domain of radiology is subject to this principle. For example, when CT was first introduced, the radiologic community had to prove its clinical efficacy or effectiveness (Manfredi, 1979). Subsequently, a large number of efficacy studies were conducted for both CT of the head and later for body CT. These studies proved that CT provided much more information on various pathologies than other conventional x-ray imaging techniques. CT has displaced routine skull x-rays and pneumoencephalography to become a well-established technique for the investigation and detection of intracranial disorders. Not only does CT outperform conventional x-ray imaging techniques, but it does so at a comparable dose of radiation.

The same holds true for magnetic resonance imaging (MRI). Clinical efficacy studies have demonstrated that MRI is superior to CT, conventional x-rays, myelography, arthrography, and angiography in the detection and management of a growing number of diseases. MRI is apparently safe in terms of biological effects because no ionizing radiation is used. Studies on the biological effects of the three fields operating in MRI (Chapter 12) suggest that currently there appear to be no harmful biological effects in humans (Bushong, 1993).

The net benefit of these two technologies (CT and MRI) to patients, and subsequently to society, is so remarkable that already we see an exponential growth in the number of MR scanners and MR examinations, as well as rapid advances in this field.

OPTIMIZATION/CONCEPT OF ALARA

The history of ALARA may be traced back to the Manhattan Project[1] of World War II (Hendee and Edwards, 1986). The NCRP's 1954 recommen-

[1] *A project was established by the United States War Department in 1942 to develop the atomic bomb. Work for this project was carried out at several different research and development facilities: in Oak Ridge, TN; Hanford, WA; Los Alamos, NM; and in laboratories at the University of Chicago and the University of California at Berkeley.*

dation that radiation exposures "be kept at the lowest practical level" was based on data collected by the scientists on the Manhattan Project. Later, in 1959, the ICRP also made similar recommendations. More recently, the ICRP (1991) has chosen to use the term *optimization of radiation protection* (ORP) and has indicated that the recommendations for ALARA and ORP are synonymous. The NCRP approach is also to recognize optimization as being synonymous with ALARA (NCRP, 1990).[2]

What does ALARA or ORP involve in diagnostic radiology? A framework suggested by the NCRP (1990) includes the following seven major actions: (1) identify problems, (2) assess problems, (3) identify responses, (4) acquire information for each response, (5) apply decision, (6) implement response, and (7) evaluate results. The NCRP (1990) stated that "the intent of this approach is to give guidance on how an individual institution might develop its own method rather than to impose a particular method on the medical radiation safety program" (p. 34).

What role does the technologist play in ALARA or in the optimization of radiation protection? Through proper education and training, the technologist is in a position to competently practice the guidelines and recommendations for the safe and prudent use of radiation in imaging patients. The technologist must apply the triad of time, shielding, and distance in keeping the dose ALARA to both patients and personnel. Understanding the factors that affect dose, dose reduction methods, and shielding requirements is vital to the radiologic technologist. This is the fundamental rationale for a course on radiation protection.

DOSE LIMITATION

The concept of dose limitation deals with doses received by an individual on a yearly basis or accumulated over a working lifetime. These doses should not be greater than those established by the ICRP and other national organizations such as the NCRP and the RPB-HC.

The recommended dose limits are intended to reduce the probability of stochastic effects and prevent detrimental deterministic effects. These dose limits are also recommended for various categories of individuals, including radiation workers and other occupationally exposed individuals, and members of the public. Dose limits are discussed in detail in Chapter 7.

Radiation Protection Actions

The second triad of radiation safety is what Wolbarst (1993) referred to as *time-distance-shielding*, primary actions which, when put into good practice, will serve to protect patients, personnel, and members of the public from the potential risks of radiation.[3]

TIME

Exposure technique factors (mA, kVp, and time) are an integral part of any x-ray examination. The time, or more precisely the exposure time, is related to radiation exposure and exposure rate (exposure per unit time) as follows:

$$\text{Exposure time} = \frac{\text{Exposure}}{\text{Exposure rate}} \quad (5\text{-}1)$$

or

$$\text{Exposure} = \text{Exposure rate} \times \text{Time} \quad (5\text{-}2)$$

These algebraic expressions simply imply that if the exposure time is kept short, then the resulting dose to the individual is small. The NCRP (1989b) suggested that the dose rate in a chest examination is high, but because of the very short exposure times utilized in chest radiography ($\leq$0.05 sec), the total dose equivalent is small [~0.2 mSv (20 mrem)].

[2] *It is not within the scope of this book to address these concerns in detail. The interested student should refer to ICRP Publication 60 (1991) and NCRP Report No. 107 (1990), for further details on optimization of protection.*

[3] *Bushong (1993) referred to this same triad as the "cardinal principles of radiation protection."*

When setting technique factors on the control panel, the technologist should always try to use short exposure times while maintaining optimum image quality.

DISTANCE

The second radiation protection action relates to the distance between the source of radiation and the exposed individual. As the individual moves farther and farther away from the radiation source, the exposure to the individual decreases inversely as the square of the distance. This is known as the *inverse square law*, stated mathematically as:

$$I \propto \frac{1}{d^2} \tag{5-3}$$

where I is the intensity of radiation and d is the distance between the radiation source and the exposed individual.

When the distance is doubled, the exposure is reduced by a factor of 4 (Fig. 5-1). This rule has applications in several situations when imaging patients. For example, in mobile radiography, where there is no fixed protective control booth, the technologist should remain at least 2 m from the patient, the x-ray tube, and the primary beam during the exposure. In this respect, the ICRP (1982), as well as the NCRP (1989a), recommended that the length of the exposure cord on mobile radiographic units be at least 2 m long. In Canada, the RPB-HC recommended that the cord length be at least 3 m long (SC-20A, 1992).

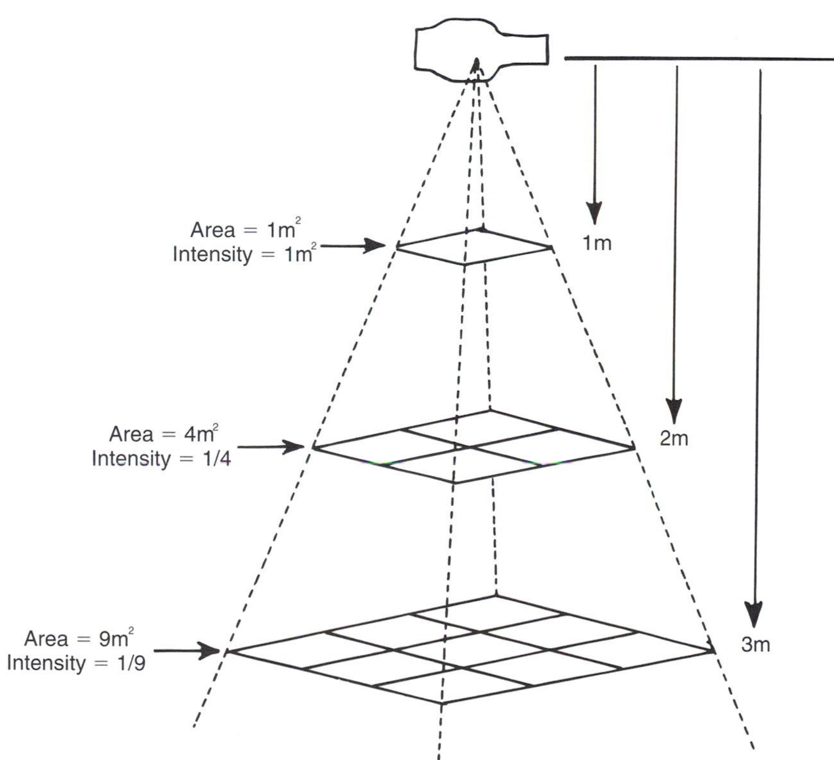

FIGURE 5-1. The inverse square law states that doubling the distance from the source decreases the exposure by a factor of 4 [From Wolbarst, A.B. (1993). *The physics of radiology*. Norwalk, CT: Appleton & Lange. Reproduced by permission.]

During mobile radiography, when other personnel (nurses and physicians) are present, the technologist should always advise these individuals to move as far away as possible from both the x-ray tube and the patient during the exposure.

In fluoroscopy, the main source of scatter is the patient, and because the radiation level for the fluoroscopy unit is high, ~87 mGy (NCRP, 1989b), the scattered radiation from the patient is potentially high. In this situation, as well as in spot-film recording, the technologist (who wears a lead apron during the procedure) should maintain a maximum distance from the patient only when it is not necessary to lend assistance to that patient.

Another important consideration with respect to distance relates to the *source-to-image receptor distance (SID)*. The appropriate SIDs for various examinations must always be maintained because an incorrect SID could mean a second exposure to the patient. For example, if the SID for an abdomen examination is 100 cm and a distance of 150 cm was used as a result of human error, the intensity (quantity) of radiation required to produce the same film density at 100 cm would have to increase according to the inverse square law. The relationship is as follows:

$$\frac{I_1}{I_2} = \frac{D_2^2}{D_1^2} \qquad (5\text{-}4)$$

where I_1 is the original intensity at the original distance D_1 and I_2 is the new intensity at the new distance D_2.

Technologists must ensure that the correct SID is always used for a particular examination, before exposing the patient.

SHIELDING

The third radiation protection action relates to shielding. Shielding implies that certain materials (concrete, lead) will attenuate radiation (reduce its intensity) when they are placed between the source of radiation and the exposed individual.

There are at least four approaches to shielding in diagnostic radiology: gonadal shielding, personnel shielding, room shielding, and x-ray tube shielding. These approaches are intended to protect patients, personnel, and members of the public from unnecessary radiation exposures.

In *gonadal shielding*, a lead apron is placed appropriately on the patient to protect the gonads from primary beam radiation exposure. This is illustrated in Figure 5-2 in which a pediatric patient is shielded by a lead apron during a lateral chest examination.

Personnel shielding refers to the use of lead apparel (gloves, aprons, and thyroid protectors) to shield individuals during examinations that require them to be present in the x-ray room (such as in fluoroscopy) rather than remain in the control booth. In addition, mobile barriers with Clear-Pb (Nuclear Associates, transparent lead-plastic shielding) can be used to shield personnel from scattered radiation as shown in Figure 5-3. This is especially useful in examinations

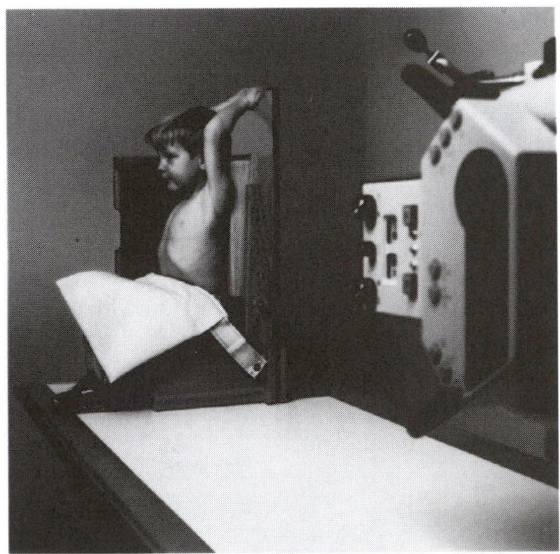

FIGURE 5-2. The use of gonadal shielding during a lateral chest x-ray examination. The lead shielding is intended to protect the patient from any unnecessary primary radiation. (Courtesy of Nuclear Associates, Carle Place, NY.)

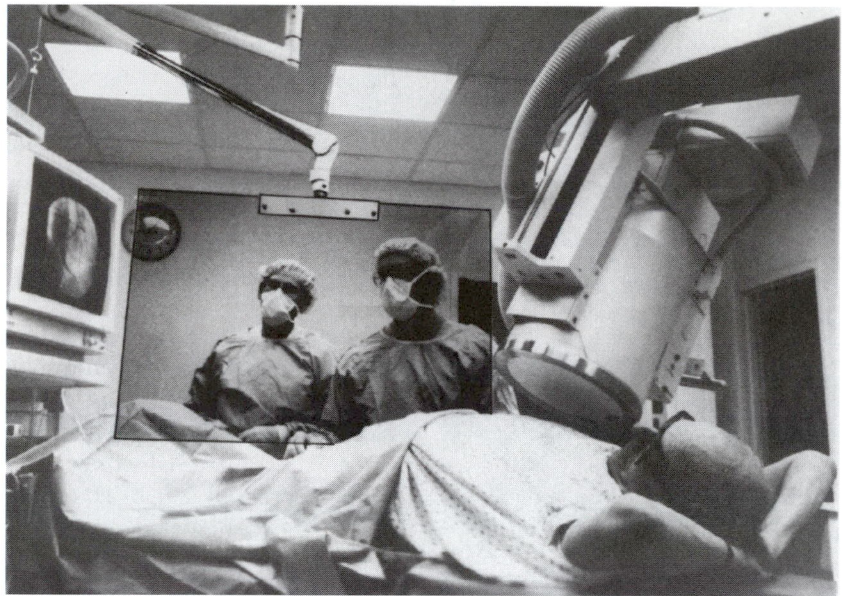

FIGURE 5-3. The use of Clear-Pb (transplant lead-plastic) in shielding personnel from scattered radiation during an angiographic examination. (Courtesy of Nuclear Associates, Carle Place, NY.)

that require personnel to be in close proximity to the patient and x-ray equipment (e.g., angiography). Figure 5-4 illustrates the use of eye wear and a lead shield to reduce exposure to the lens of the eye and thyroid, respectively.

The walls of the x-ray rooms and x-ray control booths are lined with thin sheets of lead to protect personnel and others (in adjacent rooms) essentially from scattered radiation. The view window of the control booth is generally made of Clear-Pb to enable personnel to have an unobstructed view of the patient. The bottom half of the control booth wall (Fig. 5-5) is also lined with thin lead sheets to offer the same degree of protection as the transparent panels. Room shielding will be discussed in some detail in Chapter 10.

Finally, the x-ray tube housing is lined with thin sheets of lead because x-rays produced in the tube are scattered in all directions. This shielding is intended to protect both patients and personnel from leakage radiation.

Radiation Detection and Measurement

The radiologic technologist will benefit from an understanding of radiation detection and measurement, as both of these topics are fundamental to radiation protection. The technologist who is thoroughly familiar with these concepts is able to play a more useful role in personnel and environmental radiation exposure monitoring procedures.

In order to measure radiation, it must first be detected. The instruments used to detect radiation are referred to as *radiation detection devices.* Instruments used to measure radiation are called *radiation dosimeters.*

Methods of Detection

There are several methods of detecting radiation, and they are based on physical and chemical effects produced by radiation exposure. For our purposes, these methods are ioniza-

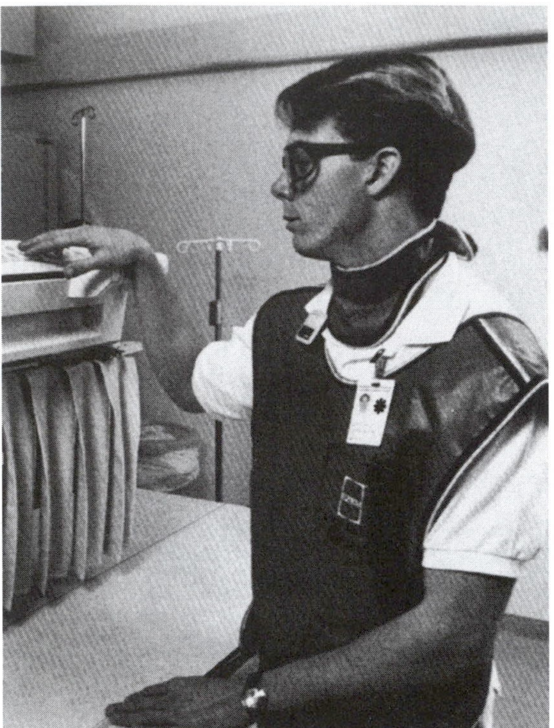

FIGURE 5-4. The use of protective eye wear and thyroid lead shield to reduce exposure to the lens of the eye and thyroid, respectively. [From Torres, L.S. (1993). *Basic medical techniques and patient care for radiologic technologists* (4th ed.). Philadelphia: J.B. Lippincott. Reproduced by permission.]

tion, the photographic effect, luminescence, and scintillation.

The ability of radiation to produce ionization (see Chapter 2) in air is the basis for some radiation detection devices. Ionization produces ion pairs in a certain volume of air, in which two electrodes (negative and positive) are carefully positioned. The negative ions (electrons) are collected by the positive electrode, while the positive ions are collected by the negative electrode. The flow of electrons (current) is a measure of the radiation intensity. Because this current is very small, a sensitive instrument called a dc (direct current) amplifier is used to measure it.

The *photographic effect*, which refers to the ability of radiation to blacken photographic films, is the basis of detectors that use film. Once the film is exposed, it is chemically processed and subsequently read by a densitometer, which measures the optical density of the film. The radiation dose can be measured using a special curve called a dose–density curve (Fig. 5-6), which is obtained by exposing a number of different films to known doses of radiation.

Luminescence describes the property by which certain materials emit light when stimulated by a physiological process, a chemical or electrical action, or by heat. When radiation strikes these materials, the electrons are raised to higher orbital levels. These electrons can return to their original state only when stimulated by one of the processes mentioned above. When they fall back to their original orbital level, light is emitted. The amount of light emitted is proportional to the radiation intensity. Lithium fluoride, for example, will emit light when stimulated by heat. This is the fundamental basis of *thermoluminescence dosimetry* (TLD), a method used to measure exposure to patients and personnel. Because TLD is used routinely in patient and personnel dosimetry, it will be described further in the next section.

Scintillation refers to a flash of light. It is a property of certain crystals such as sodium iodide to absorb radiation and convert it to light. This light is then directed to a photomultiplier tube (which is coupled to the crystal), which then converts the light into an electrical pulse. The size of the pulse is proportional to the light intensity, which is in turn proportional to the energy of the radiation.

Radiation Detectors and Measurement

The characteristics and uses of several state-of-the-art radiation detectors are shown in Table 5-1. Of the six devices listed, we focus our attention only on the ionization chamber and the scintillation detector because they are both used

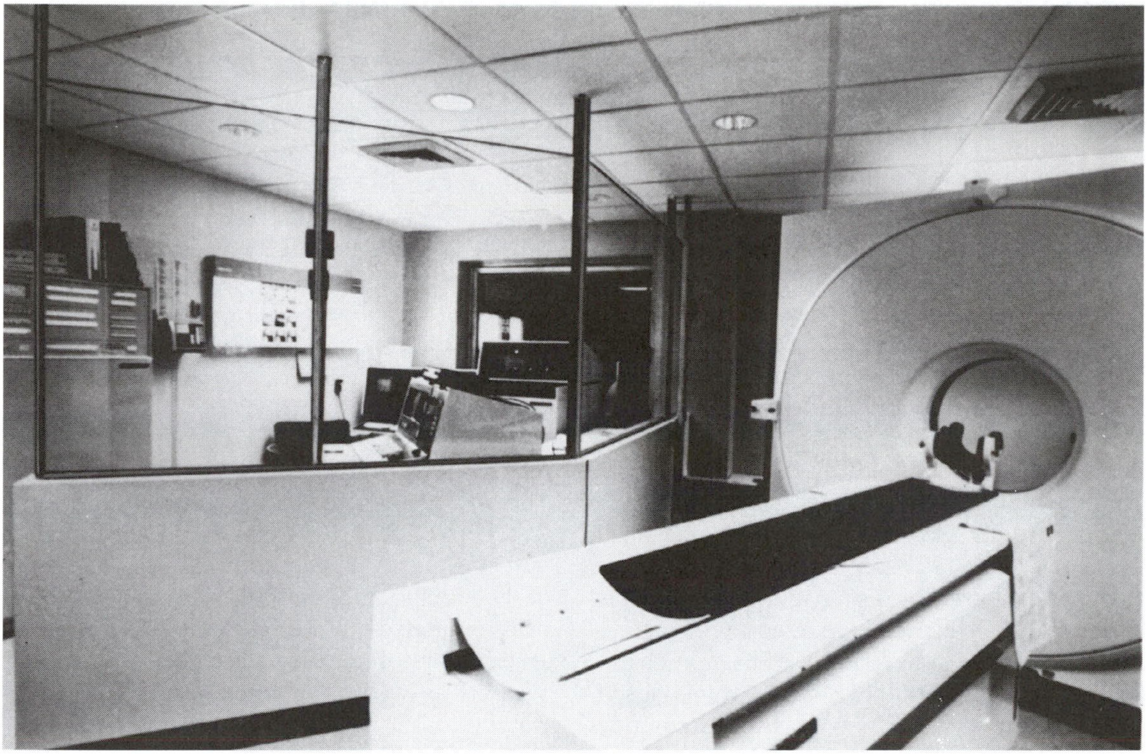

FIGURE 5-5. The walls of x-ray control booths are lined with lead to protect personnel from scattered radiation arising from the patient and equipment. In this photograph, the view window is made of Clear-Pb (transparent lead-plastic) panels, which offer the same degree of shielding as the opaque lead-lined walls. (Courtesy of Nuclear Associates, Carle Place, NY.)

in clinical radiology. The film badge detector, the pocket dosimeter, and the thermoluminescent dosimeter, all of which are used to monitor radiation exposure among personnel, will be discussed under "Personnel Dosimetry."

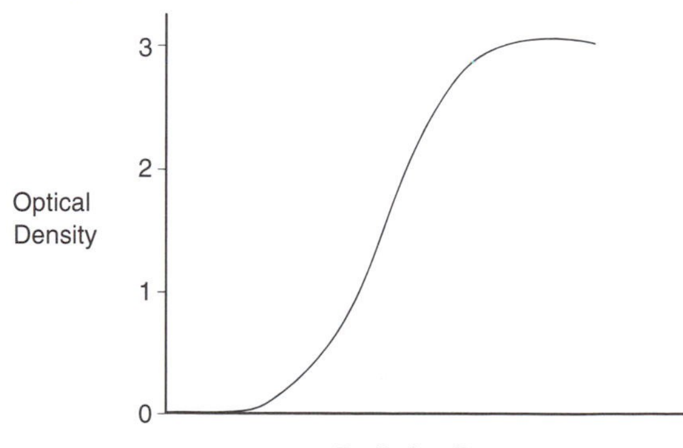

FIGURE 5-6. A dose–density curve for use in film badge dosimetry.

IONIZATION CHAMBER

The ionization chamber is a simple and useful device for measuring x-ray intensity. A typical chamber is shown in Figure 5-7. It consists of an electrode positioned in the middle of a cylinder that contains gas. When x-rays enter the chamber, they ionize the gas to form negative ions (electrons) and positive ions (positrons). The electrons

TABLE 5-1. THE CHARACTERISTICS AND USES OF SEVERAL TYPES OF RADIATION DETECTION AND MEASURING DEVICES (RADIATION DETECTORS)

Device	Characteristics and Uses
Photographic emulsion	Limited range, sensitive, energy dependent, personnel monitoring, imaging
Ionization chamber	Wide range, accurate, portable survey for fields >1 mR/hr
Proportional counter	Laboratory instrument, accurate, sensitive, assay of small quantities of radionuclides
Geiger-Müller counter	Limited to <100 mR/hr, portable survey for low fields and contamination
Thermoluminescence dosimetry	Wide range, accurate, sensitive, personnel monitoring, stationary area monitoring
Scintillation detection	Limited range, very sensitive, stationary or portable instruments, photon spectroscopy, imaging

SOURCE: Bushong, S. (1993). *Radiologic science for technologists* (5th ed.). St. Louis: Mosby–Year Book. Reproduced by permission.

are collected by the positively charged rod, while the positive ions are attracted to the negatively charged wall of the cylinder. The resulting small current from the chamber is subsequently amplified and measured. The strength of the current is proportional to the radiation intensity.

There are several types of ionization chambers such as the "Cutie Pie," an instrument used for radiation surveys as well as in fluoroscopy (Bushong, 1993); the "RadCal," which is used to measure diagnostic x-ray intensities; and the Geiger-Müller counter, which is used in nuclear medicine for the specific purpose of detecting radioactive contamination.

SCINTILLATION DETECTOR

Another major class of radiation detector is the *scintillation detector*. This detector is based on the principle that certain crystals such as sodium iodide (NaI) and cesium iodide (CsI) emit light when struck by x-rays or by charged particles.

The crystal is coupled to a photomultiplier tube (PM tube), as shown in Figure 5-8. When x-rays strike the crystal, flashes of light (scintillations) are produced. The scintillation light strikes the photocathode of the PM tube and, through the photoelectric effect, electrons are produced. These electrons are accelerated across the tube by a series of dynodes, which also play a role in increasing the number of electrons until they reach the anode of the PM tube, where they generate an electrical pulse. The size of the pulse is proportional, not only to the amount of light emitted by the scintillation crystal (which is proportional to the energy of the radiation), but also to the number of electrons emitted from the photocathode.

Scintillation detectors are used in some CT systems as well as in nuclear medicine technology.

Personnel Dosimetry

Monitoring

Personnel dosimetry refers to the monitoring of individuals who are exposed to radiation during the course of their work. Monitoring is necessary when there is a chance that an individ-

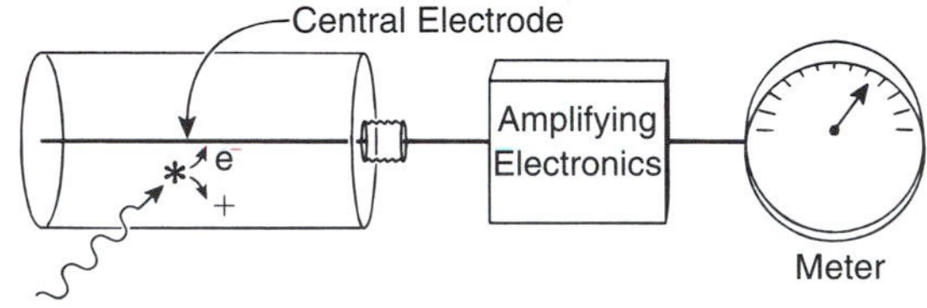

FIGURE 5-7. A typical ionization chamber for use in diagnostic radiology. [From Bushong, S. (1993). *Radiologic science for technologists* (5th ed.). St. Louis: Mosby–Year Book. Reproduced by permission.]

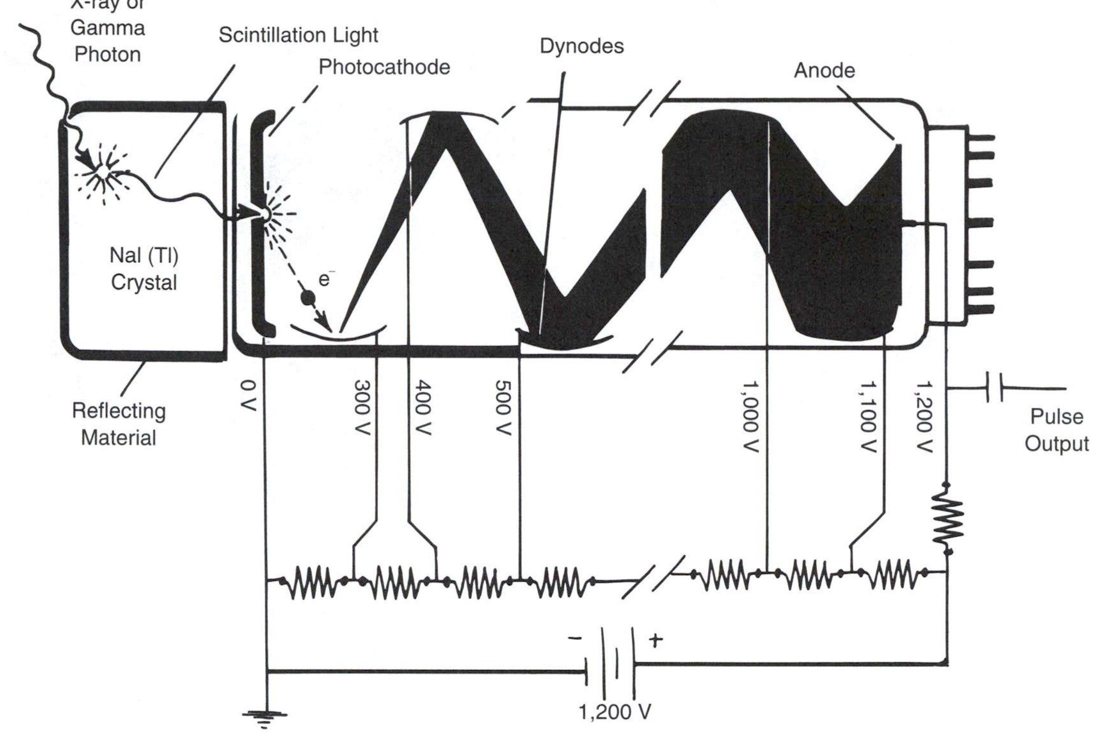

FIGURE 5-8. The characteristic features of a scintillation detector. [From Wolbarst, A.B. (1993). *The physics of radiology.* Norwalk, CT: Appleton & Lange. Reproduced by permission.]

ual may receive about one tenth of the equivalent dose.

Monitoring is accomplished through the use of personnel dosimeters (Fig. 5-9) such as the pocket dosimeter, the film badge, and the thermoluminescent dosimeter. The measurement is a *time-integrated dose,* i.e., the dose summed over a period of time, usually about 3 months. The dose is subsequently stated as an estimate of the effective dose equivalent to the whole body in mSv for the reporting period. Dosimeters used for personnel monitoring have a dose measurement limit of 0.1 to 0.2 mSv (10–20 mrem) (NCRP, 1989a).

POCKET DOSIMETER

The *pocket dosimeter* monitors dose to personnel (Fig. 5-10). It consists of an ionization chamber with an eyepiece and a transparent scale (microscope), as well as a hollow charging rod and a fixed and a movable fiber arranged as shown in Figure 5-10.

When a known standard charge is impressed upon the charging rod using the dosimeter charger (Fig. 5-11), the movable fiber is repelled from the fixed fiber. When x-rays enter the dosimeter, ionization causes the fibers to lose their charges and, as a result, the movable fiber moves closer to the fixed fiber. The movable fiber can be seen on the transparent scale, which provides some estimate of gamma or x-ray dose rate, as shown in Figure 5-12.

FILM BADGE MONITORING

Film badges have been used for personnel monitoring since the 1940s, and although film badge

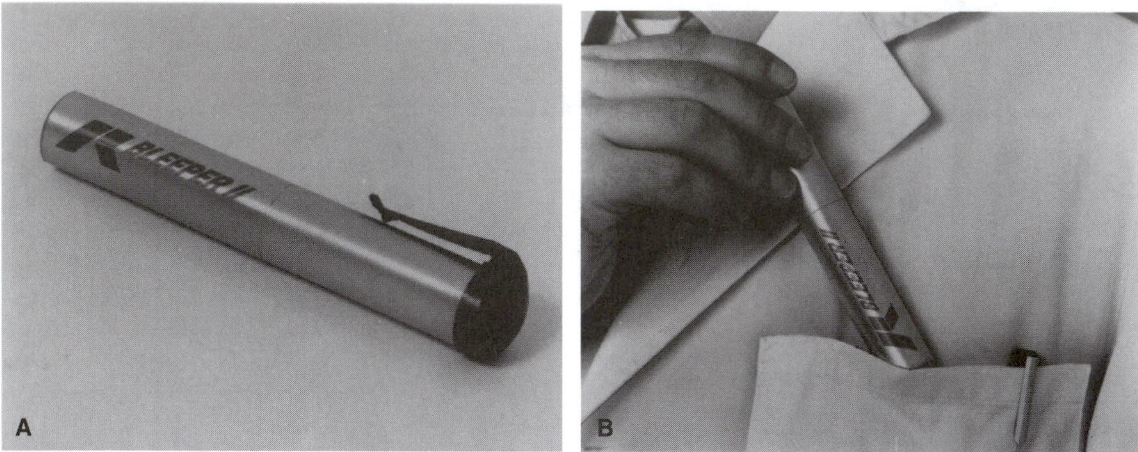

FIGURE 5-9. A pocket dosimeter that can be worn by personnel (A), or to monitor gamma x-ray dose rate (B). (Courtesy of Nuclear Associates, Carle Place, NY.)

dosimetry has been largely superseded by thermoluminescent dosimetry, film badges are still used on a limited basis in some departments. These badges use small x-ray films sandwiched between several filters to help detect beta, gamma, and x-rays. Some film badges use a two-emulsion (fast and slow) type film to record a wide range of dose measurements.

Film badges are inexpensive, easy to use, and easy to process. They do, however, have a series of limitations. Although they are useful for detecting radiation at or above about 0.1 mSv

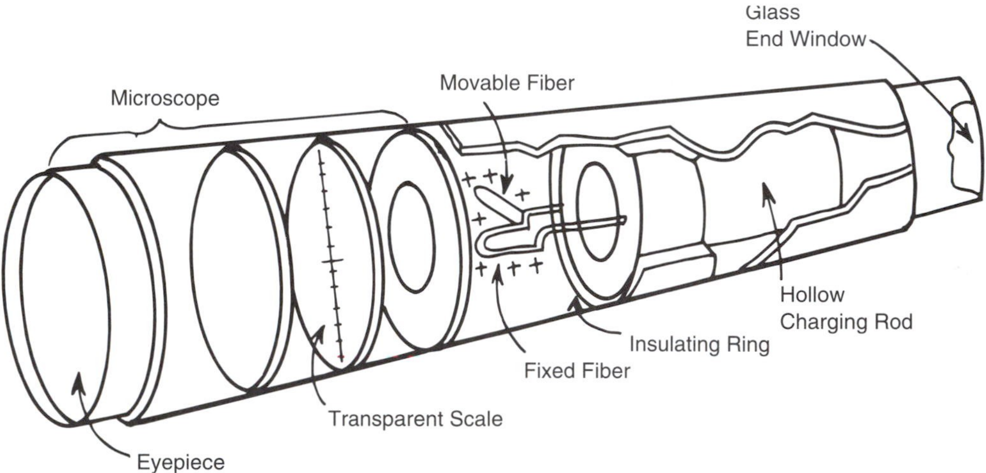

FIGURE 5-10. A diagrammatic illustration of a pocket dosimeter. [From Graham, B., & Thomas, W. (1975). *An introduction of physics for radiologic technologists*. Philadelphia; W.B. Saunders. Reproduced by permission.]

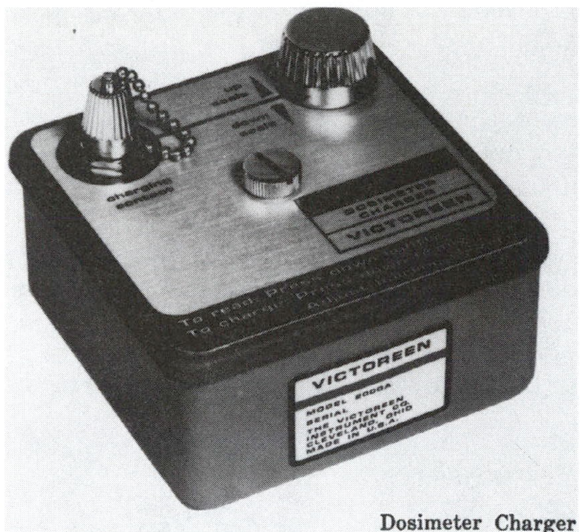

FIGURE 5-11. The charger for the pocket dosimeter. (Courtesy of Nuclear Associates, Carle Place, NY.)

(10 mrem), they are not sensitive enough to capture lower levels of radiation. Their susceptibility to fogging caused by high temperatures and light means that they cannot and should not be worn for longer than a 4-week period at a stretch. One final drawback to film badge monitoring is that it is a major task to chemically process a large number of small films and subsequently compare each to some standard test film.

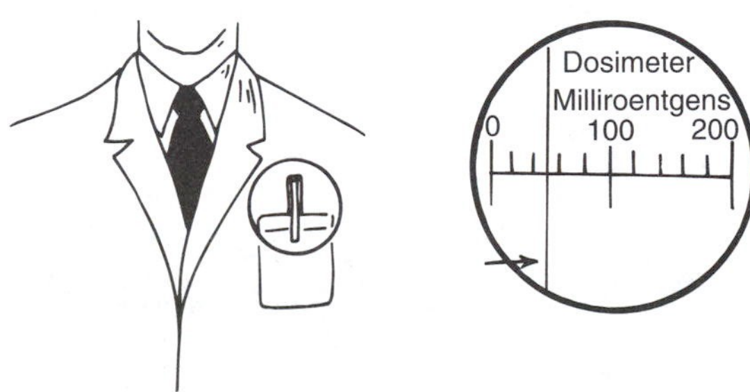

FIGURE 5-12. The appearance of the scale of a pocket dosimeter when viewed through the eyepiece. (Courtesy of Nuclear Associates, Carle Place, NY.)

THERMOLUMINESCENT DOSIMETRY (TLD) MONITORING

The limitations of the film badge are overcome by the thermoluminescent dosimeter (TLD). Before we discuss the ways in which TLD outperforms film badge dosimetry, we need to examine the ways in which thermoluminescence works.

Thermoluminescence is that property of certain materials to emit light when they are stimulated by heat. Materials such as lithium fluoride (LiF), lithium borate ($Li_2B_4O_7$), calcium fluoride (CaF_2), and calcium sulfate ($CaSO_4$) have been used to make TLDs for use in diagnostic imaging research studies ($Li_2B_4O_7$), and in environmental monitoring (CaF_2 and $CaSO_4$).

When an LiF crystal is exposed to radiation, a few electrons become trapped in higher energy levels (the number of electrons is proportional to the absorbed dose). For these electrons to return to their normal energy levels, the LiF crystal must be heated. As the electrons return to their stable state, light is emitted because of the energy difference between two orbital levels. The amount of light emitted is measured (by a photomultiplier tube) and it is proportional to the radiation dose. The device for doing this can be calibrated so that the light output is equivalent to the absorbed dose. The crystal can be reused again and again.

The measurement of the radiation is a two-step procedure, as shown in Figure 5-13. In step 1, the TLD is exposed to the radiation. In step 2, the LiF crystal is placed in a TLD analyzer, where it is exposed to heat. As the crystal is exposed to increasing temperatures, the light emission varies in an interesting fashion. When the intensity of the light is plotted as a function of the temperature, the *glow curve* results (Fig. 5-14). The glow curve can be used to find out how much radiation energy is received by the crystal because the highest peak and the area under the curve are proportional to the energy of the radiation. These parameters can be measured and converted to dose.

Whereas the TLD can measure exposures to individuals as low as 1.3 μC/kg (5 mR), the pocket dosimeter can measure up to 50 μC/kg (200 mR). The film badge, however, cannot measure exposures < 2.6 μC/kg (10 mR) (Bushong, 1993).

A typical TLD personnel dosimeter is illustrated in Figure 5-15. It consists of a plaque holder and an insert. The insert consists of an aluminum plaque (which holds two TLD chips) and an identification number. The TLD chips are usually 3 mm × 3 mm × 1 mm thick. Recently, an improved TLD service has been introduced by Landauer, Inc. These TLD badges no longer require exchange and replacement of the inserts within the plaque holder. When the badges are sent in to be read, new ones are issued and there is no need to keep track of a separate holder inventory. The badges are color-coded and bar-coded, and laser-etched identification helps to prevent fading and peeling (Fig. 5-16).

TLDs can withstand a certain degree of heat, humidity, and pressure; their crystals are reusable; and instantaneous readings are possible if the department has a TLD analyzer (Fig. 5-13). In general, TLDs are sent to a radiation protection service for analysis.

The greatest disadvantage of a TLD is its cost. In addition, some TLD crystals are energy dependent and they must be calibrated to the appropriate energy range that they will be used to measure.

Wearing the Personnel Dosimeter

As noted previously, the purpose of a personnel dosimeter is to measure occupational exposure. For radiology workers, technologists, and radiologists alike, this means exposures received from both radiography and fluoroscopy.

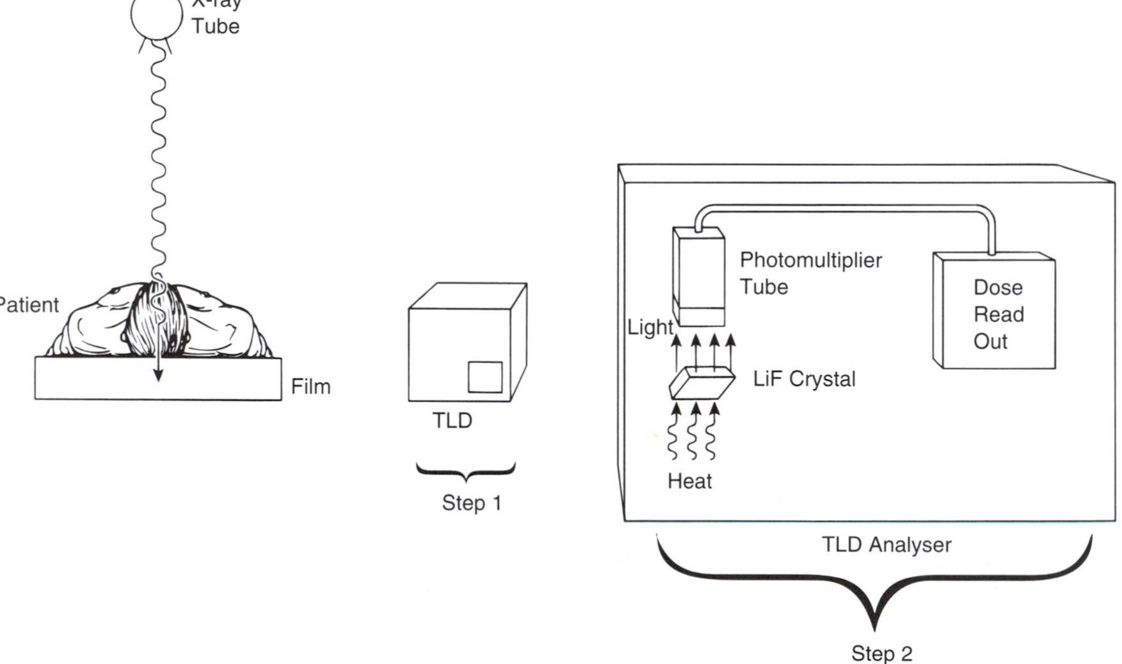

FIGURE 5-13. The basic procedure for measuring the dose from a TLD crystal.

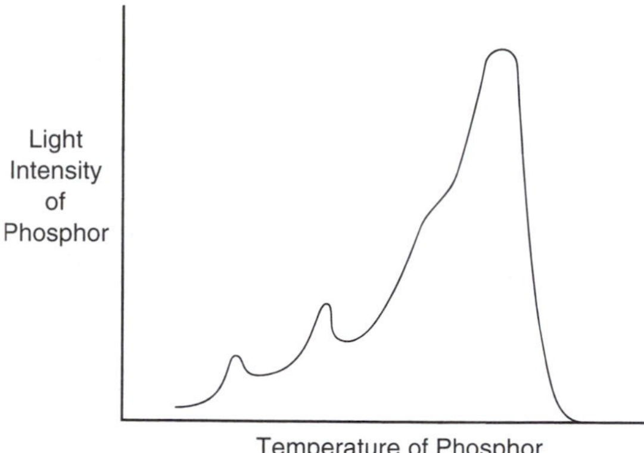

FIGURE 5-14. A typical TLD glow curve for a lithium fluoride crystal. The peaks are due to the transition of electrons from orbit to orbit.

Recall that occupational dose limits (Chapter 1) have been recommended by various radiation protection organizations such as the ICRP and the NCRP. Average annual occupational dose limits have been established for the whole body and for tissues and organs such as the lens of the eye, red bone marrow, breast, lungs, gonads, skin, and extremities. If accurate whole-body exposure readings are to be obtained, then where on the body the dosimeter is worn is important.

RADIOGRAPHY

During radiography (when no protective lead apron is worn), the personnel dosimeter is worn at one of two regions: (1) on the trunk of the body at the level of the waist, on the anterior side of the individual (NCRP, 1989a; RPB, 1992), or (2) on the upper chest region at the level of the collar area on the anterior surface of the individual.

At these positions, the dosimeter readings represent an estimate of not only exposure to the whole body but also partial body exposures to regions such as the head and neck, thorax, bone marrow, and gonads.

FLUOROSCOPY

In fluoroscopy, the situation is somewhat different because a protective apron is worn during the procedure. In this case, the NCRP (1989a) stated that:

> When the apron is worn, a decision must be made as to whether to wear one or more than one dosimeter. If only one is worn and it is worn under the apron, it can represent the dose to most internal organs but it may underestimate the dose to the head and neck (including the thyroid gland). If only one is worn and it is worn at the collar, it may represent the dose to the organs contained in the head and neck but it may overestimate the dose to the organs in the trunk of the body (p. 49).

In Canada, the Radiation Safety Code (RPB, 1992) for x-ray diagnosis simply states that:

> When a lead equivalent protective apron is worn, the personnel dosimeter must be worn under the apron. If extremities are likely to be exposed to significantly higher doses, additional extremity monitors should be worn (p. 28).

Dosimetry Report

It is important that occupational exposures be documented and that all records of individual exposures be maintained for several reasons (to be discussed subsequently).

Various radiation protection agencies that offer a personnel dosimetry service provide a report of the readings for each individual dosimeter submitted. These reports are available in different formats; however, they do provide essentially similar kinds of information. One such radiation dosimetry report is shown in Figure 5-17.

Radiation Protection Surveys

Earlier in this chapter, we introduced the concept of benefit–risk analysis. In diagnostic radiology, a radiation protection survey is the final component in the benefit–risk analysis (Krohmer, 1980).

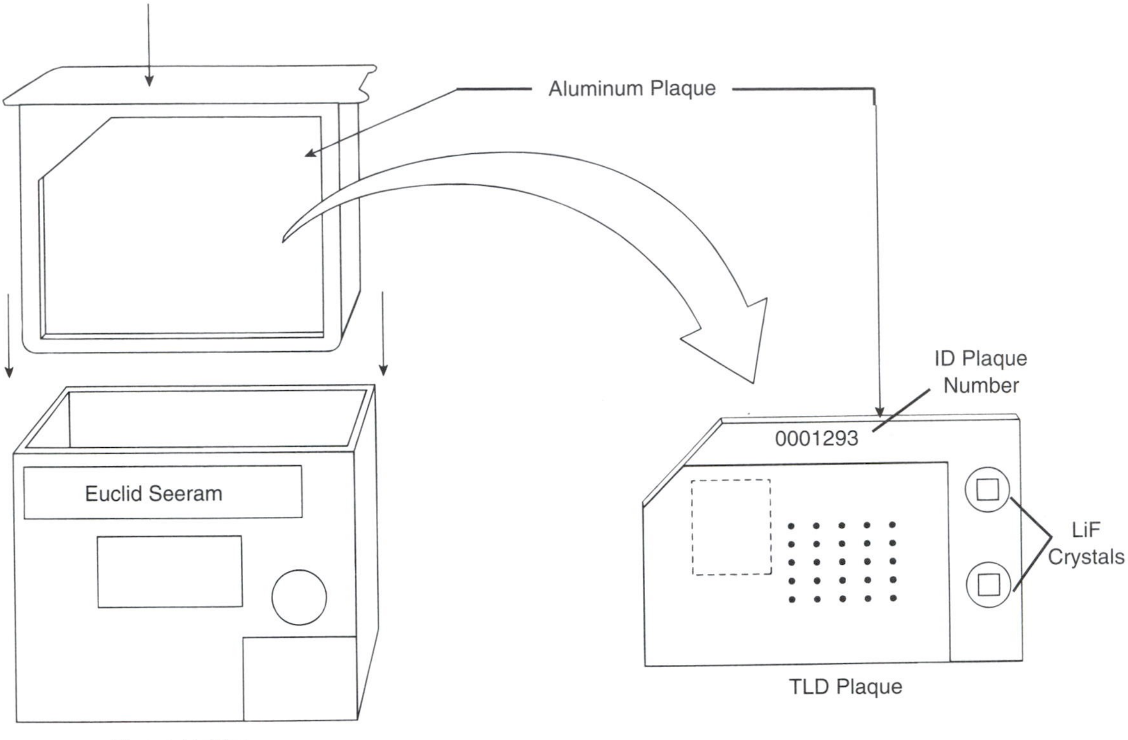

FIGURE 5-15. A typical TLD personnel dosimeter for use in radiology.

Purpose of the Survey

Radiology facilities must be surveyed on a regular basis. The purpose of these surveys is threefold:

1. To check the status of radiation safety mechanisms, procedures, and practices.
2. To ensure that the equipment is in proper working condition.
3. To ensure that the radiology department is absolutely safe not only for patients but for personnel as well.

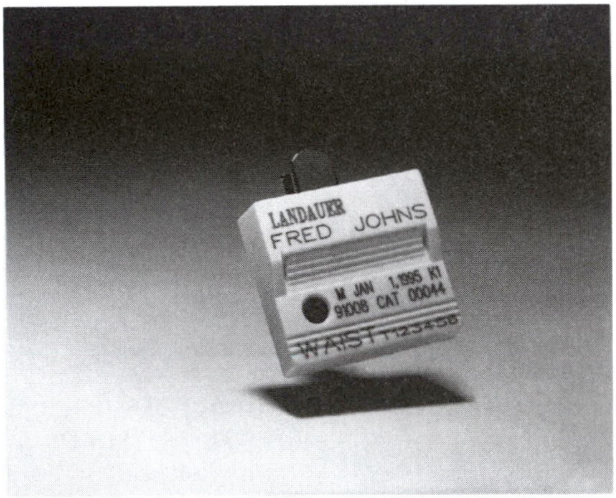

FIGURE 5-16. New TLD dosimeters, available from Landauer, Inc., offer improved service through a number of identification marks, color coding, etc. (Courtesy of Landauer, Inc., Glenwood, IL.)

Phases of a Survey

The NCRP (1989b) have identified five phases of a survey: investigation, inspection, measurement, evaluation, and recommendations. The

ACCOUNT NUMBER NUMÉRO DE COMPTE	SERIES CODE CODE DE SÉRIE

PROCESS NUMBER NUMÉRO DU PROCÉDÉ	REPORT DATE DATE DU RAPPORT	DOSIMETER RECEIVED DOSIMÈTRE REÇU	REPORT DAYS JOURS OUVR. DEPUIS RÉCEPTION	PAGE NUMBER NUMÉRO DE PAGE	QUALITY CONTROL RELEASE CONTRÔLE DE LA QUALITÉ

LANDAUER®

RADIATION EXPOSURE REPORT
RAPPORT D´EXPOSITION AUX RADIATIONS

Landauer, Inc. 2 Science Road Glenwood,Illinois 60425-1686 USA
Tel: (708)755-7000 Fax: (708)755-7016

PARTICIPANT ID NUMBER / NUMÉRO D'IDENTIFICATION DU PARTICIPANT	NAME / NOM	NOTES: (SEE ENCLOSURE) NOTES: (VOIR CI-JOINT)	DOSEMETER TYPE	TYPE DE DOSIMÈTRE	USE	UTILISATION	RADIATION QUALITY	SORTE(S) DE RADIATION	EXPOSURE TO BADGE (MILLISIEVERTS) FOR PERIOD(S) INDICATED BELOW / EXPOSITION AU DOSIMÈTRE (MILLISIEVERTS) POUR PÉRIODE(S) INDIQUÉE(S) CI-DESSOUS		CUMULATIVE TOTALS (MILLISIEVERTS) / TOTAUX CUMULATIFS (MILLISIEVERTS) — CALENDAR QUARTER / TRIMESTRE		YEAR TO DATE / CETTE ANNÉE		PERMANENT / À CE JOUR		ADJUSTMENTS	AJUSTEMENTS	NUMBER OF REPORTS / NOMBRE DE RAPPORTS		INCEPTION DATE OF PERMANENT TOTAL / DATE DU DÉBUT DES ENREGISTREMENTS	
									BODY CORPS	SKIN PEAU	BODY CORPS	SKIN PEAU	BODY CORPS	SKIN PEAU	BODY CORPS	SKIN PEAU			TO DATE À CE JOUR	QUARTER TRIMESTRE	MONTH MOIS	YEAR ANNÉE

DRAFT

USE CODE (COLUMN 5)
1-WHOLE BODY 2-LENS OF THE EYE 3-RIGHT FINGER 4-LEFT FINGER 5-RIGHT WRIST 6-LEFT WRIST 7-OTHER EXTREMITY 8-OTHER WHOLE BODY 9-MONITOR

CODE D'UTILISATION (COLONNE 5)
1-CORPS ENTIER 2-CRISTALLIN DE L'OEIL 3-DOIGT DROIT 4-DOIGT GAUCHE 5-POIGNET DROIT 6-POIGNET GAUCHE 7-AUTRE EXTRÉMITÉ 8-AUTRE CORPS ENTIER 9-MONITEUR

AN 'H' (HIGH ENERGY) DESIGNATION, WHEN ONLY LOW ENERGY EXPOSURE IS POSSIBLE MAY INDICATE THE FILM PACKET WAS EXPOSED OUT OF THE FILTERED HOLDER.

UNE DÉSIGNATION 'H' (HAUTE ÉNERGIE) LORSQUE SEULEMENT UNE BASSE ÉNERGIE EST POSSIBLE INDIQUE QUE LE PAQUET DE FILM A ÉTÉ EXPOSÉ EN DEHORS DE SON PORTEUR QUI CONTIENT LES FILTRES.

IMPORTANT: SEE EXPLANATION SHEETS FOR MORE INFORMATION.

IMPORTANT: S.V.P. VOIR LES FEUILLES D'EXPLICATIONS POUR DES INFORMATIONS PLUS COMPLÈTES.

FIGURE 5-17. An example of a radiation dosimetry report. (Courtesy of Laundauer, Inc., Glenwood, IL.)

basic requirements of each of these phases are summarized in Table 5-2. Of the five phases, the evaluation phase is the most important because it provides the foundation on which future recommendations for improvements will be based.

Quality Assurance and Quality Control

The general ideas of quality assurance (QA) were introduced in Chapter 1. In review, QA encompasses quality administration and quality control (QC). Whereas quality administration addresses management of a program intended to provide and maintain optimum image quality with the least amount of radiation, QC refers to the technical procedures that ensure that such standards of quality and dose are met.

The QC program should include the following: (1) photographic quality control, (2) radiographic quality control, (3) fluoroscopic quality control (for fixed and mobile systems), (4) conventional tomography and mammography, (5) special procedures equipment, (6) CT scanners, and (7) digital imaging systems. The QC tests are numerous and are beyond the scope of this book; however, in Chapter 13, we discuss QC and how it relates to radiation protection.

A Radiation Protection Program

The purpose of a radiation protection program is to protect patients, personnel, and members of the public from unnecessary exposure. How this is accomplished depends on the elements of the program. Programs may range from the simple to the complex, depending on the nature and size of the department. For example, a large-scale department performing a wide variety of radiological examinations (from conventional radiography and fluoroscopy to special procedures, CT, and digital imaging) and employing a number of indi-

TABLE 5-2. THE FIVE PHASES OF A RADIATION PROTECTION SURVEY AND THEIR BASIC REQUIREMENTS

Phases	Requirements
Investigation	This phase seeks to obtain information about the entire department through interviews with personnel. Information relating to workload, personnel monitoring, and records, equipment, general layout of the department, as well as equipment service records, evidence of collimation on films, and so on, is collected.
Inspection	Each diagnostic installation in the department is examined for its protection status with respect to age and mechanical operation, control booth, equipment, availability of protection devices (gonadal shields, aprons, immobilization devices, collimators, filters, timers, technique charts, automatic exposure control, and so on).
Measurement	Measurements are conducted on exposure, timers, kVp and mA controls, and so on. In addition, scattered radiation and patient dose measurements in radiography and fluoroscopy are performed.
Evaluation	Evaluation of radiation protection status of the department through an examination of records, equipment and its operation, work habits, techniques, darkroom, protective clothing, collimation, and radiation doses.
Recommendations	A report on the protection status of the department with recommendations regarding problem areas that need corrective actions. A follow-up is also recommended.

SOURCE: Krohmer, J. (1980). Radiation protection surveys. In R. Waggener, & C. Wilson (Eds.), *Quality Assurance in Diagnostic Radiology*. New York: American Association of Physicists in Medicine.

viduals with special training (such as medical or health physicists) will no doubt have a more sophisticated and elaborate program compared with a smaller, less specialized department.

Elements of a Radiation Protection Program

The elements of a radiation protection program will vary depending on the procedures done in the department as well as on the size of the institution. Regardless of these factors, however, the basic elements of a radiation protection program are illustrated in Figure 5-18.

ADMINISTRATION

The responsibility for establishing a radiation protection program stems from the administration of the facility. These individuals have the authority to staff and maintain the integrity of the programs in terms of budgets, policies, procedures, and equipment needed to implement the program.

The administration should appoint a radiation safety committee (RSC) and a radiation safety officer (RSO) and "shall ensure that a formal annual review of the entire radiation safety program is performed. The review should include operating procedures (i.e., the radiation safety manual or any other written policies dealing with radiation safety), past exposure records, results of investigations of any unusual radiation exposure incidents, inspections and recommendations of the RSO" (NCRP, 1989a, p. 34).

RADIATION SAFETY COMMITTEE

This committee assumes the responsibility for not only developing but also maintaining the effectiveness of the radiation protection program. Members of this committee must understand the principles of radiation protection, including radiation physics. In this regard, the NCRP (1989a) recommends that membership include a radiologist, a medical or health physicist, a hospital administrator, a nuclear medicine physician, a radiation oncologist, a senior nurse, as well as an internist, and someone who conducts re-

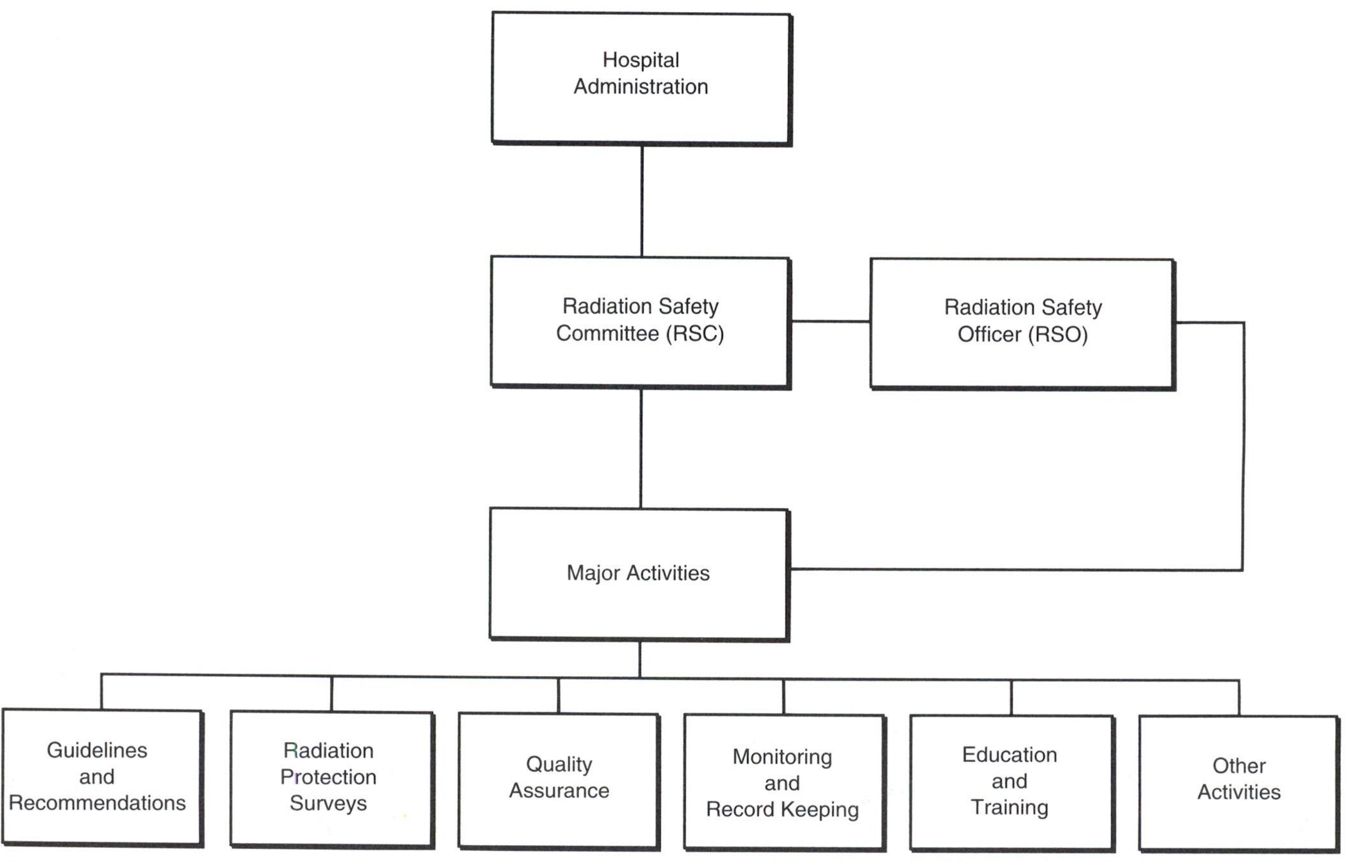

FIGURE 5-18. The basic organization and fundamental elements of a radiation protection program.

search using radiation. Although not mentioned in the NCRP (1989a) report, a senior radiological technologist, particularly one trained in QC procedures, might also serve a useful role on such a committee. In this regard, technologists should encourage hospitals to include them in matters relating to radiation protection.

RADIATION SAFETY OFFICER

The NCRP (1989a) provided a brief description of the relevant qualifications and duties of an RSO:

> The RSO should be an individual with extensive training and education in areas such as radiation protection, radiation physics, radiation biology, instrumentation, dosimetry and shielding design. The designated RSO should be a health or medical physicist, but may be a physician or other individual qualified by virtue of experience or training. The primary function of the RSO is the supervision of the daily operation of a radiation safety program to ensure that individuals are protected from radiation. To do this, the RSO *should* report directly to top management and have ready access to all levels of the organization (p. 18).

GUIDELINES AND RECOMMENDATIONS

Radiation protection programs are primarily based on guidelines, recommendations, and regulations of international and national radiation protection organizations (Chapter 6) such as the ICRP, NCRP, and RPB–Health Canada. The guidelines are recommendations that are based on the goals and philosophy of radiation protection (discussed earlier in this chapter), which define the standards of radiation protection.

Current radiation protection standards should be available to all personnel involved in radiation use and safety. In addition, all relevant radiation protection reports, particularly national safety codes and recommendations, should always be available to occupationally exposed individuals (NCRP, 1989a, c).

RADIATION PROTECTION RECORDS

Keeping accurate records is an essential part of radiation protection programs. The NCRP (1992) listed four potential uses for radiation protection records: (1) radiation safety program control and evaluation, (2) regulatory compliance, (3) epidemiological research, and (4) litigation.

This report devotes seven chapters to describing the elements necessary for maintaining accurate records. The topics covered range from guidance for generating and retaining records (program, individual, workplace, and environmental records) to radiation protection instrumentation. Although it is not within the scope of this text to address each of these elements, two points are worthy of consideration. These relate to individual records and the retention period for records.

Individual records refer to occupational radiation safety and dosimetry documentation because they are a part of the history of radiation exposure of individuals during the course of their work. Dosimetry records provide information on the magnitude of the exposures received by individuals (NCRP, 1992).

The time frame for the retention of records varies depending on these uses (Table 5-3). It is interesting to note how long one is required to retain individual and facility records for epidemiologic research and litigation.

EDUCATION AND TRAINING

It is mandatory that all individuals involved in radiation protection understand the principles underlying its practice and radiation physics. They must also demonstrate their knowledge of current radiation protection regulations, guidelines, and recommendations. A radiologic technologist is such an individual.

Continuing education programs play an important role in ensuring that workers remain current in protection principles and techniques. While a theoretical perspective is essential to radiation protection, some degree of practical training is needed so that technologists can contribute more effectively to the success of the program. For example, technologists should be trained in QC instrumentation and techniques if they are expected to perform QC tests in the de-

TABLE 5-3. THE TIME PERIOD FOR RETAINING RADIATION PROTECTION RECORDS DEPENDING ON THE POTENTIAL USE AND TYPE OF RECORD

Potential Use	Individual Records	Facility Records
Program control and evaluation	Retain until 2 yr after termination of employment	Retain for 2 yr after generation[a]
Regulatory compliance	Retention mandated by law	Retention mandated by law
Epidemiologic research	Retain until 75 yr after date of initial exposure	Retain until 75 yr after generation
Litigation	Retain until 25 yr after death, or until the 100th birth anniversary (if death date unknown)	Retain until the 100th birth anniversary of the youngest linked individual

[a] For some types of records a somewhat longer retention time may be appropriate.

SOURCE: NCRP. (1992). *Maintaining radiation protection records.* (Report No. 114). Bethesda, MD: National Council on Radiation Protection and Measurements. Reproduced by permission.

partment. The degree of practical training should depend on the responsibility of the individual. In general, medical physicists, by virtue of their higher level of training, are expected to assume higher level positions with the appropriate responsibilities, especially if they involve quantitative techniques and measurements.

REVIEW QUESTIONS

1. An effect for which the probability of occurrence increases with increasing radiation dose is referred to as:
   A. A stochastic effect.
   B. A nonstochastic effect.
   C. A deterministic effect.
   D. B and C are correct.

2. An effect for which the severity of the effect increases with increasing dose and for which a threshold dose exists is referred to as:
   A. A stochastic effect.
   B. A nonstochastic effect.
   C. A deterministic effect.
   D. B and C are correct.

3. The following are examples of deterministic effects except:
   A. Cataracts.
   B. Blood changes.
   C. Genetic effects.
   D. Impairment of fertility.

4. According to Dalrymple et al. (1984), radiation exposure may not be needed in most:
   A. Dermatologic conditions.
   B. Ophthalmologic problems.
   C. Psychiatric illnesses.
   D. All of the above.

5. The benefit–risk ratio is high in all of the following examinations except:
   A. Screening mammography of asymptomatic women younger than 33 years.
   B. Coronary angiogram in a patient with cardiovascular problems.
   C. Gastrointestinal examination in a patient with a peptic ulcer.
   D. CT of brain in a patient with cerebral hemorrhage.

6. The goal of radiation protection is to:
   A. Prevent the occurrence of deterministic effects.
   B. Keep the dose below relevant thresholds.
   C. Reduce the induction of stochastic effects.
   D. All of the above.

7. Current radiation protection standards are based on the principle(s) of:
   A. Justification.
   B. As low as reasonably achievable (ALARA).
   C. Dose limitation.
   D. All of the above.

8. Which of the following principles of radiation protection deals with a net benefit of radiation exposure to individuals?
   A. Justification.
   B. ALARA.
   C. Dose limitation.
   D. All of the above.

9. Which of the following principles of radiation protection is based on keeping exposures to a minimum and not compromising image quality?
   A. Justification.
   B. ALARA.
   C. Dose limitation.
   D. All of the above.

10. The principle of radiation protection that addresses the issue of doses established for individuals on a yearly basis is:
    A. Justification.
    B. Dose limitation.
    C. ALARA.
    D. All of the above.

11. If the exposure time for an x-ray examination is reduced, the dose to the patient:
    A. Increases.
    B. Decreases.
    C. Remains unchanged.
    D. The amount of dose a patient receives is not related to the exposure time.

12. The inverse square law states that the intensity of radiation is:
    A. Directly proportional to the square of the exposure time.
    B. Directly proportional to the square of the distance.
    C. Inversely proportional to the square of the distance.
    D. Inversely proportional to the square of the exposure time.

13. The NCRP recommends that in mobile radiography, the exposure cord length be at least:
    A. 2 m long.
    B. 3 m long.
    C. 5 m long.
    D. 1 m long.

14. Which of the following is used to protect the patient's reproductive organs?
    A. Distance.
    B. The inverse square law.
    C. Room shielding.
    D. Gonadal shielding.

15. Instruments used to measure radiation are called:
    A. Radiation detectors.
    B. Radiation dosimeters.
    C. Ionization timers.
    D. All of the above.

16. Radiation detection methods include:
    A. Ionization.
    B. Luminescence.
    C. Scintillation.
    D. All of the above.

17. The property of luminescence is used in:
    A. The film badge dosimeter.
    B. The TLD monitor.
    C. Scintillation devices.
    D. Ionization chambers.

18. The most popular form of personnel dosimetry is the:
    A. Film badge.
    B. Pocket dosimeter.
    C. TLD.
    D. Scintillation detector.

19. Which of the following uses lithium fluoride (LiF)?
    A. TLD.
    B. Pocket dosimeter.
    C. Film badge.
    D. None of the above.

20. The personnel dosimeter is intended to:
    A. Measure the occupation exposure of the individual.
    B. Give a time-integrated dose over a period of about 3 months.
    C. Monitor individuals exposed to radiation during the course of their work.
    D. All of the above.

21. The film badge cannot measure exposures less than:
    A. 1.3 μC/kg.
    B. 50 μC/kg.
    C. 2.6 μC/kg.
    D. 2.6 C/kg.

22. During radiography, the personnel dosimeter should be worn on the:
    A. Trunk of the body at the level of the waist on the posterior surface of the technologist.
    B. Upper chest region at collar level on the anterior surface of the technologist.
    C. Trunk of the body at waist level on the anterior surface of the technologist.
    D. B and C are correct.

23. During fluoroscopy, when an apron is worn and when the dose to the organs contained in the head and neck is of concern, the dosimeter should be worn at the:
    A. Level of the waist under the apron.
    B. Collar level outside the apron.
    C. Collar level under the apron.
    D. Waist level outside the apron.

24. The purpose of a radiation survey includes all of the following except:
    A. To ensure that the equipment is in proper working condition.
    B. To ensure the safety of individuals working in the radiology department.
    C. To determine which technologists are observing proper radiation protection practices.
    D. To check the status of radiation protection practices in a department.

25. In which phase of a radiation protection survey are tests conducted on the equipment to ensure that it is safe?
    A. Investigation.
    B. Inspection.
    C. Measurement.
    D. Evaluation.

26. Which is the most important phase of a radiation protection survey?
    A. Inspection.
    B. Investigation.
    C. Evaluation.
    D. Measurement.

27. The purpose of a radiation protection program is to protect:
    A. Personnel.
    B. Patients.
    C. Members of the public.
    D. All of the above.

28. The elements of a radiation protection program include all of the following except:
    A. Radiation safety office.
    B. Radiation safety committee.
    C. Guidelines and recommendations.
    D. Technologists with good protection practices.

29. A radiation safety officer:
    A. Is a medical physicist.
    B. Is trained in radiation physics, radiation biology, dosimetry, and shielding design.

C. Supervises the daily operation of a radiation safety program.
D. All of the above.

30. Radiation protection records are used for the following except:
 A. Radiation safety control.
 B. Regulatory compliance.
 C. Litigation.
 D. Keep track of technologists with poor protection practices.

REFERENCES

Bushong, S. (1993). *Radiologic science for technologists* (5th ed.). St. Louis: Mosby-Year Book.

Dalrymple, G., Baker, M., & Holder, J. (1984). Benefits of radiation. In W. Hendee (Ed.), *Health Effects of Low Level Radiation.* East Norwalk, CT: Appleton-Century Crofts.

Edwards, M. (1991). Development of radiation protection standards. *Radiographics, 11,* 699–712.

Fabrikant, J. (1983). Radiation and health. *Western Journal of Medicine, 3,* 387–390.

Feig, S., & Ehrlich, S. (1990). Estimation of radiation risk from screening mammography: Recent trends and comparison with expected benefits. *Radiology, 174,* 638–647.

Health and Welfare Canada. (1992). *Safety code-SC20A, x-ray equipment in medical diagnosis. Part A: Recommended safety procedures for installation and use.* Ottawa: Ministry of Supply and Services.

Hendee, W. (1991). Personal and public perceptions of radiation risks. *Radiographics, 11,* 1109–1119.

Hendee, W., & Edwards, M. (1986). ALARA and an integrated approach to radiation protection. *Seminars in Nuclear Medicine, 16,* 142–150.

International Commission on Radiological Protection. (1991). *Recommendations of the International Commission on Radiological Protection* (Publication No. 60). Elmsford, New York: Pergamon Press.

International Commission on Radiological Protection. (1982). *Protection of the Patient in Diagnostic Radiology.* Elmsford, NY: Pergamon Press.

Krohmer, J. (1980). Radiation protection surveys. In R. Waggener, & C. Wilson (Eds.), *Quality Assurance in Diagnostic Radiology.* New York: American Association of Physicists in Medicine.

Manfredi, O.L. (1979). Cost effectiveness of CT and ultrasound. *Applied Radiology, 2,* 73–76.

NCRP. (1989a). *Medical x-ray, electron beam and gamma ray protection for energies up to 50 MeV: Equipment design, performance and use* (Report No. 102). Bethesda, MD: National Council on Radiation Protection and Measurements (NCRP).

NCRP. (1989b). *Radiation protection for medical and allied health personnel* (Report No. 105). Bethesda, MD: National Council on Radiation Protection and Measurements (NCRP).

NCRP. (1992). *Maintaining radiation protection records* (Report No. 114). Bethesda, MD: National Council on Radiation Protection and Measurements (NCRP).

NCRP. (1993). *Limitation of exposure to ionizing radiation* (Report No. 116). Bethesda, MD: National Council on Radiation Protection and Measurements (NCRP).

Radiation Protection Bureau–Health Canada (1992). *Safety Code SC20A, X-ray equipment in medical diagnosis, Part A.* Ottawa: Health Protection Branch, Environmental Health Directorate.

Seeram, E. (1982). *Computed tomography technology.* Philadelphia: W.B. Saunders.

Tabar, L. (1990). Control of breast cancer through screening mammography. *Radiology, 174,* 655–656.

Wolbarst, A.B. (1993). *The physics of radiology.* Norwalk, CT: Appleton & Lange.

APPENDIX 5–1

An example of the benefit/risk concept in radiation protection of occupationally exposed individuals. This extract is taken from an article by Marc Edwards, Ph.D.[1]

. . . .

Figure 1 illustrates the basic philosophy of radiation protection and the linkage of risks and benefits to occupational exposure. The figure shows the benefits and lack of benefits (i.e., detriments) of the use of radiation plotted versus occupational exposure to the operator of a computed tomographic (CT) scanner (in units of dose equivalent). The operator is protected from the x-ray source by the shielded control station of the scanner (a simple planar barrier).

If the CT scanner were operated in a totally unshielded environment, the operator would receive a dose equivalent of 80 mSv per year. This exposure to the operator would result in a detriment to the individual and to society due to resources expended as a result of radiation-induced diseases and genetic effects. In Figure 1, the line labeled radiation detriment shows the cost of radiation-induced detriment in arbitrary units as a function of dose equivalent. Theoretically, detriment can be expressed in monetary units (i.e., dollars), although other units such as productivity or life span are also possible. As resources are expended for radiation protection, the dose to the worker decreases and the detriment due to radiation exposure decreases. In the case shown here, a linear dose–response, and hence a linear dose–detriment, model is used. At zero dose to the worker, no cancer or genetic effects are induced and thus the radiation detriment is zero. If radiation detriment is quantified in monetary terms, the slope of the radiation detriment line, which has units of dollars per sievert, is the product of risk per dose equivalent (in units of excess deaths per sievert) and the value of loss of life (in units of dollars per death).

Radiation detriment is reduced by buying more shielding. In Figure 1, the resources expended to provide shielding (i.e., the cost of radiation protection) are labeled shielding detriment. In the unshielded environment (that results in a dose of 80 mSv per year), no resources are expended and the shielding detriment is zero. To decrease worker exposure, the thickness of the protective barrier must be increased. In the case of exponential attenuation of x-rays through a planar barrier as shown here, a linear decrease in worker exposure results in a logarithmic increase in the thickness, and hence the cost, of shielding. Absolute safety (i.e., zero radiation exposure) is obtained only with an infinitely thick barrier and thus an infinite expenditure of resources.

The use of radiation in the performance of an imaging examination results in some gross benefit to the institution and the imaging technician in the form of profit collected for the procedure and wages paid to the worker. For simplicity, gross benefit is assumed to be independent of the amount of radiation exposure received by the worker. (The worker is not paid differently nor does the institution charge differently based on the level of occupational exposure.) Thus, the gross benefit line in Figure 1 is the same for all levels of occupational exposure.

The net benefit is the sum of gross benefit, radiation detriment, and shielding detriment. The principles of radiation protection require that there be a positive net benefit from any activity in which radiation is used. In the example illustrated in Figure 1, for exposure greater than about 65 mSv, the net benefit is negative due to excessive radiation detriment. No radiation-utilizing activity is appropriate beyond that point.

For occupationally exposed individuals, a minimum level of resource expenditure is necessary to meet required dose limitations. This level is labeled dose limit in Figure 1. For example, it may be necessary to spend $10,000 on shielding to assure that no one receives more than 50 mSv per year of whole-body effective dose equivalent. Even if dose limits are met, the net benefit may not be positive. Use of fluoroscopy to fit shoes is a classic example of a use of radiation for which there is no net benefit, regardless of whether dose limitations are met. In Figure 1, a positive net benefit is provided at the dose limit; hence, this use of radiation is appropriate.

The level of resource expenditure required to meet dose limitations does not necessarily provide the optimal level of radiation protection. In the example in Figure 1, a further expenditure of resources beyond that required by dose limits continues to yield increased net benefit until a maximum is reached. At this point, the exposure to personnel

[1]*From Edwards, M. (1991). Development of radiation protection standards.* Radiographics, 11, *699. Extract reprinted by permission of the Radiological Society of North America and Dr. Edwards.*

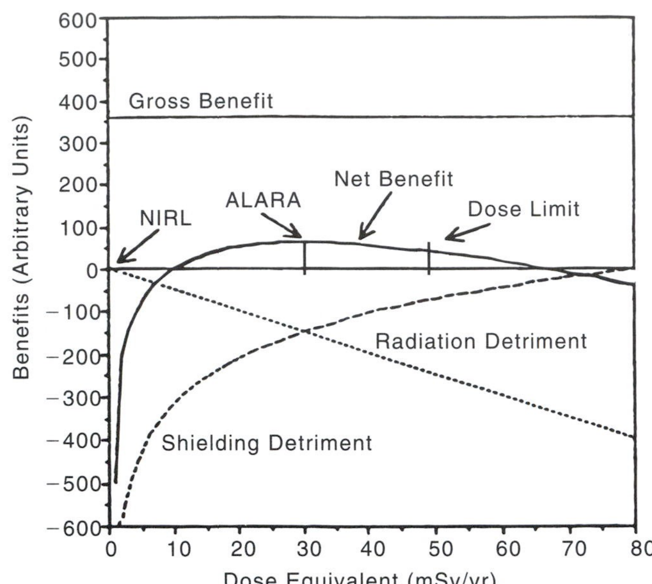

FIGURE 1. Risks and benefits in radiation protection of occupationally exposed individuals (see text for explanation). *NIRL* = negligible individual risk level.

is lower than that required by dose limits. Further expenditure of resources to provide a still lower level of exposure results in lowering net benefit. The point at which the net benefit is maximized defines the exposure level that is as low as reasonably achievable. The ALARA requirement is thus seen as a requirement that radiation protection be optimized to provide the greatest net benefit to society.

Negligible individual risk level (NIRL) is a dose limit beneath which further protection activities are unwarranted. In Figure 1, the net benefit becomes negative before the NIRL is reached because of the large shielding detriment. Thus, even though the radiation detriment has been reduced to a very low level, the net benefit to society is negative because of the cost of the shielding required for that dose reduction.

CHAPTER SIX

Radiation Protection Organizations

Learning Objectives

Upon completion of this chapter, the reader should be able to:

1 ■ List six international organizations dealing with radiation protection issues.

2 ■ State the operating philosophy of the International Commission of Radiological Protection (ICRP).

3 ■ Explain the role of the ICRP in radiation protection matters as they relate to diagnostic radiology.

4 ■ List several publications of the ICRP of importance to the technologist.

(continued)

5 ■ Explain the fundamental role of the United Nations Committee on the Effects of Atomic Radiation (UNSCEAR) and the Biological Effects of Ionizing Radiation Committee (BEIR).
6 ■ List four national radiation protection organizations.
7 ■ Explain the role and objectives of the United States Food and Drug Administration (USFDA) and the National Council on Radiation Protection and Measurement (NCRP), in radiation as applied to diagnostic radiology.
8 ■ List several reports of the NCRP of importance to the radiologic technologist.
9 ■ State the objectives of the Canadian Safety Code for diagnostic radiology.
10 ■ Define the terms "shall" and "should" as used by the ICRP and the NCRP.
11 ■ Define the terms "must" and "should" as used by the Canadian Radiation Protection Bureau.

Introduction

The safety standards, recommendations, and guidelines cited in this book for the prudent use of radiation in medicine are based on the work of dedicated, knowledgeable persons who are members of various radiation protection organizations throughout the world. Because we cite the work of several of these organizations in this book, it is important that we become familiar with the activities and contributions of these various groups.

In this chapter, we explore the nature of these organizations in terms of their contributions to radiation protection. In particular, we state the overall goals and describe briefly the major activities of groups relevant to radiology. Finally, we identify the major reports dealing with radiation protection considerations for radiology and define the meanings of the words "should," "shall," and "must" as used in the reports.

In general, organizations are divided into those that operate at an international level and those that serve a national function. In addition, some of these bodies deal primarily with biological effects of radiation, while others concentrate on radiation protection.

International Organizations

There are several important international organizations of relevance to radiation protection; however, only six of them will be discussed in this section. These are:

- International Commission on Radiological Protection (ICRP)
- United Nations Scientific Committee on the Effects of Atomic Radiation (UNSCEAR)
- Radiation Effects Research Foundation (RERF)
- Biological Effects of Ionizing Radiation Committee (BEIR)
- International Commission on Radiological Units and Measurements (ICRU)
- International Radiation Protection Association (IRPA)

International Commission on Radiological Protection (ICRP)

For radiology, the ICRP is an important body because it makes recommendations on radiation protection based on information provided by organizations concerned primarily with the biological effects of radiation, such as BEIR and UNSCEAR.

The ICRP was formed in 1928 by the Second International Congress of Radiology and was called the International X-ray and Radium Protection Committee. Its primary activity at that time was to ensure radiation safety standards in radiology. The ICRP assumed its present name in 1950 to reflect more accurately its expanded role in radiation protection. The ICRP bases its recommended radiation protection measures on fundamental principles and it leaves to the various national protection bodies the task of devising the safety standards, regulatory procedures, and practice guidelines that best address that country's needs (Berry, 1987).

The ICRP is made up of individuals who are experts in radiology, physics, biology, health physics, radiation protection, genetics, biochemistry, and biophysics. This commission is actively involved with several other organizations including the ICRU, the World Health Organization (WHO), the International Atomic Energy Agency, the International Labor Organization, UNSCEAR, and IRPA, to mention but a few.

The first recommendations of the ICRP were published in the *British Journal of Radiology* in 1928. These recommendations addressed x-ray and radium protection. This was followed by subsequent recommendations until 1959, when the first report, that is, Publication 1, entitled "Recommendations of the International Commission on Radiological Protection," was published by Pergamon Press in Oxford. Later, these general recommendations were published in 1964 (Publication 6), 1966 (Publication 9), 1977 (Publication 26), and 1990 (Publication 60); each publication reflected the changes in radiation protection philosophy.

In 1977, Publication 26, Recommendations of the ICRP, *Annals of the ICRP* introduced the current system of radiation protection, which is based on the three concepts of justification, optimization, and dose limitation. This publication was also significant for its introduction of the terms *stochastic* and *nonstochastic* to describe the genetic and somatic effects of radiation. (See Chapters 1 and 4 for discussions of these terms.)

In accordance with this new system of radiation protection, the goals of the ICRP were intended to avoid completely the nonstochastic effects and to limit the stochastic effects to an acceptably low level of risk.

In 1991, the ICRP revised its recommendations once again and Publication 26 was superseded by Publication 60, 1990R recommendations of the International Commission on Radiological Protection, *Annals of the ICRP*. In this publication, some major changes were made based on the results of BEIR Committee Report V, *Health effects of exposure to low levels of ionizing radiation*. In this ICRP report, the risks of radiation are recognized to be about three to four times greater than had been previously estimated. This major finding prompted the ICRP to make several recommendations of importance on radiation protection. One such recommendation relates to reducing the dose limit to occupationally exposed individuals from 50 mSv (5 rems) to 20 mSv (2 rems) per year, averaged over defined periods of 5 years.

The ICRP has been very active in radiation protection endeavors. They have not only kept pace with the trends in setting safety standards, but they also "improve the presentation of the recommendations" and "maintain as much stability in the recommendations as is consistent with the new information" (ICRP, 1991, p. vii).

The system of radiation protection recommended by the ICRP does affect the reduction of dose to both patients and workers and is intended to ensure that the dose is kept to a minimum (Berry, 1987).

The ICRP has made available numerous reports on radiation protection, of which the following (in addition to Publication 60) are important to the radiologic technologist:

1. ICRP Publication 34: Protection of the patient in diagnostic radiology, *Annals of the ICRP*. Vol. 9, No. 213, 1982.
2. ICRP Publication 33: Protection against ionizing radiation from external sources in medicine, *Annals of the ICRP*. Vol. 9, No. 3, 1982a.
3. ICRP Publication 57: Radiologic protection of the worker in medicine and dentistry, *Annals of the ICRP*. Vol. 20, No. 3, 1989.
4. Summary of the current ICRP principles for protection of the patient in diagnostic radiology, *Note in the Annals of the ICRP*. Vol. 22, No. 3, 1989.

Finally, the ICRP works in conjunction with its "sister body," the ICRU, and has "official relationships" with organizations such as UNSCEAR, WHO, and IRPA, among others.

United Nations Scientific Committee on the Effects of Atomic Radiation (UNSCEAR)

UNSCEAR, which was established in 1955, is made up of expert radiobiologists from around the globe. According to Brown (1989), this committee has the task of examining all of the available data on the risks of natural and artificial radiation from sources as diverse as RERF, major epidemiological studies, and animal studies. UNSCEAR also makes it a priority to stay abreast of developments in basic radiology as a means of keeping track of biological effects at both the animal and cellular level. Finally, this committee makes predictions about the incidence of biological effects among the general population.

Major UNSCEAR reports have been published in 1977, 1982, 1986, and 1988. Generally, the purpose of these reports was to assess the risk of exposure from the available biological evidence. These reports are entitled:

1. United Nations Scientific Committee on the Effects of Atomic Radiation (UNSCEAR), *Sources and effects of ionizing radiation*, 1977.
2. United Nations Scientific Committee on the Effects of Atomic Radiation (UNSCEAR), *Ionizing radiation: Sources and biological effects*, 1982.
3. United Nations Scientific Committee on the Effects of Atomic Radiation (UNSCEAR), *Genetic and somatic effects of ionizing radiation*, 1986.
4. United Nations Scientific Committee on the Effects of Atomic Radiation (UNSCEAR), *Sources, effects and risks of ionizing radiation*, 1988.

Radiation Effects Research Foundation (RERF)

The RERF group is run by the government of Japan and obtains half its funding from the United States. RERF was formed in the 1950s, and one of its major tasks was to study the survivors of the atomic bomb explosions at Hiroshima and Nagasaki. These 100,000 survivors represent the most extensively studied group of humans ever to have been exposed to radiation.

Brown (1989) was careful to point out that the data provided in RERF studies are purely statistical in nature. Once RERF publishes its data, other organizations pore over it in an effort to evaluate new risk models and predictions with the ultimate aim of devising new recommendations for radiation protection procedures.

Biological Effects of Ionizing Radiation Committee (BEIR)

The BEIR Committee was formed by the National Research Council (NRC), organized by the U.S. National Academy of Sciences (NAS), and in this regard, the BEIR Committee is not "strictly" an international committee (Brown, 1989).

The BEIR Committee has evolved from BEIR I to the most recent BEIR V, with each committee charged with the specific responsibility of advising the United States government on the health effects of radiation exposures. In 1986, the BEIR V Committee was formed "to conduct a comprehensive review of the biological effects of ionizing radiations focusing on the information that had been reported since the conclusion of the BEIR III study and, to the extent that available information permitted, provide new estimates of the risks of genetic and somatic effects in humans due to low-level exposures of ionizing radiation" (NRC, 1990, p. vi).

Using information provided by RERF, the BEIR V report concluded that the risks of radiation are about three to four times greater than had been previously estimated in the BEIR III report (NRC, 1990).

The results of this BEIR study, as presented in the BEIR V report entitled *Health effects of exposure to low levels of ionizing radiation*, have significant implications for radiation protection. It is with these results that the ICRP made its most recent recommendations on standards and guidelines for radiation protection.

International Commission on Radiological Units and Measurements (ICRU)

The ICRU was established in 1925 with the goal of developing recommendations that would be accepted internationally. The ICRU deals primarily with establishing radiation quantities and units, measurement procedures, and the use of data to ensure uniform reporting. While the ICRU encourages national organizations to develop their own procedures for standards, it also recommends that countries pay careful attention to the universal concepts relating to quantities and units for radiation protection.

International Radiation Protection Association (IRPA)

The IRPA is made up of national organizations from all over the globe, and its primary goal is to deal with recommendations for nonionizing radiation.

National Organizations

There are several national organizations on medical radiation protection that provide recommendations for their own countries. The major organizations to be described briefly in this section are those of the United States, Canada, and the United Kingdom.

The U.S. organizations include the National Council on Radiation Protection and Measurements (NCRP), the Center for Devices and Radiological Health (CDRH), and the Food and Drug Administration (FDA). The Canadian organization of importance is the Radiation Protection Bureau–Health Canada (RPB-HC).

An important point to note is that there are additional organizations such as the United States Nuclear Regulatory Commission (USNRC) and the Canadian Atomic Energy Control Board (AECB). Because these two organizations deal with all aspects of nuclear safety, they will not be considered further in this text.

United States Food and Drug Administration (USFDA)

The design and manufacture of x-ray equipment in the United States is regulated by the FDA. Various performance specifications of x-ray equipment are established by the FDA, for both radiographic and fluoroscopic equipment. These regulations are in *Title 21 of the Code of Federal Regulations* published in 1992.

National Council on Radiation Protection and Measurements (NCRP)

The NCRP is a nonprofit organization chartered by Congress in 1964 to replace the Advisory Committee on X-Ray and Radium Protection, the original agency that was founded in 1929.

The NCRP is organized into a main committee and more than 60 scientific subcommittees and is made up of expert scientists in radiation protection. These subcommittees study and prepare reports on specific radiation protection issues and then submit them to the main committee for approval and publication.

The objectives of the NCRP are as follows:

1. Collect, analyze, develop and disseminate in the public interest information and recommendations about (a) protection against radiation and (b) radiation measurements, quantities, and units, particularly those concerned with radiation protection;
2. Provide a means by which organizations concerned with the scientific and related aspects of radiation protection and of radiation quantities, units and measurements may cooperate for effective utilization of their combined resources and to stimulate the work of such organizations;

3. Develop basic concepts about radiation quantities, units, and measurements about the application of these concepts, and about radiation protection;
4. Cooperate with the International Commission on Radiological Protection, the International Commission on Radiation Units and Measurements, and other national and international organizations, governmental and private, concerned with radiation quantities, units and measurements and with radiation protection (NCRP, 1990, p. 108).

The NCRP is not a government organization; however, its recommendations on radiation protection are often considered by local, state, and federal governments.

The NCRP has published quite a large number of proceedings, Lauriston S. Taylor lectures, commentaries, and reports. Recent important reports of relevance to the radiologic technologist are as follows:

1. Report No. 82: *SI units in radiation protection and measurements* (1985).
2. Report No. 85: *Mammography—a user's guide* (1986).
3. Report No. 99: *Quality assurance for diagnostic imaging* (1988).
4. Report No. 102: *Medical x-ray, electron beam and gamma-ray protection for energies up to 50 MeV (equipment design, performance and use)* (1989).
5. Report No. 105: *Radiation protection for medical and allied health personnel* (1989).
6. Report No. 107: *Implementation of the principle of as low as reasonably achievable (ALARA) for medical and dental personnel* (1990).
7. Report No. 116: *Limitation of exposure for ionizing radiation* (1993).

Center for Devices and Radiological Health (CDRH)

The CDRH was created by merging the Bureau of Radiological Health (BRH) and the Bureau of Medical Devices (BMD) to assume responsibility for all medical devices including radiation-producing equipment. The CDRH is of interest to radiologic technologists because it is a federal organization (U.S. Public Health Service) that also plays a major role in evaluating population exposure to x-rays, as well as other diagnostic imaging modalities and radiation therapy.

The CDRH aims to minimize unnecessary exposure to radiation by assuming regulatory control of the performance of x-ray equipment, and by providing technical and biological background information and advice to the medical profession to the general public (Whalen and Balter, 1984).

Radiation Protection Bureau–Health Canada (RPB-HC)

Radiation protection in Canada is dealt with by two major federal government organizations, the RPB-HC and AECB. Because the AECB is responsible for the nuclear industry and has no direct applicability to medical radiation practices, it will not be discussed any further.

The RPB-HC is involved in several aspects of radiation protection, of which x-ray protection is but one. Two other activities include the operation of a National Dosimetry Service (mainly for thermoluminescent dosimeters [TLDs]), and a National Dose Registry, a computer-based system that monitors radiation dose to radiation workers (Letourneau, 1982).

The RPB has an x-ray section and a nonionizing radiation section. While the x-ray section addresses safety procedures and presents equipment and installation guidelines, the nonionizing radiation section looks after issues related to microwaves, radiowaves, and lasers.

A major publication of the x-ray section of the RPB is *Safety Code-20A: X-Ray equipment in medical diagnosis. Part A: Recommended safety procedures for installation and use.* The major objectives of this important safety code for Canadian diagnostic radiology departments are as follows:

1. To minimize patient exposure in medical diagnostic radiology.
2. To ensure adequate protection of personnel operating or using x-ray equipment.
3. To ensure adequate protection of the general public in the vicinity of areas where diagnostic procedures are in progress (RPB-Health Canada, 1992, p. 10).

Canadian Radiation Protection Association (CRPA)

The CRPA was incorporated in 1982 with several objectives in mind. Apart from the objectives of developing scientific knowledge, encouraging research, and promoting educational opportunities in the discipline of radiation protection, the CRPA also "assists in the development of professional standards . . ." and "supports the activities of other societies, associations or organizations, both national and international, having any activities or objectives relevant to the foregoing" (CRPA, 1992, p. 1).

Definition of Terms

In selected radiation protection reports of the ICRP, NCRP and the RPB, the terms "*shall*," "*should*," and "*must*" are used in specific recommendations. In Table 6-1, the terms used by each of these three organizations are given. Each of these terms, as defined by each organization, has a special meaning.

TABLE 6-1. TERMS USED BY THREE RADIATION PROTECTION ORGANIZATIONS TO INDICATE THE NATURE OF THEIR RECOMMENDATIONS

ICRP	NCRP (US)	RPB (Canada)
Shall	Shall	Must
Should	Should	Should

ICRP's Definitions

The meanings of the terms *shall* and *should* as defined by the ICRP (1982) are as follows:

Shall: Necessary or essential for protection against radiation;

Should: To apply, whenever reasonable, in the interests of improving radiation protection (p. 1).

Likewise, the negatives of these terms carry distinct meanings.

An example of the use of these terms with respect to the recommendation of holding patients during radiological procedures is as follows:

"No person *should* normally hold patients during diagnostic examinations. Motion-restricting devices *shall* be used as much as practicable, and cassettes *should not* be hand-held during exposure. When patients must be held during an examination, the individual holding should be chosen so that his cumulative doses will be held within local, authorized limits. No pregnant women nor persons under the age of 18 years *should* be permitted to hold patients. Those holding the patients *shall* wear protective aprons and gloves and *should* ensure, as far as practicable, that no part of their body, even if covered by protective clothing, is in the path of the primary beam (ICRP, 1982, p. 14).

NCRP's Definitions

In the NCRP's reports, the meanings of the terms *shall* and *should* are stated as follows:

Shall and *shall not* are used to indicate that adherence to the recommendation is considered necessary to meet accepted standards of protection.

Should and *should not* are used to indicate a prudent practice to which exceptions may occasionally be made in appropriate circumstances (NCRP, 1989, p. 2).

With respect to the recommendation of holding patients during x-ray examinations, the NCRP (1989) stated that:

No person *should* routinely hold patients during diagnostic examinations; when a patient must be held in position for radiography, a mechanical support or restraining device *should* be

> used. If such use of mechanical means is not possible and human support or restraint must be used, the individual holding the patient *should* be chosen so that the cumulative doses will be held within acceptable limits. Pregnant women or persons under the age of 18 years *should not* be permitted to hold patients. If a patient must be held by someone, that individual *shall* be protected with appropriate shielding devices such as protective gloves and aprons. Positioning *should* be arranged so that no part of the holder's torso, even if covered by protective clothing, will be struck by the useful beam, and so that the holder's body is as far as possible from the useful beam (p. 9).

RPB-HC's Definitions

> In Canada, the RPB-HC defines the terms *must* and *should* as follows:
>
> *Must* indicates a recommendation that is essential to meet the currently accepted standards of protection, while
>
> *Should* indicates an advisory recommendation that is highly desirable and that is to be implemented where applicable (RPB, 1992, p. 7).

With regard to the recommendation of holding patients during x-ray examinations, the terms *must* and *should* are used as follows:

> When there is a need to support children or weak patients, holding devices *should* be used. If parents, escorts or other personnel are called to assist, they *must* be provided with protective aprons and gloves and positioned so as to avoid the useful beam. No one person *should* regularly perform these duties (RPB, 1992, p. 28).

Recommendations: Common Elements

With respect to recommendations, the ICRP, NCRP, and RPB essentially state the same guiding principles. For example, with respect to the above recommendations, the guiding principles are as follows:

1. Restraining devices *should* be used to immobilize patients during examinations.
2. Individuals holding patients *shall* and *must* be protected by lead aprons and gloves.
3. No part of the shielded body of those who hold patients is in the direct path of the primary beam.

In this particular example, holding patients, it appears that both national organizations, the NCRP and RPB-HC, have adopted the recommendation of the ICRP. In situations in which the recommendation of the national organization differs from what is proposed by the international organization, the recommendation must be more stringent and definitely not below the guidelines stated by the ICRP. For example, the ICRP recommends a total filtration of 2.5 mm aluminum equivalent for machines operating above 70 kVp. National organizations must either adopt this recommendation or provide a more stringent one, in which case the total filtration at the same kVp will be greater than 2.5 mm but not less.

Throughout this book, most notably Chapters 7, 10, and 11, we cite several recommendations, guidelines, and standards for radiography, fluoroscopy, mammography, and computer-assisted imaging modalities such as computed tomography and magnetic resonance imaging. The citations will reflect those of the ICRP, the NCRP, and the RPB-HC, with an emphasis on those of the NCRP.

Although our primary goal is to know the major recommendations, guidelines, and standards of the safe use of radiation in imaging patients, our secondary goal is to become familiar with the common elements inherent in these radiation protection guidelines and recommendations.

REVIEW QUESTIONS

1. The following are international organizations concerned with radiation protection except:

A. ICRP.
B. ICRU.
C. UNSCEAR and BIER.
D. CDRH.

2. Which of the following makes recommendations regarding radiation protection?
   A. ICRP.
   B. BEIR.
   C. UNSCEAR.
   D. RERF.

3. Which of the following represents the "overall operating philosophy" of the ICRP?
   A. Radiation protection recommendations are based on basic principles and quantitative analysis.
   B. Formulation of specific advice for countries.
   C. Establishment of codes of practice or regulations for individual countries.
   D. All of the above.

4. The new ICRP system of radiation protection is based on:
   A. Justification.
   B. ALARA.
   C. Dose limitation.
   D. All of the above.

5. Which of the following major findings of the BEIR Committee prompted the ICRP to revise its dose limits for radiation workers?
   A. Radiation effects are stochastic.
   B. Radiation effects are nonstochastic.
   C. Radiation risks are three to four times greater than previously predicted.
   D. Radiation risks are deterministic.

6. Which of the following committees' major task is to study the survivors of the Hiroshima and Nagasaki bombings?
   A. ICRP.
   B. RERF.
   C. BEIR.
   D. UNSCEAR.

7. The committee that deals essentially with radiation quantities is the:
   A. ICRP.
   B. NCRP.
   C. ICRU.
   D. RPB-Health Canada.

8. The international committee that deals with nonionizing radiation recommendations is the:
   A. ICRP.
   B. ICRC.
   C. UNSCEAR.
   D. IRPA.

9. The design and manufacture of x-ray equipment in the United States is regulated by the:
   A. USFDA.
   B. NCRP.
   C. CDRH.
   D. AECB.

10. Which of the following plays a role in evaluating population exposure to x-rays and other diagnostic imaging modalities?
    A. USFDA.
    B. NCRP.
    C. CDRH.
    D. AECB.

11. The ________ is not a government organization.
    A. NCRP.
    B. USFDA.
    C. USNRC.
    D. CDRH.

12. The goal of the Canadian radiation protection Safety Code (SC-20A) for diagnostic radiology is to:
    A. Protect the patient.
    B. Protect personnel.
    C. Protect members of the public.
    D. All of the above.

13. Which of the following organizations played a role in developing the first guidelines for exposure to the magnetic fields and radiowaves in magnetic resonance imaging?
    A. NCRP.
    B. ICRP.
    C. RPB-Canada.
    D. NRPB.

14. The term "shall" as defined by the ICRP refers to:
    A. As essential for radiation protection.
    B. Apply, whenever reasonable, to improve radiation protection.
    C. A practice to which exemptions apply.
    D. Apply to all radiation protection recommendations.

15. The term "should" as defined by the ICRP refers to:
    A. As essential for radiation protection.
    B. Apply whenever reasonable to improve radiation protection.
    C. A practice to which exemptions apply.
    D. Apply to all radiation protection guidelines.

REFERENCES

Berry, R.J. (1987). The international commission on radiological protection: An historical perspective. In J. Rusell, & R. Southwood (Eds.), *Radiation and Health*. New York: John Wiley and Sons.

Brown, D. (1989). International bodies of importance for radiation protection practices in Canada. *Bulletin of the Canadian Radiation Protection Association, 10*, 9–15.

CRPA. (1992). Objectives of the association. *Bulletin of the Canadian Radiation Protection Association: Membership Handbook, 2*, 1.

International Commission on Radiological Protection. (1991). *1990 recommendations of the ICRP* (Publication No. 60). Elmsford, New York: Pergamon Press.

Letourneau, E.G. (1982). Radiation protection in Canada. In *Radiation Protection and New Medical Diagnostic Approaches*. Washington, DC: National Academy of Sciences/NCRP.

National Council on Radiation Protection and Measurements. (1990). *Implementation of the principles of as low as reasonably achievable (ALARA) for medical and dental personnel.* Bethesda, MD: National Council on Radiation Protection and Measurements.

National Council on Radiation Protection and Measurements. (1989). *Medical x-ray, electron beam and gamma ray protection for energies up to 50 MeV: Equipment design, performance and use.* Bethesda, MD: National Council on Radiation Protection and Measurements.

NRC BEIR Committee. (1990). *The effects on populations of exposure to low levels of ionizing radiations.* Washington, DC: National Academy of Sciences/National Research Council.

RPB. (1992). *Safety code-SC 20A. X-ray equipment in medical diagnosis. Part A. Recommended safety procedures for installation and use.* Ottawa: Health Protection Branch, Environmental Health Directorate.

Whalen, J.P., & Balter, S. (1984). *Radiation risks in medical imaging.* Chicago: Year Book Medical Publishers.

CHAPTER SEVEN

Dose Limits

Learning Objectives

Upon completion of this chapter, the reader should be able to:

1. Trace the history of the concept of dose limits for radiation workers.
2. Explain each of the following terms: skin erythema dose, tolerance dose, maximum permissible dose, and dose equivalent limit.
3. State the categories of individuals for whom dose limits have been established.
4. State the ICRP and NCRP recommended dose limits for whole body exposure for radiation workers.
5. State the ICRP and NCRP recommended dose limits for the lens of the eye, skin, and extremities for radiation workers.
6. State the ICRP and NCRP recommended dose limits for pregnant radiation workers.
7. State the NCRP recommended dose limit for the embryo-fetus.
8. State the ICRP and NCRP recommended dose limits for members of the public as well as for the lens of the eye and skin for members of the public.

(continued)

9 ■ Compare the NCRP and the Canadian dose limits for radiation workers and members of the public.

10 ■ Discuss occupational dose trends.

11 ■ List three magnetic resonance imaging fields for which exposure limits have been established.

Introduction

It is the goal of radiation protection to prevent deterministic effects and to decrease the probability of stochastic effects. This goal can be achieved by adhering to the three fundamental principles of radiation protection, explored in Chapter 5, that is, net benefit, ALARA, and dose limits. Because dose limits continue to receive much attention in the literature, they will be treated here in some detail.

The first order of business in this chapter is to identify the categories of individuals for whom dose limits have been established and to state the recommended limits. Particular attention is paid to examining dose limits for both stochastic and deterministic effects, not only for occupationally exposed individuals and members of the public, but also for pregnant women as well as the embryo and fetus.

Dose Limitation: A Brief History

The first sign that there was a limit to how much radiation exposure an individual could sustain without ill effects surfaced in the 1900s. At that time, the dose limitation was labeled the *skin erythema dose* by Mutscheller and Sievert. It was defined as a dose of x-rays strong enough to produce a reddening of the skin 10 to 14 days following the exposure. The erythema dose was thought to be ~6000 mSv (600 rem), and the dose limit for occupationally exposed individuals was 600 mSv (60 rem) per year (Edwards, 1991).

In 1928, the ICRP was formed and it was at this time that formal radiation protection standards were introduced. The establishment of dose limits was one of the primary activities of the ICRP at that time. From the period between 1928 and 1990, several dose limitation terms emerged (Fig. 7-1).

The term *tolerance dose* was used to describe an acceptable level of exposure and appeared to suggest a threshold dose below which no radiation damage would occur. Later, the term tolerance dose was replaced by another term, the *maximum permissible dose* (MPD), the largest allowable dose that is *not* expected to result in significant radiation effects (Bushong, 1993, p. 602). In other words, although doses below the MPD would produce neither somatic nor genetic responses, doses at the level of the MPD would be associated with a small risk. This small risk is outweighed by the potential benefits to be gained.

The MPD could be calculated using the following formula:

$$\text{MPD} = (N - 18)\ \text{rem} \qquad (7\text{-}1)$$

where N = age in years.

Since it was the practice not to train individuals under 18 years of age, the MPD was computed to be 5 rem (5000 mrem), or 50 mSv, with regard to student training in radiologic technology. Currently, this rule has been replaced by a cumulative dose equivalent of 10 mSv × age in years (NCRP, 1987).

In 1977, the ICRP recommended a new term to replace the MPD. This was the *dose equivalent limit*, or effective dose equivalent (H_E) which is a part of a more comprehensive system of radiation protection identified in Chapter 1.

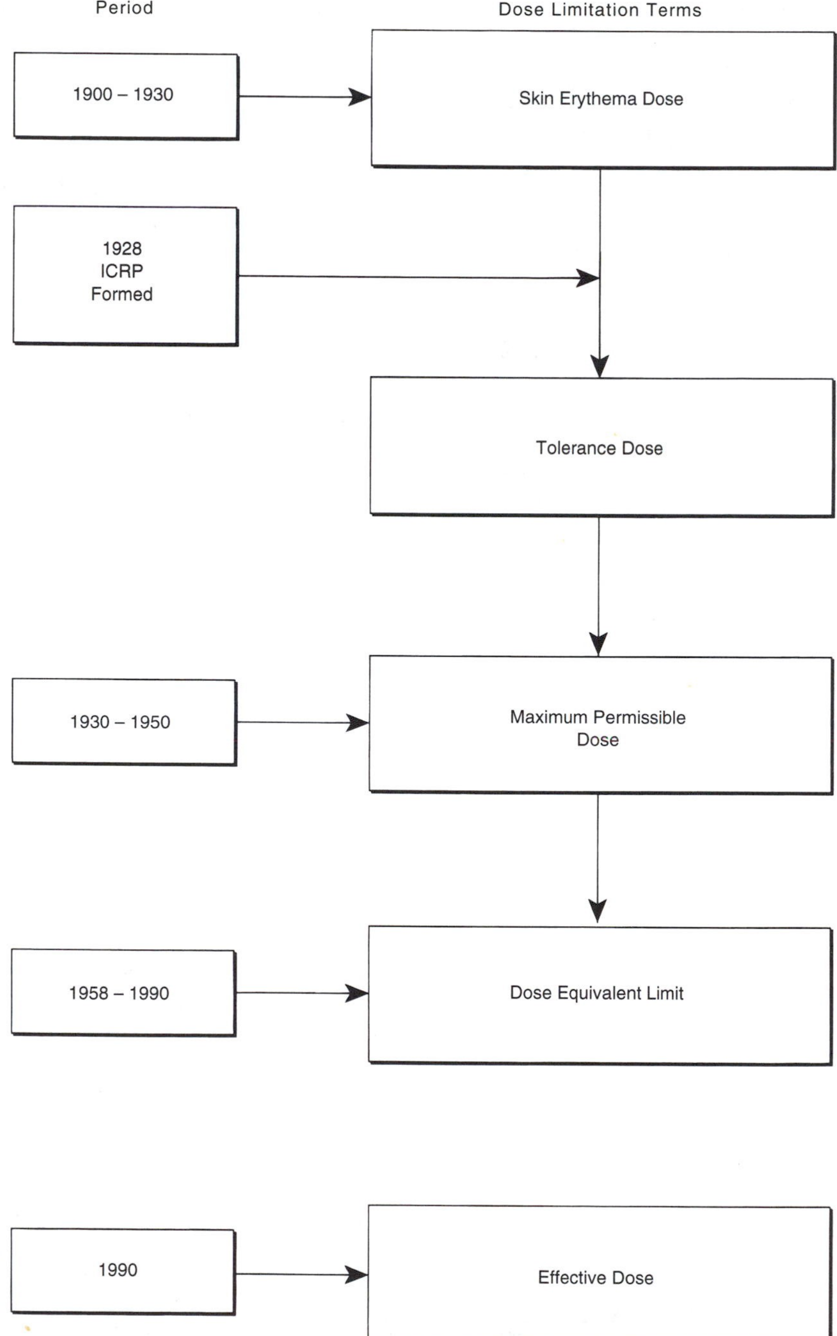

FIGURE 7-1. Dose limitation terms and the periods in which they were introduced. The current term, effective dose, has been introduced by the ICRP to relate the risk from partial body exposure to that from an equivalent whole-body exposure.

REVIEW BOX:

- *Net benefit*: There must be a benefit associated with each exposure.
- *ALARA*: All exposures should be kept as low as reasonably achievable.
- *Dose limits*: Doses should not exceed recommended limits per year.

The terms *justification* (net benefit), *optimization* (ALARA), and *dose and risk limits* (dose limits), which are integral to the characterization of these concepts, are defined in current ICRP language.

The most recent recommendations for occupational dose limits established by both the ICRP and NCRP are stated in terms of the *effective dose, E.* (It should be noted that the NCRP dose limits published in 1987 are stated in terms of effective dose equivalent because the term effective dose was not adopted until 1991.) This term is used to relate the risk of exposure of a portion of the body to that of exposure of the whole body (Zankl et al., 1992). It should be noted that the terms effective dose equivalent (H_E) and effective dose (E) are essentially similar concepts.

In 1991, the ICRP made several changes to their radiation protection recommendations based on new data obtained from the Hiroshima and Nagasaki radiation survivors. They found that the risk of radiation is three to four times greater than previously estimated (BEIR V, 1990). As a result of this significant finding, the ICRP reduced the dose limits for occupationally exposed individuals from 50 to 20 mSv (5 to 2 rem). The NCRP, on the other hand, has not adopted this limit as yet, and still recommends 50 mSv/year.

Additional details of the history of these recommendations are reviewed in Table 7-1.

Categories of Exposed Individuals

Dose limits are specified for whole-body exposure, partial-body exposure, organ exposure, and the general population exposure.

These limits apply to each of the following:

1. *Occupational exposures*: Those individuals who are exposed at work. These include (a) women who are not pregnant and men, and (b) pregnant women.
2. *Public exposures*: These include members of the general population, excluding those who undergo medical exposure.
3. *Education and training exposures*: Individuals who receive radiation exposure during a course of study or apprenticeship.
4. *Embryo-fetus exposures*: Exposures that occur when the embryo or fetus is directly or indirectly exposed to radiation in utero.

Recommended Dose Limits: ICRP

Table 7-2 summarizes the ICRP's recommended dose limits which, if carefully observed, should reduce the probability of stochastic effects and prevent detrimental deterministic effects. These limits exclude exposure from natural background and medical exposure.

Individual Limits for Occupational Exposure

EFFECTIVE DOSE

The effective dose is used to estimate the risks accompanying whole-body exposure; it is equal to the sum of all equivalent doses, or those values deemed safe for irradiating discrete organs and areas of tissue.

The ICRP recommends an effective dose limit of 20 mSv per year averaged over 5 years (100 mSv in 5 years) to limit the probability of stochastic effects. In addition, the effective dose should not exceed 50 mSv in any given year.

LENS OF THE EYE, SKIN, AND HANDS AND FEET

For the prevention of detrimental deterministic effects to the lens of the eye (cataracts), skin (reddening or ulceration), and hands and feet,

TABLE 7-1. A REVIEW OF THE EVENTS RELATING TO DOSE LIMITATION RECOMMENDATIONS

Year	Recommendation	Approximate Daily Dose (mrem)	Recommender
1902	Dose limited by fogging of a photographic plate following 7-minute contact exposure	10,000	Rollins
1915	Lead shielding of tube needed (no numerical exposure levels given)		British Roentgen Society
1921	General methods to reduce exposure		British X-Ray and Radium Protection Committee
1925	"It is entirely safe if an operator does not receive every thirty days a dose exceeding 1/100 of an erythema dose."	200	Mutscheller
1925	10% of an SED[a] per year	200	Sievert
1926	1 SED per 90,000 working hours	40	Dutch Board of Health
1928	0.00028 of an SED per day	175	Barclay and Cox
1928	0.001 of an SED per month; 5 R per day permissible for the hands	150	Kaye
1931	Limit exposure to 0.2 R per day	200	Advisory Committee on X-ray and Radium Protection of the United States
1932	0.001 of an SED per month	30	Failla
1934	5 R per day permissible for the hands		Advisory Committee on X-Ray and Radium Protection of the United States
1936	0.1 R per day	100	Advisory Committee on X-Ray and Radium Protection of the United States
1941	0.02 R per day	20	Taylor
1943	200 mR per day is acceptable	200	Patterson
1959	5 rem per year, 5($N - 18$) rem accumulated	20	National Council on Radiation Protection and Measurements
1987	50 mSv per year, 10 × N mSv accumulated	20	National Council on Radiation Protection and Measurements
1991	20 mSv per year	8	International Commission on Radiation Protection

[a] Skin erythema dose.

SOURCE: Bushong, S. (1993). *Radiologic science for technologists* (5th ed.). St. Louis: Mosby–Year Book. Reproduced with permission.

the ICRP recommends a yearly equivalent dose (absorbed dose × radiation weighting factor) of 150, 500, and 500 mSv, respectively.

OCCUPATIONAL LIMIT FOR PREGNANT WOMEN

There are no special considerations for women in general. However, women who are pregnant should have a supplementary equivalent dose limit of 2 mSv applied to the surface of her abdomen for the remainder of the pregnancy (ICRP, 1991).

This recommendation is intended to protect the fetus by reducing the risk of mental retardation and perhaps childhood leukemia.

Individual Limits for Members of the Public

EFFECTIVE DOSE

The effective dose limit for members of the public is 1 mSv per year to limit the probability of stochastic effects.

LENS OF THE EYE AND SKIN

The ICRP recommends an annual equivalent dose limit of 15 mSv to the lens of the eye and 50 mSv average over any 1 cm^2 area of skin, so that detrimental deterministic effects can be prevented. This is an arbitrary reduction factor of 10.

Recommended Dose Limits: NCRP

In keeping with the recent ICRP changes in radiation dose limits, the NCRP has also revised its recommended limits for stochastic and deterministic effects for various categories of individuals, including occupationally exposed individuals and members of the public.

The new recommendations are given by the NCRP (1993) and are shown in Table 7-3.

Individual Limits for Occupational Exposure

To limit the probability of stochastic effects, the effective dose equivalent for occupationally-exposed individuals is 50 mSv per year for whole-body exposure; it is 150 mSv per year for the lens of the eye and 500 mSv per year for all other organs to prevent detrimental deterministic effects.

The cumulative exposure is governed by the following formula:

$$\text{Cumulative exposure} = 10 \text{ mSv} \times \text{age in years} \quad (7\text{-}2)$$

Individual Limits for Members of the Public

To limit the probability of stochastic effects, the annual effective dose equivalent limits for frequent and infrequent exposures are 1 and 5 mSv, respectively. To prevent detrimental deterministic effects, an annual effective dose equivalent limit of 15 mSv is recommended for the lens of the eye, and 50 mSv for the skin and extremities.

Table 7-3 also indicates dose equivalent limits in other situations. For example, for a pregnant woman, the NCRP recommends a monthly dose limit of 0.5 mSv for the embryo-fetus exposures.

TABLE 7-2. A SUMMARY OF THE RECOMMENDED DOSE LIMITS OF THE ICRP

	Dose Limit[a] (mSv)	
Application	Occupational	Public
Effective dose	20 mSv per year, averaged over defined periods of 5 years[c]	1 (in a year)[d]
Annual equivalent dose in		
Lens of the eye	150	15
Skin[b]	500	50
Hands and feet	500	—

[a] The limits apply to the sum of the relevant doses from external exposure in the specified period and the 50-year committed dose (to age 70 years for children) from intakes in the same period.

[b] The limitation on the effective dose provides sufficient protection for the skin against stochastic effects. An additional limit is needed for localized exposures to prevent deterministic effects.

[c] In special circumstances, a higher value of effective dose could be allowed in a single year, provided that the average over 5 years does not exceed 1 mSv per year.

[d] With the further provision that the effective dose should not exceed 50 mSv in any single year. Additional restrictions apply to the occupational exposure of pregnant women.

SOURCE: International Commission on Radiological Protection. (1991). *1990 recommendations of the ICRP* (ICRP Publication No. 60). Elmsford, New York: Pergamon Press. Reproduced by permission.

TABLE 7-3. A SUMMARY OF DOSE-LIMITING RECOMMENDATIONS OF THE NCRP

Occupational exposures[a]	
Effective dose limits	
Annual	50 mSv
Cumulative	10 mSv × age
Equivalent dose annual limits for tissues and organs	
Lens of eye	150 mSv
Skin, hands, and feet	500 mSv
Guidance for emergency occupational exposure[a]	
Public exposures (annual)	
Effective dose limit, continuous or frequent exposure[a]	1 mSv
Effective dose limit, infrequent exposure[a]	5 mSv
Equivalent dose limits for tissues and organs[a]	
Lens of eye	15 mSv
Skin, hands, and feet	50 mSv
Remedial action for natural sources	
Effective dose (excluding radon)	>5 mSv
Exposure to radon decay products	$>7 \times 10^{-3}$ J·hr m^{-3}
Education and training exposures (annual)[a]	
Effective dose limit	1 mSv
Equivalent dose limit for tissues and organs	
Lens of eye	15 mSv
Skin, hands, and feet	50 mSv
Embryo-fetus exposures[a] (monthly)	
Equivalent dose limit	0.5 mSv
Negligible individual dose (annual)[a]	0.01 mSv

[a] Sum of external and internal exposures but excluding doses from natural sources.

SOURCE: National Council on Radiation Protection and Measurements. (1993). *Limitation of exposure to ionizing radiation* (Report No. 116). Bethesda, MD: NCRP. Reproduced by permission.

Another special case relates to education/training situations, in which case the effective dose equivalent limit is 1 mSv per year and 15 mSv for the lens of the eye. For the skin and extremities, it is 50 mSv per year.

Recommended Dose Limits: RPB–Health Canada

The Radiation Protection Bureau (RPB)–Health Canada also has dose-limiting recommendations for radiation workers, members of the public, and individuals who fall into the special cases category.

The Canadian dose limits are listed by the Radiation Protection Bureau–Health Canada (1992). The dose limits are those that were originally published in the ICRP's 1977 Publication No. 26. At the time of writing this book, the dose limits were as follows:

1. A dose equivalent limit (whole-body) of 50 mSv per year is recommended for radiation workers, that is, occupationally exposed individuals. In addition, the average weekly limit for this group is 1 mSv.

2. The dose limit to members of the public is 5 mSv per year with the average weekly limit being 0.1 mSv.
3. For the lens of the eye, the dose limit is 0.15 Sv per year and 0.5 Sv per year for all other tissues to prevent detrimental deterministic effects.
4. For women of reproductive capacity, a dose equivalent to the abdomen of not >13 mSv per 13 weeks is recommended.
5. For a pregnant woman, the dose equivalent to the abdomen for the rest of the pregnancy should not be >15 mSv.
6. For students in training who are <18 years old, the dose equivalent should not exceed 15 mSv per year.

The revision of this code is now in progress (1993) and will reflect the recent recommendations of the ICRP (1991) with respect to dose limits (Chaloner, 1993).

Occupational Exposure Trends

Several studies have examined occupational radiation doses and trends (Hendee, 1991; Huda et al., 1991a, b; Kumazawa et al., 1984; NCRP, 1989; Nicklason et al., 1993).

The purpose of these studies is usually fourfold:

1. To verify whether occupationally exposed individuals generally exceed the recommended annual dose limits.
2. To determine the effectiveness of radiation protection programs.
3. To relate dose to risk.
4. To assist in developing regulations not only in classifying but also in monitoring radiation workers.

Early Studies

The NCRP (1989) reviewed the data from several major studies, such as the X-ray Exposure Studies of 1964 and 1970; Johnson and Associates Survey of 1973, 1979, and 1980; Radiation Experience Data, a study done in 1980 and 1981; Radiation Experience Data Study 2, conducted in 1982; and the more popular Nationwide Evaluation of X-ray Trends (NEXT). These studies are described further in Chapter 11. In this section, we shall report only the effective dose equivalent limits.

The NCRP (1989) reported an annual per capita effective dose equivalent for the U.S. population from diagnostic x-rays to be ~0.40 mSv (40 mrem) compared with 1.3 mSv (130 mrem) for Japan, 0.3 mSv (30 mrem) for the United Kingdom, and 1.4 mSv (140 mrem) for the USSR.

Another study done in the United States (Kumazawa et al., 1984), which surveyed occupationally exposed individuals in hospitals, private clinics, and dental offices, reported an average whole-body dose equivalent of 0.7 mSv (70 mrem) per year. This study also showed that 88% of the workers received <1 mSv (100 mrem) for the year with only <0.05% whose dose limit was greater than the recommended 50 mSv (5 rem) per year.

Recent Studies

Although no comprehensive U.S. survey on effective dose equivalents has been conducted recently, several investigators continue to examine occupational dose equivalents.

An interesting study is one by Huda et al. (1991a), who examined the whole-body occupational dose equivalent to medical radiation technologists in Manitoba, Canada, between the period of 1978–1988, using data from the Canadian National Dose Registry. Figure 7-2 shows the mean dose equivalent to Manitoban radiation technologists, and Table 7-4 summarizes the distribution of whole-body dose equivalent among diagnostic x-ray technologists, nuclear medicine technologists, and radiotherapy technologists.

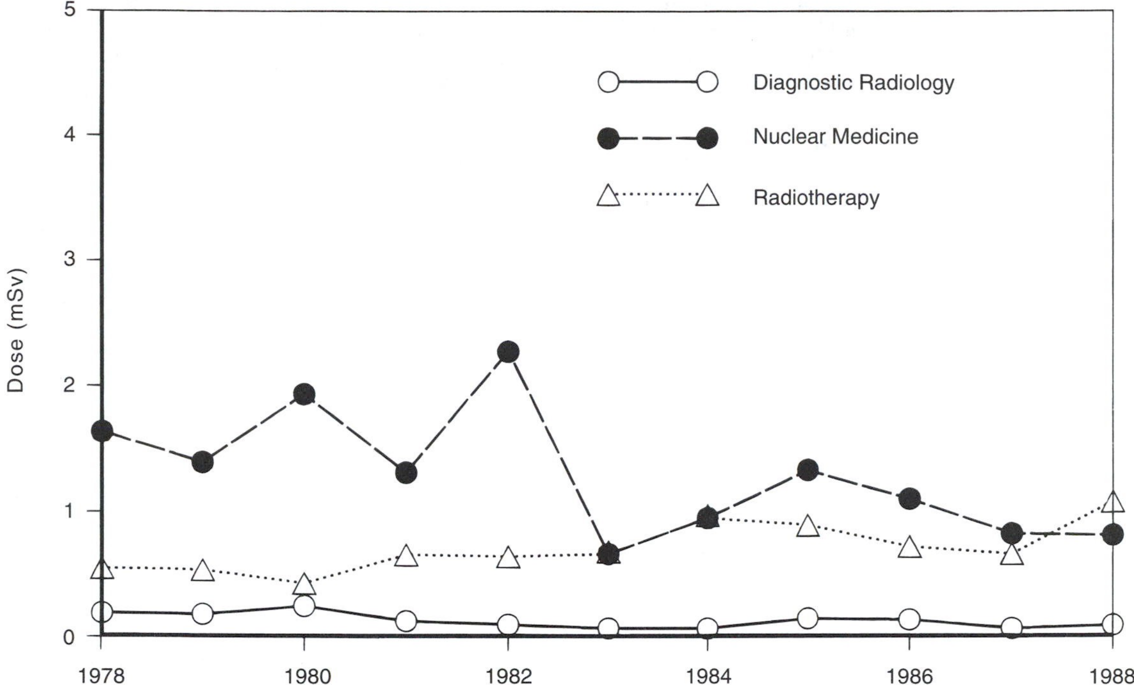

FIGURE 7-2. The mean occupational dose equivalent (whole-body) to technologists in the Canadian province of Manitoba. [From Huda, W., Bews, J., Gordon, K., Sutherland, M.D., Sont, W.N., & Ashmore, J.P. (1991a). Occupational doses to medical radiation technologists in Manitoba (1978–1988). *Canadian Journal of Medical Radiation Technology, 22,* 23. Reproduced by permission.]

These results indicate the following:

1. The average yearly dose equivalent for technologists in diagnostic radiology, nuclear medicine, and radiotherapy was 0.13, 1.30, and 0.70 mSv, respectively.
2. A total of 79% of diagnostic radiology technologists receive a dose equivalent below the minimum whole-body dose equivalent of 0.2 mSv reported by the National Dose Registry based on four dosimeter readings for 1 year.
3. A total of 13% received a yearly dose equivalent between 0.2 and 0.5 mSv.
4. No technologists received the recommended annual dose equivalent of 50 mSv.

Another study by Huda et al. (1991b) examined the occupational doses to Canadian radiologic technologists between 1978 and 1988, using data from the National Dose Registry. The researchers reported the following:

1. The minimum dose equivalent reported by RPB (Canada) was 0.2 mSv.
2. The mean annual dose equivalent for diagnostic radiology technologists, nuclear medicine technologists, and radiotherapy technologists varied around 0.2, 1.18, and 1.1 mSv, respectively, over the 11-year period.
3. No technologists received the recommended dose equivalent of 50 mSv per year.
4. The mean annual occupational whole-body dose equivalent for x-ray technologists for the last 3 years (0.14 mSv in 1986 to 0.12 mSv in 1988) was lower than for the first 3 years (0.36 mSv in 1978 to 0.28 in 1980). This

TABLE 7-4. THE DISTRIBUTION OF WHOLE-BODY DOSE EQUIVALENT RECEIVED BY RADIOTHERAPY TECHNOLOGISTS (RTs) IN DIAGNOSTIC RADIOLOGY IN THE CANADIAN PROVINCE OF MANITOBA DURING THE PERIOD OF 1978–1988[a]

Whole-Body Dose Equivalent (mSv)	X-Ray	NM	RX
0.0–0.19	3771 (78.8)	120 (36.1)	270 (45.8)
0.2–0.49	622 (13.0)	36 (10.8)	84 (14.2)
0.5–0.99	227 (4.7)	53 (16.0)	78 (13.2)
1.0–1.99	105 (2.2)	47 (14.2)	95 (16.1)
2.0–4.99	56 (1.2)	70 (21.1)	61 (10.3)
5.0–29.9	7 (0.1)	6 (1.8)	2 (0.3)
30–49.9	0 (0.0)	0 (0.0)	0 (0.0)
>50.0	0 (0.0)	0 (0.0)	0 (0.0)

[a] The values in parentheses refer to the percentage of the total number of RTs in a particular category.

NM = Nuclear Medicine; RX = Radiation Therapy.

SOURCE: Huda, W., Bews, J., Gordon, K., Sutherland, M.D., Sont, W.N., & Ashmore, J.P. Occupational doses to medical radiation technologists in Manitoba (1978–1988). *Canadian Journal of Medical Radiation Technology, 22*, 23. Reproduced by permission.

reduction could have been attributed to several improvements in radiation protection practices, such as improved shielding and adherence to the ALARA principle.

Feygelman et al. (1992) conducted a study to investigate the effective dose equivalent (H_E) to patients undergoing cerebral angiography. They examined contributions from fluoroscopy, cut film, and digital subtraction angiography (DSA) and subsequently compared the doses with plain film skull radiography, CT, and nuclear medicine.

The study showed that the average H_E was 10.6 mSv, with values ranging from 2.7 to 23.4 mSv; contributions from fluoroscopy, cut film, and DSA to the total H_E were 67, 26, and 7%, respectively. The investigators concluded that patients undergoing diagnostic cerebral angiography and those involved in nuclear medicine brain studies have comparable radiation doses typically of ~10 mSv. They also noted that a patient receiving a plain skull x-ray receives a much lower dose of radiation (~0.15 mSv) than a patient undergoing CT (2 mSv).

Yet another study examined the annual effective dose received by interventional radiologists. This study was done by Niklason et al. (1993), who studied 35 interventional radiologists from 17 institutions. The radiologists wore dosimeters over the lead apron at the level of the collar and under the apron at waist level, for a 2-month period.

The mean effective dose is reported in Table 7-5. The mean annual effective dose ranged from 0.37 to 10.1 mSv, with an average annual effective dose of 3.16 mSv. This dose is well below the limit of 50 mSv per year currently recommended by the NCRP.

As Low as Reasonably Achievable (ALARA)

The studies just cited demonstrate that recommended dose limits for occupationally exposed individuals are being met. It would appear that technologists and radiologists alike give careful consideration to the three principles of radiation

TABLE 7-5. THE MEAN EFFECTIVE DOSE TO 35 INTERNATIONAL RADIOLOGISTS[a]

Region	Effective Dose (mSv)	
	With Thyroid Shield[b]	Without Thyroid Shield[c]
Head and neck	0.40 (0.02–0.97)	2.61 (0.14–6.34)
Extremities	0.63 (0.03–1.53)	0.63 (0.03–1.53)
Under apron (whole-body)	0.88 (0.22–4.11)	0.88 (0.22–4.11)
Total	1.91 (0.37–5.75)	4.12 (0.48–10.1)

[a] Values in parentheses are ranges.

[b] Values are for all 28 radiologists assuming all participants wear a thyroid shield.

[c] Values are for all 28 radiologists assuming none of the participants wears a thyroid shield.

SOURCE: Nicklason, L. T., Marx, M. V., & Chan, H.P. (1993). Interventional radiologists: Occupational radiation doses and risks. *Radiology, 187*, 729. Reproduced by permission.

protection in an effort to protect themselves as well as their patients.

Although technologists and radiologists take care to justify all patient exposure to radiation based on the expectation of a positive net benefit, as well as observe recommended dose limitations, it is their rigorous commitment to keeping exposure ALARA that is by and large responsible for success of their efforts.

To uphold the ALARA standard, the technologist and the radiologist must ensure that the lowest possible exposures are used to image patients without compromising image quality. Technical factors such as correct collimation and exposure technique factors (mAs and kVp), for example, are optimized to produce diagnostic quality images.

Magnetic Resonance Imaging: Exposure Limits

The basic principles of magnetic resonance imaging (MRI) were introduced in Chapter 1. (See Chapter 12 for an in-depth treatment of the safety aspects of MRI.) In MRI, the patient is exposed to three fields: a static magnetic field, a changing (or time-varying) magnetic field, and radiowaves [radiofrequency (RF) energy]. The technologist, on the other hand, is exposed when preparing the patient for a scan in the MRI room.

Although there are no current adverse biological effects in patients undergoing MR examinations using established protocols and exposure factors, safety considerations and exposure limits for guidelines have been issued.

The safety limits of concern relate to the exposure to all three physical fields operating in MRI. The static magnetic field is measured in Tesla (T), the time-varying gradient magnetic field is measured in Tesla per second (T/s), and radiowaves are measured in watts per kilogram (W/kg).

The limits of exposure to these fields have been issued to allay concerns that biological effects may be produced. For example, membrane permeability and nerve conduction may be altered when exposed to strong magnetic fields. In addition, some patients have experienced flashes of light when exposed to the time-varying gradient magnetic field. Exposure to this field may also cause cardiac fibrillation. Finally, radiowaves can cause tissue heating depending on the exposure. Such heating can be described by the *specific absorption rate* (SAR), which is measured in *watts per kilogram* (W/kg).

Exposure limits have been recommended by the U.S. National Center for Devices and Radiological Health as well as other radiation protection agencies in Canada, the United Kingdom, and the Federal Republic of Germany. In the United States, for example, the exposure limits for the static magnetic field, the changing gradient magnetic field, and radiowaves are 2 T, 3 T/s and 0.4 W/kg, respectively, to the whole body with a maximum of 2 W/kg. These will be discussed in some detail in Chapter 12.

REVIEW QUESTIONS

1. Which of the following is defined as a dose of x-rays that would produce a reddening of the skin in 10 to 14 days following exposure to radiation?
   A. Erythema dose.
   B. Tolerance dose.
   C. Maximum permissible dose.
   D. Dose equivalent.

2. Which of the following suggests a threshold dose below which no radiation damage would occur?
   A. Erythema dose.
   B. Tolerance dose.
   C. Maximum permissible dose.
   D. Dose equivalent.

3. The tolerance dose was replaced by the term:
   A. Erythema dose.
   B. Maximum permissible dose.
   C. Dose equivalent.
   D. Effective dose.

4. The formula for computing the maximum permissible dose (MPD) knowing the age (N), in years, of the individual is:
   A. MPD = N − 18 rem.
   B. MPD = 5N − 18 rem.
   C. MPD = 5(N + 18) rem.
   D. MPD = 5(N − 18) rem.

5. Which of the following has replaced the maximum permissible dose formula?
   A. 10 Sv × age in years.
   B. 10 Sv + age in years.
   C. 10 mSv × age in years.
   D. 10 mSv − age in years.

6. In 1977, the ICRP replaced the term maximum permissible dose with the term:
   A. Justification.
   B. Effective dose.
   C. Optimization.
   D. Dose equivalent limit.

7. The more comprehensive system of radiation protection of the ICRP includes all of the following except:
   A. Justification (net benefit).
   B. Optimization (ALARA).
   C. Maximum permissible dose.
   D. Dose limitation.

8. Which of the following terms is used to relate the risk of exposure of a portion of the body to that of exposure to the whole body?
   A. Roentgen.
   B. Gray.
   C. Effective dose.
   D. Tolerance dose.

9. The most recent terminology of the ICRP and NCRP used to relate to occupational dose limits is the:
   A. Equivalent dose.
   B. Dose equivalent.
   C. Optimization.
   D. Effective dose.

10. Dose limits have been established for:
    A. Whole-body exposure.
    B. Partial-body, as well as organ, exposures.
    C. Population exposure.
    D. All of the above.

11. Dose limits have been established for:

A. Occupationally exposed individuals.
B. Members of the public.
C. Students in training and the embryo-fetus.
D. All of the above.

12. The effective dose limit of the ICRP for occupationally exposed individuals is:
    A. 50 Sv per year.
    B. 20 mSv per year averaged over 5 years.
    C. 20 Sv per year averaged over 5 years.
    D. 50 mSv per year.

13. The ICRP effective dose limit for members of the public is:
    A. 1 mSv in a year.
    B. 20 mSv in a year.
    C. 50 mSv in a year.
    D. None of the above is correct.

14. The annual equivalent dose limit (ICRP) to the lens of the eye is:
    A. 150 mSv.
    B. 150 Sv.
    C. 500 Sv.
    D. 500 mSv.

15. The annual equivalent dose limit of the ICRP to the skin of members of the public is:
    A. 50 Sv.
    B. 150 mSv.
    C. 500 mSv.
    D. 50 mSv.

16. The annual effective dose limit of the NCRP for occupationally exposed individuals is:
    A. 20 mSv.
    B. 50 mSv.
    C. 50 Sv.
    D. 10 mSv × age in years.

17. The cumulative effective dose limit of the NCRP for occupationally exposed individuals is:
    A. 20 mSv.
    B. 50 mSv.
    C. 150 mSv.
    D. 10 mSv × age in years.

18. The NCRP annual equivalent dose limit for the skin, hands, and feet of occupationally exposed individuals is:
    A. 50 mSv.
    B. 10 mSv.
    C. 150 mSv.
    D. 500 mSv.

19. The NCRP effective dose limit for members of the public is:
    A. 20 mSv per year.
    B. 1 mSv per year.
    C. 5 mSv per year for continuous or frequent exposure.
    D. 50 mSv per year.

20. The monthly equivalent dose limit of the NCRP for the embryo-fetus is:
    A. 5 mSv.
    B. 5 Sv.
    C. 0.5 mSv.
    D. 0.01 mSv.

21. The Canadian annual dose equivalent limit for occupationally exposed individuals is:
    A. 20 Sv.
    B. 50 Sv.
    C. 50 mSv.
    D. 150 mSv.

22. The annual dose equivalent limit to members of the public in Canada is:
    A. 5 Sv.
    B. 5 mSv.
    C. 0.5 mSv.
    D. 0.15 Sv.

23. To prevent detrimental deterministic effects to the lens of the eye, the Canadian dose equivalent limit is:
    A. 0.15 Sv per year.
    B. 0.15 mSv per year.
    C. 150 mSv per year.
    D. 0.5 Sv per year.

24. In Canada, the annual dose equivalent limit for all other tissues except the lens of the eye is:
    A. 0.15 Sv.
    B. 0.15 mSv.
    C. 10 mSv.
    D. 0.5 Sv.

25. In Canada, the dose equivalent limit to the abdomen of women of reproductive capacity is not more than ℞ per 13 weeks:
    A. 13 Sv.
    B. 130 mSv.
    C. 13 mSv.
    D. 20 mSv.

26. The Canadian dose equivalent limit for students in training who are younger than 18 years:
    A. Should not exceed 15 mSv per year.
    B. Should not exceed 0.15 Sv per year.
    C. Should not exceed 20 mSv per year.
    D. Should add up to 50 mSv per year.

27. Occupational dose and trends studies are done to:
    A. Verify whether dose limits are exceeded.
    B. Determine the effectiveness of radiation protection programs.
    C. Relate dose to risk.
    D. All of the above.

28. The annual effective dose equivalent for the U.S. population from diagnostic x-rays as reported by the NCRP in 1989 is:
    A. 1.3 mSv.
    B. 0.40 mSv.
    C. 0.30 mSv.
    D. 1.4 mSv.

29. The concern for safety in magnetic resonance imaging (MRI) stems from exposure to:
    A. Static magnetic field.
    B. Time-varying gradient magnetic fields.
    C. Radiowaves.
    D. All of the above.

30. The units of specific absorption rate (SAR) are:
    A. Watts per kilogram (W/kg).
    B. Coulombs per kilogram (C/kg).
    C. Tesla per second (T/s).
    D. Watts per meter squared (W/m^2).

31. In the United States, the exposure limit for the static magnetic fields used in MRI is:
    A. 2 T.
    B. 3 T.
    C. 10 T.
    D. 4 T.

32. In the United States, the exposure limit for changing gradient magnetic fields used in MRI is:
    A. 1 T/s.
    B. 2 T/s.
    C. 3 T/s.
    D. 10 T/s.

33. In the United States, the exposure limit for radiowaves used in MRI is:
    A. 40 W/kg.
    B. 0.4 W/m^2.
    C. 0.4 W/kg.
    D. 0.04 W/kg.

REFERENCES

Biological Effects of Ionizing Radiations Committee. (1990). *Health effects of exposures to low levels of ionizing radiation* (BEIR V). New York: National Academy Press.

Bushong, S. (1993). *Radiologic science for radiologic technologists* (5th ed.). St. Louis: Mosby-Year Book.

Chaloner, P. (1993). *Personal communications.* Ottawa: Radiation Protection Bureau–Health Canada.

Edwards, M. (1991). Development of radiation protection standards. *Radiographics, 11,* 699.

Feygelman, V.M., Huda, W. & Peters, K.R. (1992). Effective dose equivalents to patients undergoing cerebral angiography. *American Journal of Neuroradiology, 13,* 845.

Hendee, W.R. (1991). Personal and public perceptions of radiation risks. *Radiographics, 11*, 1109.

Huda, W., Bews, J., Gordon, K., et al. (1991a). Occupational doses to medical radiation technologists in Manitoba (1978–1988). *Canadian Journal of Medical Radiation Technologists, 22*, 23.

Huda, W., Bews, J., Gordon, K., Sutherland, M.D., Sont, W.N. & Ashmore, J.P. (1991b). Doses and population irradiation factors for Canadian radiation technologists. *Canadian Association of Radiologists Journal, 42*, 247.

International Commission on Radiological Protection. (1977). Recommendations of the ICRP. (ICRP Publication No. 26). Elmsford, NY: Pergamon Press.

International Commission on Radiological Protection. (1991). *1990 recommendations of the ICRP* (ICRP Publication No. 60). Elmsford, New York: Pergamon Press.

Kumazawa, S., Nelson, D.R., & Richardson, A.C. (1984). Occupational exposure to ionizing radiation in the United States: A comprehensive review for the year 1980 and a summary of trends for the years 1960–1985 (Environmental Protection Agency 520/1-84-005). Springfield National Technical Information Service.

National Council on Radiation Protection and Measurements. (1987). Recommendations on Limits for Exposure to Ionizing Radiation (NCRP Report No. 91). Bethesda, MD: NCRP.

National Council on Radiation Protection and Measurements. (1989). *Exposure of the U.S. population from diagnostic medical radiation* (Report No. 100). Bethesda, MD: NCRP.

National Council on Radiation Protection and Measurements. (1993). *Limitation of exposure to ionizing radiation* (Report No. 116). Bethesda, MD: NCRP.

Nicklason, L. T., Marx, M.V., & Chan, H.P. (1993). International radiologists: Occupational radiation doses and risks. *Radiology, 187*, 729.

Radiation Protection Bureau–Health Canada. (1992). *Safety code SC20A: X-ray equipment in medical diagnosis, Part A: Recommended safety procedures for installation and use.* Ottawa: Health Protection Branch, Environmental Health Directorate.

Zankl, M., Petoussi, N., & Drexler, G. (1992). Effective dose and effective dose equivalent. The impact of the new ICRP definition for external photon irradiation. *Health Physics, 62*, 395.

CHAPTER EIGHT

Factors Affecting Dose in X-ray Imaging

Learning Objectives

Upon completion of this chapter, the reader should be able to:

1. Identify the basic exposure components of a radiographic system that affect dose.
2. Identify the basic components of exposure of a fluoroscopic system that affect dose.
3. Identify the exposure components of a computed tomography (CT) system that affect dose.
4. Discuss the responsibilities of radiation workers when conducting radiographic examinations on patients.
5. List 16 major factors affecting dose in radiography and explain how each of these affect the dose to the patient.
6. Explain one strategy for minimizing errors during radiologic examinations.
7. Describe the elements of shielding radiosensitive organs during radiography.
8. Explain the major elements of a fluoroscopic examination.
9. State the range of kVp and mA used in fluoroscopy.
10. Explain the meaning of the following terms and how each affects dose in fluoroscopy: pulsed fluoroscopy, high-level-control fluoroscopy, grids, magnification, last image hold, image recording techniques, and C-arm fluoroscopy.
11. Explain how the technologist can reduce dose during a fluoroscopic examination.
12. List the factors affecting dose in CT.
13. Explain the influence of each of the following on dose in CT: kVp and mAs, filtration, collimation, tube motion, detector efficiency, spatial resolution, and slice thickness.
14. Explain the influence of each of the following on dose in mammography: technique factors, tube target, filtration, image receptor type, thickness and shape of the breast, and source-to-image receptor distance.

Introduction

Radiation protection in diagnostic radiology is concerned with minimizing radiation dose to patients, personnel, and members of the public. To accomplish this goal, it is necessary for the technologist to have a firm understanding of each of the following: (1) the factors affecting radiation dose and (2) the guidelines and recommendations for the safe use of radiation in diagnostic radiology.

This chapter addresses the former, specifically the clinical and general technical factors affecting dose. Additionally, specific factors affecting dose in radiography, fluoroscopy, mammography, and computed tomography (CT) are highlighted. The guidelines and recommendations for the safe use of radiation in diagnostic radiology are discussed in Chapter 9.

Imaging System Exposure Components Affecting Dose

Components of Exposure in Radiographic Systems

The basic components of patient exposure in a radiographic imaging system are illustrated in Figure 1-3. The important considerations with respect to radiation dose are as follows:

1. The technologist selects exposure technique factors (kVP, mA, and exposure time in seconds) for the appropriate radiographic examination.
2. The radiation beam emanating from the x-ray tube is a broad beam (open beam geometry), which is first filtered and subsequently collimated to the area of interest on the patient.

3. During the exposure, the beam is fixed in one position (area of interest) on the patient.
4. The beam passes through the patient, tabletop, and grid and subsequently falls upon the image receptor (film/screen combination), the sensitivity of which affects the dose to the patient.
5. Patient positioning varies. The patient may assume the anterior-posterior (AP), posterior-anterior (PA), or oblique positions during the examination.
6. The exposed films are processed in a chemical processor.

Components of Exposure in Fluoroscopic Systems

The components of patient exposure in a fluoroscopic imaging system are shown in Figure 8-1. In terms of radiation dose to the patient during a fluoroscopic examination, the following points are to be noted:

1. Fluoroscopic technique factors (kVp, mA) must be selected for the examination.
2. The radiologist first performs the examination by collimating the beam and moving it along and across the patient, to image the anatomy of interest (e.g., the upper and lower gastrointestinal tract). Patient positioning may range from PA, AP, to lateral positions. During the fluoroscopic portion of the examination, the radiologist records several spot films of the anatomy. These types of spot films are exposed using radiographic technique factors. The system switches from fluoroscopic technique factors (low tube currents and high kVp) to radiographic technique factors (higher tube currents and high kVp) and subsequently back to the fluoroscopic mode of operation. (See Major Elements of a Fluoroscopic Examination for a sequential listing of the necessary steps.)

   In performing the examination, the radiologist may also choose to use the magnification technique to enhance recording of anatomical details.
3. After completion of the fluoroscopic portion of the examination, the technologist then performs a radiographic examination by exposing several large format "overhead" films. In this case, radiographic exposure technique factors are used.
4. While the image receptor in fluoroscopy is the image intensifier tube, the radiographic portion of the examination utilizes a film-screen image receptor.
5. The films obtained in a fluoroscopic examination are processed in a chemical processor.

Components of Exposure in CT Systems

The scheme for exposing the patient in CT is shown in Figure 1-5. There are several noteworthy points regarding this method of exposure:

1. The x-ray beam is highly collimated (narrow beam geometry) to pass through a thin cross section of the patient.
2. The x-ray tube rotates around the patient to collect transmission measurements (attenuation data) for computer reconstruction of images.
3. Radiographic exposure technique factors (kVp, mAs) are used to image the patient.
4. The beam emanating from the x-ray tube is shaped, filtered, and collimated before passing through the patient.
5. On passing through the patient, the x-ray beam falls upon special detectors whose properties differ from those of film-screen image receptors.
6. Generally, the patient assumes an AP position for most examinations.
7. Several sections of the patient may be scanned for one complete examination.
8. Images are recorded onto magnetic tapes or disks and laser optical disks, or they may be recorded onto x-ray films. These films are then processed in a chemical processor.

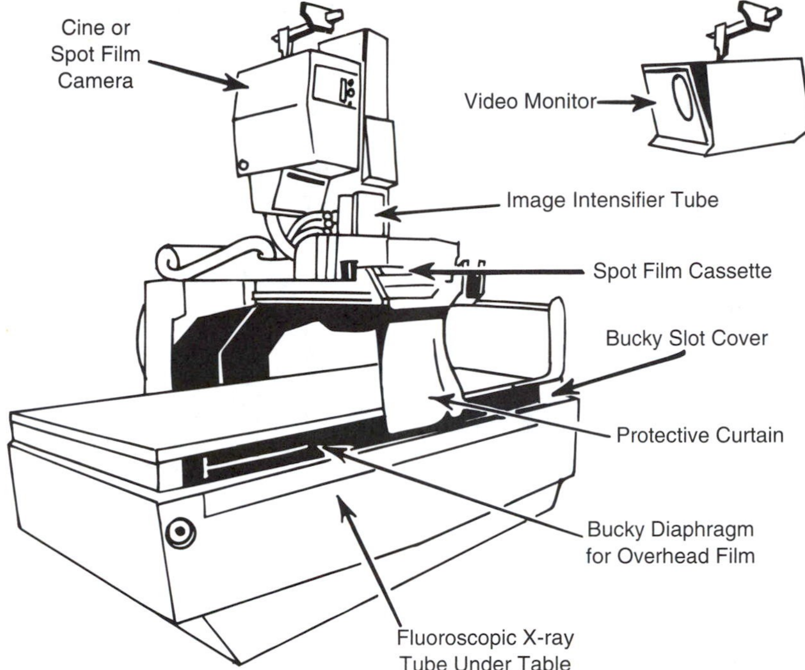

FIGURE 8-1. The components of fluoroscopic equipment. In this system, the x-ray tube is under the table. The spot film device contains a film cassette that is exposed to radiographic exposure technique factors. The images displayed on the video monitor and those recorded by cine and/or the spot film camera are based on exposure to fluoroscopic technique factors. [From Bushong, S. (1993). *Radiographic science for technologists* (5th ed.). St. Louis: Mosby–Year Book. Reproduced by permission.]

Clinical Factors

Clinical factors refer to the overall responsibilities of the individuals involved in exposing patients to radiation. These responsibilities relate not only to the prescription of the x-ray examination but also to the nontechnical procedural aspects such as patient care, communications, and comfort. The individuals who shoulder the responsibility for determining the nature and extent of a patient's radiologic examination are the referring physician, the radiologist, and the technologist. The patient first sees the referring physician (family physician or the emergency physician), who prescribes the x-ray examination based on a physical/clinical examination of the patient. Next, the patient arrives in the radiology department and, depending on the type of procedure, may come in contact with the technologist and/or radiologist, or both. While the technologist is responsible for performing the radiographic examination, the radiologist, with the assistance of the technologist, assumes the responsibility for performing examinations that require fluoroscopy.

Responsibility of Referring Physicians

Having examined the patient clinically, the referring physician prescribes the x-ray examination. Generally, the physician indicates on a requisition form the clinical justification for the x-ray examination. For example, a chest x-ray is justified if the patient suffers from an inflammatory disease (pneumonia), a traumatic problem (pneumothorax), or a neoplastic disease (bronchogenic carcinoma) of the respiratory system. It is important that the physician provide enough clinical data regarding the patient's condition because this information enables both the radiologist and technologist to carry out the appropriate x-ray procedure.

Role of the Technologist

The role of technologists in medical radiography is clear. They must be trained in the art and science of radiography and maintain an understanding of new instrumentation and procedures. Technologists apply a knowledge of anatomy and physiology, physics, instrumentation, radiobiology and radiation protection, pathology, and radiographic technique and positioning to the successful completion of an x-ray examination. Communication and interpersonal skills are also vital to the technologist for successful completion of the daily activities that accompany radiologic procedures. In summary, the technologist is responsible for performing the radiographic examination on the patient, as well as for using the clinical information provided by the patient's physician and the protocols established by the radiology department.

Role of the Radiologist

Radiologists perform fluoroscopic examinations with the assistance of the technologist. Radiologists communicate with the patient's physician to tailor the x-ray examination to the needs of the patient. They also communicate to the patient all details related to the procedure. The radiologist and technologist work together to expedite the examination and to ensure patient safety and comfort before, during, and after the examination.

The responsibilities of the radiologist, the patient's physician (referring physician), and the role of the technologist are further elaborated in Appendix 8-1.

Responsibility of the Patient

The patient must also assume some degree of responsibility for ensuring that the examination is conducted expeditiously. This means that:

1. Patients must first understand the instructions provided by the technologist.
2. Patients must follow all instructions during the conduct of the examination.
3. Patients should cooperate with personnel to ensure successful completion of the examination.

The technologist should ensure that patients understand the significance of these requirements before and during the examination.

Factors in Radiography

There are several factors affecting patient dose in radiography. However, only the major technical factors are discussed in this chapter. These factors are illustrated in Figure 8-2 and include exposure technique factors, x-ray generator waveform, filtration, collimation and beam alignment, source-to-skin distance, source-to-image receptor distance, patient thickness and density, tabletop material, grids, image receptor sensitivity, and film processing.

Each of these are now explained briefly.

Exposure Technique Factors

Recall that during x-ray production electrons are "boiled off" the filament of the cathode and are accelerated across the x-ray tube to strike the target of the anode. Upon striking the target, a beam of x-rays is produced. This beam, the useful beam, is a heterogeneous beam of radiation that is transmitted through the patient to produce an image.

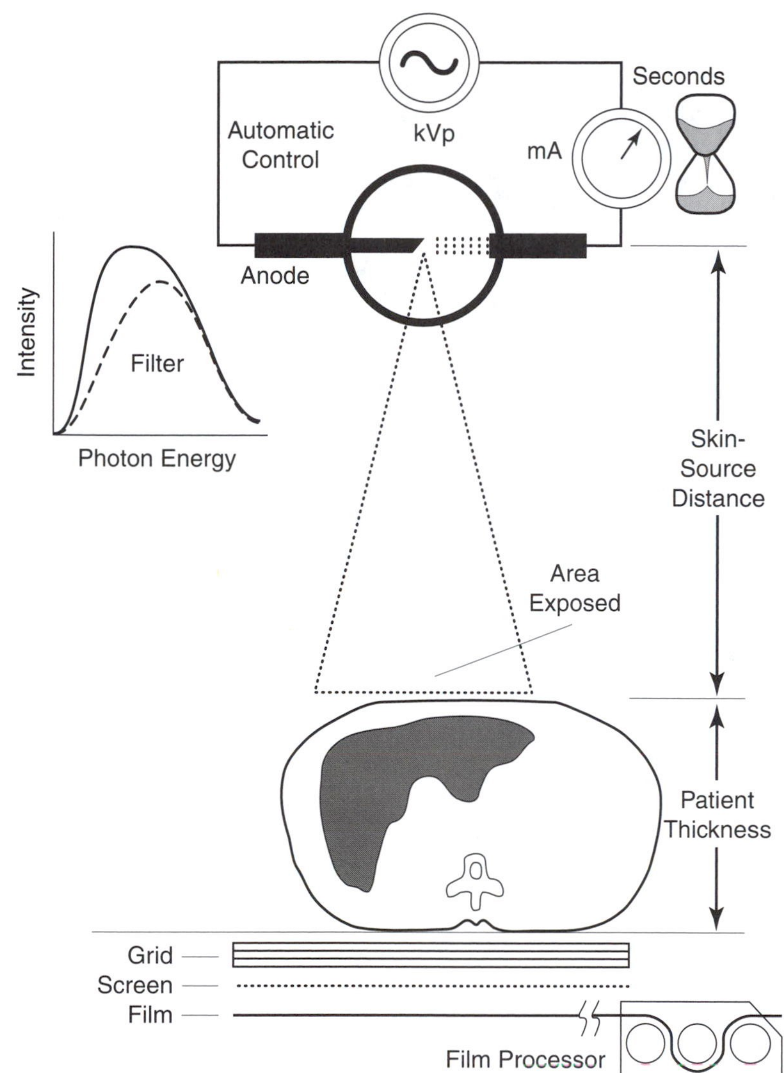

FIGURE 8-2. Major technical factors affecting patient dose in diagnostic radiology. [From Myers, M.F. (1993). Radiation doses: The ranges of radiation dose that are given to a patient with a particular procedure, the principal factors that affect the dose, and the methods of measuring sub-doses. In: Wooten, R. (ed.). Radiation Protection of Patients. Cambridge University Press: Cambridge, England. Reproduced by permission.]

The photons of a heterogeneous beam have different energies ranging from low to high. Whereas the high-energy photons pass through the patient to strike the image receptor and produce the image, the low-energy photons do not have enough energy to penetrate the patient. They are absorbed by the patient and subsequently contribute to patient dose.

Exposure technique factors are characterized by the tube potential, defined by the kilovolts (kVp); the tube current, defined by the milliamperage (mA); and the exposure time in seconds (s). The kilovoltage not only determines the speed of the electrons striking the target but also the energy of the photons (quality of the radiation beam) emanating from the x-ray tube. The mA, which is the flow of electrons across the tube, is the primary determinant of the quantity of photons falling on the patient. The exposure time, on the other hand, refers to the duration (in seconds) of exposing the patient to the radiation beam.

These three technique factors (kVp, mA, and time) not only determine the quality and quantity of the radiation beam needed to produce an image, but they also affect the radiation dose to the patient. In addition, these factors are under the direct control of the technologist, who must be able to optimize image quality while minimizing the radiation dose to the patient. This can be accomplished through the selection of the best combination of kVp and mAs (mA × s) needed for a particular examination.

kVp

The kVp affects the penetrating power of the radiation beam. A beam produced by a high kVp is much more penetrating than a beam produced by a low kVp. This affects the dose deposited in the patient as shown in Figure 8-3. Wolbarst (1993) has two arguments for explaining the differential in deposited dose as a function of the penetrating power of the beam. The first is that with low kVp techniques more dose is deposited in a larger area of the patient (Fig. 8-3B) because the photons do not have enough energy to penetrate the entire thickness of the patient. On the other hand, as shown in Figure 8-3A, high kVp techniques result in less dose deposited in the tissues because the photons have a high enough energy to penetrate the tissues and get to the film. He also explains that of the two interactions of radiation with matter that are of importance in radiology, the photoelectric effect predominates at lower kVP techniques, particularly in tissues with high atomic numbers, such as bone. As a result, there is more absorption of the radiation beam (dose) in tissues with high atomic numbers.

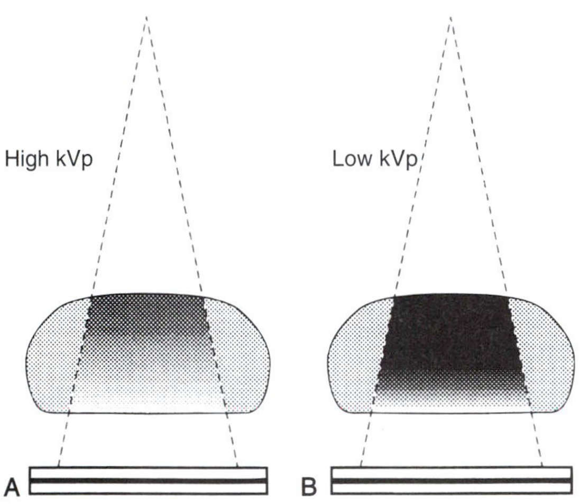

FIGURE 8-3. The influence of kVp on the dose deposited in the patient: high kVp (A) and low kVp (B). [From Wolbarst, A.B. (1993). *Physics of radiology*. Norwalk, CT: Appleton & Lange. Reproduced by permission.]

mA

mA primarily affects the quantity of radiation coming from the tube. Because the quantity of radiation is directly proportional to the mA, doubling the mA doubles the radiation quantity (hence dose) to the patient.

EXPOSURE TIME

The dose delivered to the patient during a radiographic examination is directly proportional to the exposure time. Recall the relationship:

$$\text{Exposure} = \text{Exposure rate} \times \text{Time}$$

Thus, if the exposure time is doubled, the exposure (dose) to the patient will also be doubled.

mAs

mAs is the product of mA and time, in seconds (s). The quantity of radiation is influenced by the mAs of the exposure technique. Such quantity is directly proportional to the mAs; hence, if the mAs is doubled, the quantity of radiation (dose to the patient) doubles. Techniques based on high kVp require a subsequent reduction in the mAs; hence, high kVp techniques result in a reduced dose to the patient.

AUTOMATIC EXPOSURE CONTROL

Automatic exposure control timing systems were developed to solve exposure technique problems experienced with manual exposure timing systems. Such problems arise as a result of variations in patient types, patient pathologies, and tube aging, for example. Automatic exposure control (AEC) ensures that a preselected amount of radiation reaches the film and in this manner provides correct exposures regardless of the problems mentioned earlier. Repeat exposures are subsequently minimized. AEC devices are not completely "fail-safe" and therefore require that the technologist be trained in the correct use during radiography employing AEC.

X-Ray Generator Waveform

In Figure 8-4, the voltage across the x-ray tube and the relative x-ray intensity and energy are shown. It is clear that as the voltage rises from zero to some maximum (in this case, 100 kVp), the x-ray intensity and energy also rise from zero to some maximum value. This production can be characterized by the voltage waveform of the x-ray generator. In Figure 8-5, five different waveforms are illustrated. An important characteristic of a voltage waveform is its *ripple*, or the way in which the voltage is supplied to the x-ray tube. As the percentage ripple decreases, the generator is said to be more effi-

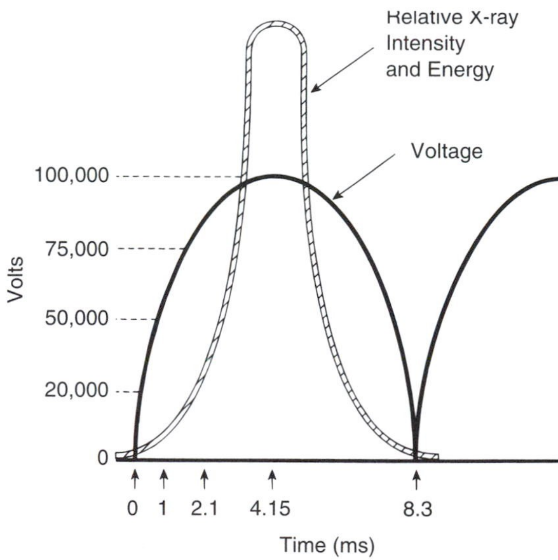

FIGURE 8-4. The voltage waveform across the x-ray tube rises from zero to some maximum value (100,000 volts) and results in x-ray production, which is at its maximum only when the voltage reaches its maximum value. [From Bushong, S. (1993). *Radiologic science for technologists* (5th ed.). St. Louis: Mosby–Year Book. Reproduced by permission.]

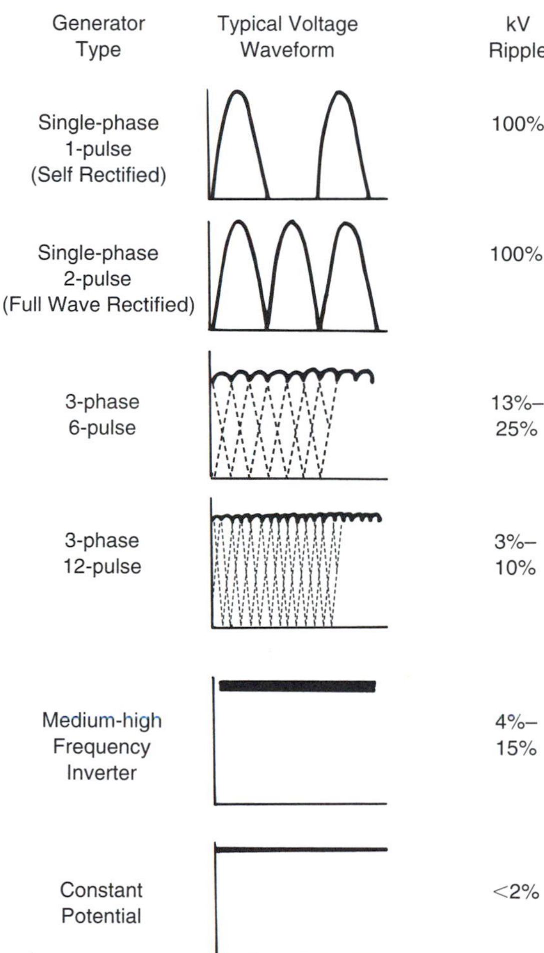

FIGURE 8-5. Several x-ray generator types and their associated voltage waveform and percentage ripple. [From Bushberg, J.T., Siebert, J.A., Leidholdt, Jr., E.M., & Boone, J.M. (1994). *The essential physics of medical imaging*. Baltimore: Williams & Wilkins. Reproduced by permission.]

cient in terms of x-ray production. A ripple of 4% indicates that the x-ray tube voltage never drops below 96% of the maximum value. A ripple of $<2\%$ indicates that the tube voltage is almost constant.

This efficiency implies that patient dose and hence exposure technique factors (kVp and mAs) are related to the type of voltage waveform. Three-phase and high frequency generators are much more efficient at x-ray production than single-phase generators (see Chapter 2). The high frequency generator, however, produces greater x-ray intensity and greater effective energy compared with single-phase and three-phase x-ray generators. This means that shorter exposure times (hence mAs) are possible with high frequency generators. For example, the exposure techniques (kVp and mAs) for an abdomen examination using single-phase equipment and three-phase (6-pulse) units are 74 kVp/40 mAs and 72 kVp/34 mAs, respectively. With a high frequency generator, the equivalent technique is 70 kVp/24 mAs (Bushong, 1993).

Filtration

The x-ray beam emerging from the x-ray tube is a heterogeneous beam. This means that the beam consists of low-energy photons and high-energy photons. Whereas the high-energy photons penetrate the patient to form the image, the low-energy photons do not contribute to image formation. They are merely absorbed by the tissue, thus increasing the dose to the patient.

These low-energy photons can be selectively removed by inserting metal absorbers (e.g., aluminum) in the beam before it strikes the patient. These absorbers are called *filters* and the absorption or removal of the low-energy photons is referred to as *filtration.*

There are two types of filtration: inherent and added. The former type of filtration is accomplished by the x-ray tube itself, which consists of the glass envelope and insulating oil; the latter is so named to acknowledge the addition of a specified thickness of aluminum outside the x-ray tube (close to the tube port). The total filtration is computed as follows:

$$\text{Total filtration} = \text{Inherent filtration} + \text{Added filtration}$$

Recommendations for total permanent filtration are presented in Chapter 10.

Filtration is the selective removal of low-energy photons from the radiation beam, and it is intended to protect the patient from radiation. The result of filtration is a reduction of the x-ray intensity and an increase in the effective energy of the beam (the beam becomes harder and therefore more penetrating). Specifically, filtration reduces patient skin dose (Wootton, 1993). This reduction has been demonstrated in a study by Burns and Renner (1993), who investigated the use of a molybdenum/aluminum filter to reduce entrance skin dose. Their results are shown in Table 8-1.

Collimation and Field Size

The term collimation refers to a method of defining the size and shape of the primary beam so that it covers only the region of anatomical interest. The area covered by the beam falling on the patient is the *field size* or more specifically the *field of view* (FOV) (Fig. 1-3).

The purpose of collimation is to protect the patient from unnecessary radiation by limiting the field size to the anatomy of interest (Fig. 8-6). Limiting the field size to the smallest practicable area results in a decrease in the total radiation energy to the patient because the surface integral exposure (total radiation) is directly proportional to the size of the irradiated area, as illustrated in Figure 8-7. Even though both patients are exposed to 100 mR of radiation, the patient to the right is exposed to 10 times more radiation than the patient on the left, simply because the dose is delivered over a larger surface area (Sprawls, 1995). In describing an examination of the lumbosacral junction, Dowd (1994)

TABLE 8-1. THE REDUCTION OF ENTRANCE SKIN EXPOSURE FOR DIFFERENT TYPES OF FILTERS: SINGLE AND THREE-PHASE GENERATORS AT 80 kVp FOR NIOBIUM AND NIOBIUM (Nb)/ALUMINUM (Al) STACKS COMPARED WITH 2.5 mm ALUMINUM

	Single-Phase (%)		Three-Phase (%)	
	ESE	Tube Load	ESE	Tube Load
Nb only	+9	+5	+5	+5
Nb + 1 mm Al	−23	+18	−20	+10
Nb + 2 mm Al	−27	+33	−28	+21
Nb + 3 mm Al	−40	+44	−36	+26

SOURCE: Burns, C.B., Renner, J.B., Gratale, P., & Moyle, L.A. (1993). Niobium/aluminum filters reduce patient exposure. *Radiologic Technology, 63*, 170–174. Reproduced by permission.

reported that simply collimating the beam down from a field size of 8″ × 10″ to a field size of 6″ × 6″ decreases the surface exposure by >50%. Collimation also decreases not only the bone marrow and gonadal doses but reduces the genetically significant dose by about 65% (Travis, 1989). Last, but not least in terms of protecting the patient, collimation is an effective means of assuring that the dose meets the all-important ALARA standard.

Beam Alignment

To avoid unnecessary radiation of the patient, the light-field of the collimator and the radiation beam must be in perfect alignment. If these two fields do not coincide, the anatomical region of interest may not be included because of beam "cut off," and the patient receives unnecessary radiation because of beam "overlap."

Source-to-Image Receptor Distance/Source-to-Skin Distance

The *source-to-image receptor distance* (SID) is the distance from the focal spot of the x-ray tube to the film cassette. For most radiographic examinations, the SID is set at 101 cm (40″). As the SID [and source-to-skin distance (SSD)] decrease, the divergence of the beam increases. (See Fig. 8-8 for a graphic comparison of beam divergences for short and long SIDs.) This effect has an impact on the concentration of photons on the surface of the patient. A short SID increases the photon concentration, thus increas-

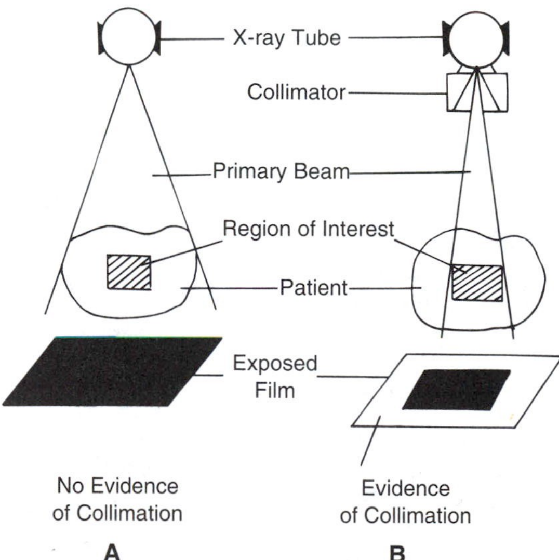

FIGURE 8-6. The use of collimation to prevent unnecessary irradiation of structures surrounding the regions of interest: no evidence of collimation (A) and evidence of collimation (B). [From Seeram, E. (1985). *X-ray imaging equipment: An introduction*. Springfield, IL: Charles C Thomas. Reproduced by permission.]

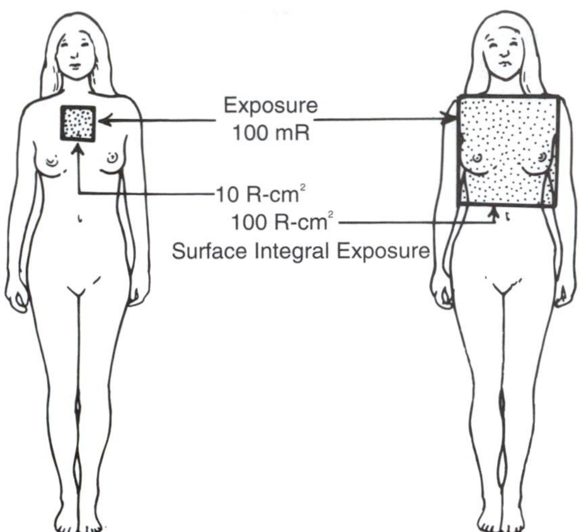

FIGURE 8-7. A comparison of the effect of two different field sizes on the surface integral exposure for the same dose of 100 mR. A larger field size results in 10 times more radiation to the patient. [From Sprawls, P. (1995). *Physical principles of medical imaging* (2nd ed.). Decatur, IL: Perry Sprawls and Associates, Inc. Reproduced by permission.]

ing the surface exposure (entrance dose) to the patient. This is clearly illustrated in Figure 8-9.

In conducting x-ray examinations, the technologist should pay particular attention to proper use of the correct SID for the particular anatomical area of interest. The recommended SIDs for fluoroscopic and radiographic examinations have been obtained by maintaining a balance between image quality and patient dose.

Patient Thickness and Density

The patient thickness and density (mass per unit volume) also affect dose. In general, as the thickness and density increase, more radiation is needed for image formation (Bushong, 1993; Wootton, 1993). The exposure, of course, depends on whether a fixed or variable kVp technique is applied in the imaging process. For example, for a technique fixed at 80 kVp, the mAs values for a 16, 20, 24, and 30 cm patient thickness are 12, 22, 45, and 120 mAs, respectively (Bushong, 1993). In addition, Sprawls (1995) indicated that "if the point of interest or organ is not located at the exit surface of the body, the attenuation in the tissue layer between the organ and exit surface will further increase the exposure" (p. 594).

Tabletop

Because the purpose of the tabletop is to support the patient during an examination, it must be constructed of materials that can withstand the weight of heavy patients. These materials must also allow a good proportion of the beam to be transmitted through the tabletop to reach the image receptor. The ratio of patient-to-receptor exposure will increase if the tabletop attenuates a greater fraction of the beam transmitted through the patient (Sprawls, 1995). For

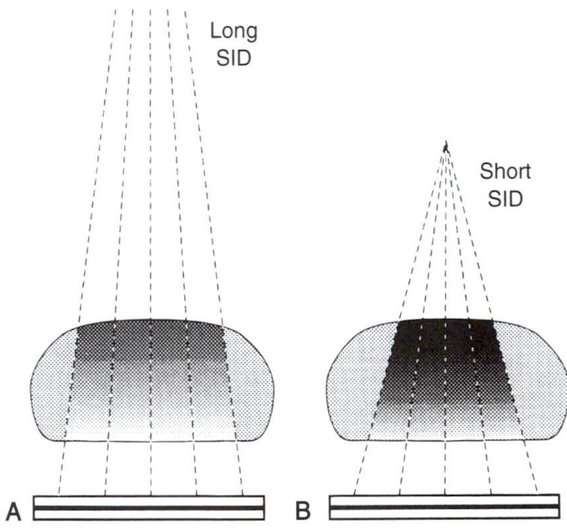

FIGURE 8-8. The divergence of two beams with different SIDs. A: The long SID results in a less divergent beam and a decrease in the concentration of photons in the patient. B: The short SID results in a more divergent beam, which increases the concentration of photons (or surface exposure) in the patient. The short SID is equivalent to a low kVp technique in terms of dose to the patient. [From Wolbarst, A. (1993). *Physics of radiology*. Norwalk, CT: Appleton & Lange. Reproduced by permission.]

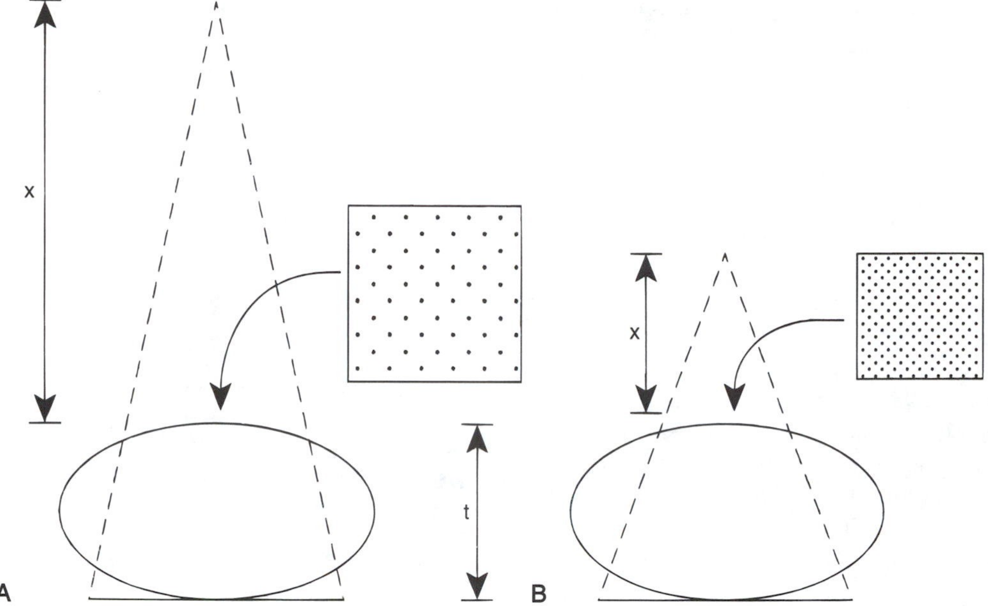

FIGURE 8-9. The concentration of photons (surface exposure) on the patient increases as the SID decreases. A: At a long SID, the concentration decreases on the patient surface. B: The concentration of photons increases on the patient's surface when short SIDs are used. [From Sprawls, P. (1995). *Physical principles of medical imaging* (2nd ed.). Decatur, IL: Perry Sprawls and Associates. Reproduced by permission.]

this reason, materials are carefully chosen in the design of tabletops.

Tabletops used in radiology are made of carbon-fiber materials because they allow a high transmission of the beam. As a result, the absorbed dose in the skin of the patient is reduced. For example, at 80 kVp, the absorbed dose in the skin of the patient is reduced by 3–15% when carbon fiber materials are used in tabletops (ICRP, 1993).

Antiscatter Grids

A radiographic *grid* is positioned between the tabletop and the image receptor (Fig. 1-3) for the purpose of improving radiographic contrast. It does this by absorbing radiation scattered from the patient and preventing it from reaching the film. Grids are designed in such a way that their lead strips allow the transmission of primary radiation but prevent scattered radiation (which degrades image contrast) from reaching the film.

Once a grid is introduced into the imaging process, the radiation dose to the patient will increase. The characteristics of the grids responsible for this dose increase are grid ratio, grid frequency, interspace material, selectivity, and the Bucky factor. Each of these will now be described.

The *grid ratio* is the ratio of the height of the lead strip to the distance between the strips. The grid ratios used in clinical imaging are 6:1, 8:1, 12:1, and 16:1; 12:1 is the most commonly used in Bucky mechanisms. As the grid ratio increases, the dose to the patient increases. Additionally, a moving grid (grid in the Bucky mechanism) requires ~15% more radiation than a stationary grid with the same design features (Seeram, 1985).

The number of lead strips per centimeter of the grid is referred to as the *grid frequency*, or grid lattice or strip density. Grid frequencies range from about 24 to 43 lines per centimeter, although higher strip densities are available. As the grid frequency increases, the relative patient exposure increases because there is more lead to absorb a small proportion of the primary beam (Seeram, 1985).

The *interspace material* of the grid supports the lead strips and provides an equal amount of separation between them. The interspace material is usually aluminum or plastic fiber. While each of these has its advantages, aluminum, with its higher atomic number, absorbs more radiation than the plastic fiber, especially with low kVp techniques. This will result in an increase in patient dose by about ≥20% (Bushong, 1993).

The *selectivity* of a grid is yet another factor that affects patient dose. It is the ratio of primary radiation transmission to scattered radiation transmission. Selectivity depends on not only the grid ratio but also on the amount of lead used in the construction of the grid. In general, grids with high selectivity will result in higher patient dose because of an increase in the thickness of the lead strips.

The *Bucky factor* (B) (or *grid factor*, as it is sometimes referred to), influences the dose to the patient during an x-ray examination. B is defined as in Figure 8-10. It is the ratio of the incident total radiation striking the grid (primary photon scatter) to the total radiation transmitted through the grid. B is related to the grid ratio as well as the kVp. As the grid ratio and kVp increase, B increases. For example, the B for a 12:1 grid is 3.5, 4, and 5 at 70, 90, and 120 kVp, respectively. The B for a 16:1 grid is 4, 5, and 6 at 70, 90, and 120 kVp, respectively. As B increases, patient dose (hence exposure technique) increases proportionately (Bushong, 1993).

Finally, the material that encases the grid strips and interspace material has some effect on patient dose due to its radiation transmission properties. At 80 kVp, carbon-fiber grids will reduce the absorbed dose to the skin by 20–30% (ICRP, 1993).

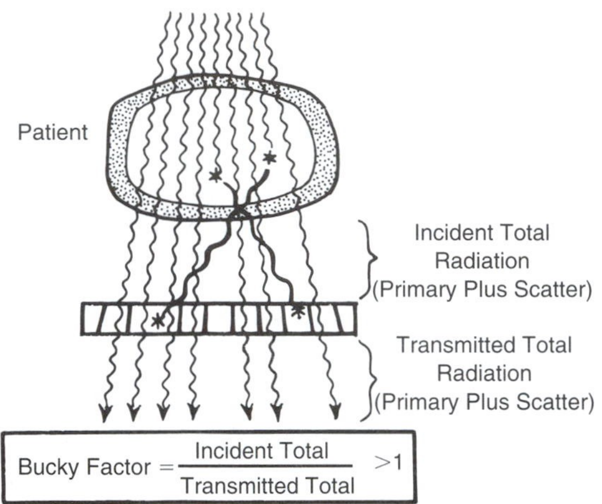

FIGURE 8-10. The Bucky factor is a factor by which the output of the x-ray tube must be increased to return the cassette to its pregrid level of exposure. [From Wolbarst, A.B. (1993). *Physics of radiology*. Norwalk, CT: Appleton & Lange. Reproduced by permission.]

Image Receptor Sensitivity

The *image receptor* captures the radiation transmitted through the patient and is used to record images. In the case of radiography, the image receptor can be film or a film-screen combination (film cassette); however, in fluoroscopic systems, the image intensifier tube is considered the image receptor (specifically, it is the input screen of the image intensifier tube). The *image receptor sensitivity*, however, accounts for the amount of radiation needed to produce an image. In particular, sensitivity refers to the speed of the receptor and it relates to film speed as well as screen speed. High speed film (fast film) requires much less radiation to produce images than low speed film. By the same token, high speed (fast) screens require less radiation than low speed (slow) screens. For example, an image receptor speed of 400 can reduce the entrance skin exposures by 20–50% compared with a 200 speed system (Dowd, 1994).

The sensitivity of image receptors with screens depends on the phosphors used in the construction of the screens. Screens made of rare earth phosphors (gadolinium, lanthanum, and yttrium) have much higher speeds than do conventional screens made of calcium tungstate. The speed of the screen is related to the x-ray absorption efficiency (ability of the screen to absorb photons), as well as to the conversion efficiency (ability of the screen to convert x-ray photons to light photons). While calcium tungstate screens absorb ~30% of the photons incident upon them, rare earth screens absorb about five times more x-rays in the energy range between the rare earth K-shell electron binding energy and the K-shell binding energy for tungsten. In addition, the conversion efficiencies of rare earth screens are about three to four times (15–20%) that of conventional calcium tungstate screens (Bushong, 1993). These characteristics of rare earth screens result in exposure reductions of >50% vs. calcium tungstate image receptors.

Another important characteristic of the image receptor that affects dose is that of the material used in the front (side facing the x-ray tube) of the cassette. Materials made of carbon fiber (graphite fibers in a plastic matrix) reduce patient exposure because they absorb only about half as many x-ray photons as conventional cassettes with aluminum fronts. An overall reduction of absorbed dose to the skin of the patient in the range of ~6–12% can be achieved with carbon-fiber fronts (ICRP, 1993).

Film Processing

Radiographic film processing is an integral part in the chain of factors affecting dose to the patient. A film exposed with the correct technique for a particular examination may not necessarily provide optimum diagnostic information if it is subject to poor processing. Correct processing techniques are mandatory, not only to produce films of optimum quality but also to reduce the radiation dose to the patient by eliminating the need to repeat examinations, which can increase the patient dose by a factor of 2 (ICRP, 1993).

In an effort to minimize problems in processing films and maintain the integrity of the processor, a quality control program for radiographic film processors is essential. Such a program includes a wide range of activities, all intended to ensure films of optimum diagnostic quality (NCRP, 1990).

Repeat Radiographic Examinations

Why are radiographic examinations repeated? What are the rates of repeats and what are the reasons for them? The answers to these questions have been explored in the literature (Dowd, 1994; Statkiewicz-Sherer et al., 1993; ICRP, 1993). The ICRP (1993), for example, reported that repeat rates (based on a number of surveys) varied from 3% to 15% and that the major causes of repeats were due to patient positioning errors and exposure technique errors. Other possible causes of repeated examinations include the following:

- Poor processing of films.
- Incorrect use of the automatic exposure system.
- Inaccurate measurement of patient anatomy (body part).
- Collimation errors.
- Incorrect SID.
- Incorrect placement of markers (right, left, and other descriptive numbers).
- Not including all of the anatomy of interest.
- Incorrect angulation of the x-ray tube.
- Incorrect centering to the anatomy as well as to the cassette.
- Poor or incomplete instructions to the patient.
- Not observing the patient during the exposure.
- Poor placement of the gonadal shield.
- Uneducated and untrained radiologic workers.

- Incorrect interpretation of the requisition (request for an x-ray examination).
- Incorrect identification of the patient.

In view of the wide variety of the sources of errors, technologists must always be alert when performing radiographic procedures. To minimize errors and ensure that the best possible images will be obtained with the least amount of radiation, the technologist should have a carefully planned strategy for conducting the examination. One such strategy might include the following sequence of steps:

1. Obtain and correctly interpret the patient's requisition.
2. Prepare the room for the particular examination.
3. Correctly identify the patient.
4. Explain the examination to the patient, emphasizing the need to follow all instructions including the admonition against movement during the exposure. Breathing instructions should also be clearly explained as well.
5. Measure the patient correctly, particularly if the exposure technique chart is based on a measurement. If automatic exposure systems are used, the patient size must also be correctly assessed. Note also whether patient pathology might have an effect on the exposure technique.
6. Establish and set up the correct exposure technique factors for the particular examination based on the assessment.
7. Position the patient correctly.
8. Check for proper collimation, SID, marker placement, proper placement of the cassette in the Bucky, and proper alignment of the cassette with the useful beam.
9. Check that the gonads are shielded correctly.
10. Expose and observe patients during the exposure to ensure that they follow instructions.
11. After exposure, process all films. Check that the processor is in good working order.
12. Check all films for acceptability.
13. If the film is acceptable, dismiss the patient.
14. Clean up the room and prepare for the next examination.

These steps, if carefully executed, should assist the technologist in conducting the examination in a smooth and orderly fashion to ensure films of optimal quality. Avoiding repeat exposures can reduce the genetically significant dose (GSD) by ~10%. Additionally, improved techniques and education could also result in a 50% decrease in the GSD (Travis, 1989).

Shielding Radiosensitive Organs

Shielding is yet another factor affecting the dose to the patient during an examination. Shielding very radiosensitive organs such as the gonads and eyes is especially important because of the respective risks of genetic effects and cataracts. For the gonads, shielding will reduce the gonadal dose. For example, the correct use of a 1-mm lead equivalent shield will reduce the gonadal dose by ~50% for females and 90–95% for males (Statkiewicz-Sherer et al., 1993). Shielding the eyes (depending upon the examination) can result in a dose reduction of 50–75% (Wootton, 1993).

Two types of shields have been described in the literature (Bushong, 1993; Dowd, 1994; Statkiewicz-Sherer et al., 1993; Thompson et al., 1994): *contact shields* and *shadow shields*. While contact shields are flat or shaped (Fig. 8-11), shadow shields (Fig. 8-12) are constructed so that they attach to the x-ray tube by means of a ring. The shadow of the radiopaque sector-like portion of the shield is positioned over the patient's gonads. Shadow shields are perhaps best used in examinations where it is important to maintain a sterile field.

Gonadal shielding is intended to protect the gonads from primary radiation and, as such, the thickness of the shield must be at least 0.5 mm lead equivalent.

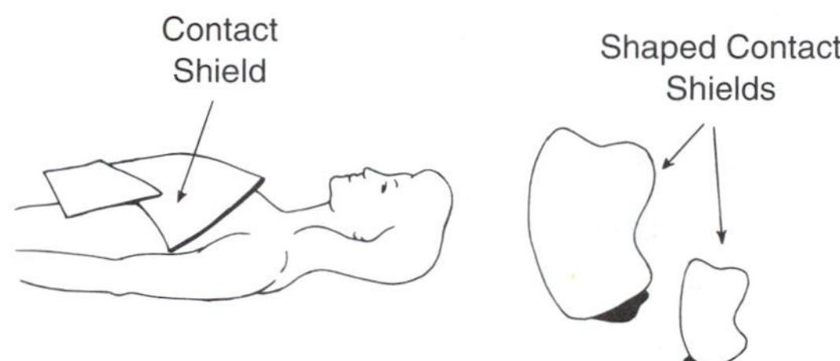

FIGURE 8-11. Flat and shaped contact shields used in gonadal protection. While the flat shield can be used to protect the gonads, it can also provide shielding of the breasts, a highly radiosensitive organ. The shaped contact shield shown in the figure is specifically used to shield male gonads. [From Thompson, M.A., Hattaway, M.P., Hall, J.D., & Dowd, S.B. (1994). *Principles of imaging sciences and protection.* Philadelphia: W.B. Saunders. Reproduced by permission.]

In addition, the ICRP (1993) stated that "the gonads should be shielded when, of necessity, they are directly in the x-ray beam or within 5 cm of it, unless such shielding excludes or degrades important diagnostic information" (p. xviii). In Chapter 9, other recommendations and guidelines for the use of gonadal shielding are discussed.

If gonadal shielding is to be effective, placement of the lead shield on the patient must be accurate to ensure protection of the gonads. For males, it is useful to use the symphysis pubis as the external landmark to guide the placement of the shield. For females, the external landmark 2.5 cm medial to the anterior superior iliac spines can be used for accurate placement of the shield to protect the ovaries from radiation.

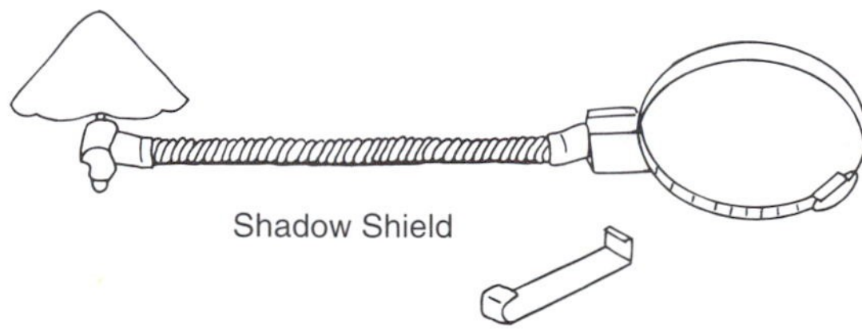

FIGURE 8-12. A diagrammatic representation of a shadow shield. [From Thompson, M.A., Hattaway, M.P., Hall, J.D., & Dowd, S.B. (1994). *Principles of imaging sciences and protection.* Philadelphia: W.B. Saunders. Reproduced by permission.]

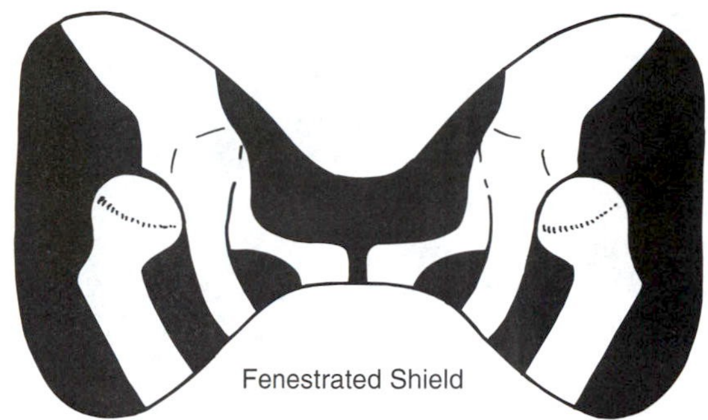

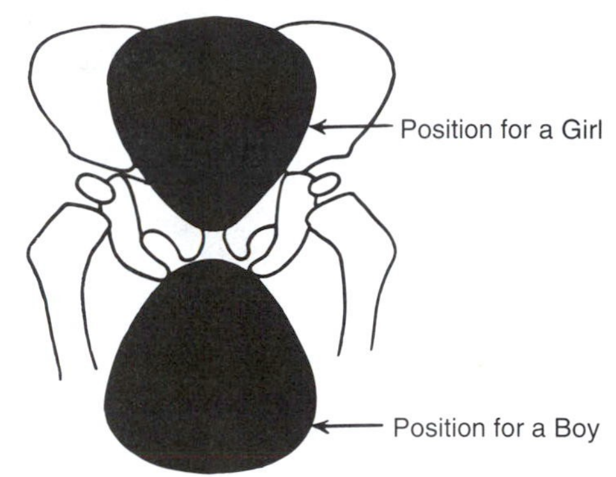

FIGURE 8-13. The methods of shielding the gonads in children. [From Plaut, S. (1993). *Radiation protection in the x-ray department.* Oxford: Butterworth-Heinemann. Reproduced by permission.]

Finally, gonadal shielding of children can best be accomplished through the methods shown in Figure 8-13.

Shielding the breasts during certain x-ray examinations has been advocated by some authors (Plaut, 1993; Bushong, 1993) due to the extreme radiosensitivity of the breasts. Shielding is suggested especially when the x-ray field is in close proximity to the breasts (such as in urinary tract examinations, upper humerus, shoulder girdle, thoracic spine, clavicle, abdomen, and scoliosis examinations in children).

Patient Orientation

The position of the patient during an examination is another factor affecting patient dose. Several authors have reported a reduction of the dose to specific organs, depending upon patient positioning. For example, Wootton (1993) reported that positioning the skull PA will reduce the dose to the eyes by ~95% compared with the AP position. Similarly, the dose to the female breast is reduced by ~95% with PA positioning compared with AP positioning. Additionally, Bushong (1993) reported a breast dose reduction of ~1% of the AP projection when children's scoliosis examinations are done in the PA projection.

Heriard et al. (1993) found that the PA projection in lumbar spine radiography resulted in a dose reduction of 17% to the thyroid and 200% to the eyes, ovaries, uterus, and testes, compared with the AP projections. In addition, the PA projection also resulted in an entrance skin exposure 52% lower than the AP projection. These results lead the authors to suggest that lumbar spine examinations be done in the prone position rather in the supine position.

Factors in Fluoroscopy

The NCRP (1989) pointed out that fluoroscopic examinations result in higher doses to patients than most radiographic examinations. In addition, Bushong (1993) reported that occupational exposure of personnel is highest in fluoroscopy because the exposure levels are relatively high. For these reasons, it is mandatory that the technologist have a good understanding of the factors affecting dose in fluoroscopy.

Major Elements of a Fluoroscopic Examination

Fluoroscopy is a dynamic imaging procedure that allows the radiologist to evaluate not only anatomical details but physiological ones as well. A fluoroscopic examination involves at least three major elements: fluoroscopy, radiography, and fluorography. (The procedural elements are shown in Fig. 8-14.) While *fluoroscopy* is used to display images in real-time on a television monitor and requires continuous x-ray production, *radiography* includes two components. The first involves recording images radiographically (film-screen cassette) using the spot film device. In this situation, a film cassette is introduced into the exposure field of the spot film device and the system switches from fluoroscopic factors (low tube currents) to radiographic factors (high tube currents), which are used to create the image on a large format film. The second component of radiography is that of the "overheads" generally taken by the technologist after the radiologist has completed the fluoroscopic portion of the examination. These overheads are taken on large format film using the Bucky and radiographic exposure technique factors. Fluorography, on the other hand, refers to recording images (during a fluoroscopic examination) onto cine film (35 mm film) or photospot film (100–105 mm roll or cut film) with a cine camera or a photospot camera, respectively, using fluoroscopic exposure factors. In summary, these three elements of a fluoroscopic examination, by virtue of their imaging characteristics (e.g., exposure requirements, beam geometries, image receptor sensitivities) contribute to the overall dose to patients undergoing fluoroscopy.

The fundamental imaging differences between fluoroscopy and radiography have been described previously. Essentially, all of the general factors affecting dose in radiography (e.g., collimation, filtration, SID, processing, grids, gonadal shielding) apply equally as well to fluoroscopy; however, there are other factors specific only to fluoroscopy. These include fluoroscopic exposure factors, fluoroscopic instrumentation factors, and factors relating to the conduct of the examination. Each of these is now described.

Fluoroscopic Exposure Factors

Fluoroscopic exposure technique factors are used to produce images that can be displayed for viewing on a television monitor and

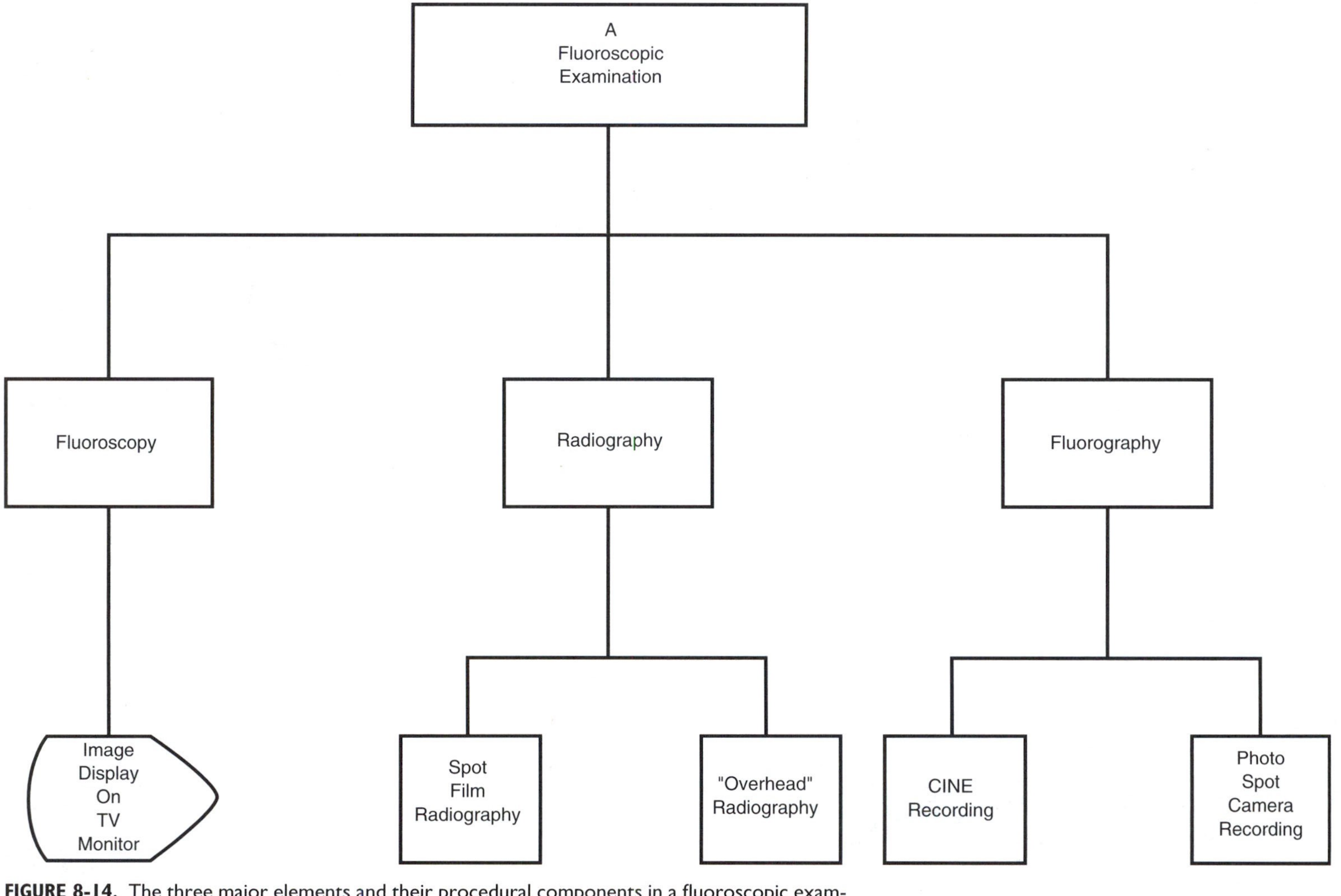

FIGURE 8-14. The three major elements and their procedural components in a fluoroscopic examination.

recorded onto cine film (35 mm roll film) or onto photospot film (100 mm or 105 mm cut film or roll film). In these situations, the images are recorded off the output screen of the image intensifier tube by means of the image distributor. These factors are generally low mA and high kVp, with a range of 1–3 mA and 65–120 kVp, depending upon the examination. For example, a single-contrast barium enema requires a range of 110–120 kVp, while a range of 50–90 kVp is acceptable for a double-contrast (air contrast) barium enema (Bushong, 1993).

The exposure time in fluoroscopy can range from minutes to hours (Pattee et al., 1993) depending on the examination. For example, cardiac catheterizations done by cardiologists can take up to 5 hours of fluoroscopy (Bieze, 1993). This exposure time can result in a wide range of dose to the skin and internal organs. A recent study of radiation risks to patients undergoing percutaneous transluminal coronary angioplasty found that the average patient skin entrance exposure per angioplasty was 32.0 mC/kg (124 R). In light of these high exposures, it is important to limit the "beam-on" time (fluoroscopy time) through the practice of *intermittent fluoroscopy* (short bursts of "beam-on" time) rather than continuous fluoroscopy. Additionally, every fluoroscopic unit is equipped with a *cumulative timer* not only to keep track of the fluoroscopic exposure time but to remind the radiologist of each 5-minute time period of exposures by producing an audible sound and by interrupting the production of x-rays at the end of 5 minutes of radiation exposure. State-of-the-art fluroscopic units now allow a maximum of 3 minutes.

Fluoroscopic Instrumentation Factors

These factors refer to fluoroscopic equipment factors affecting dose, including general technical factors (e.g., collimation, filtration, source-to-tabletop distance) and specific factors (e.g., pulsed fluoroscopy, automatic dose rate control). In this section, only the following specific factors are highlighted: pulsed fluoroscopy, high-level-control fluoroscopy, magnification, last-image-hold, image recording techniques (such as cine fluorography, photospot camera recording, videotape recording), and C-arm fluoroscopy.

PULSED FLUOROSCOPY

Pulsed fluoroscopic systems allow for the radiation to be produced in short bursts (pulses) rather than continuously. Systems that can pulse the beam to <10 pulses per second can result in up to 90% less exposure compared with non-pulsed systems (Bieze, 1993).

HIGH-LEVEL-CONTROL FLUOROSCOPY

High-level-control (HLC), a feature of most state-of-the-art fluoroscopic machines, provides a higher dose rate than can be achieved with conventional exposure. The higher dose rate is intended to improve image quality by reducing quantum noise. The higher dose rate selection just about doubles the patient dose compared with a low-dose rate selection (Wootton, 1993).

The Food and Drug Administration in Title 21 of the Federal Regulations Code specifies a maximum exposure rate of 2.58 mC/kg/min (10 R/min) for fluoroscopic units with automatic brightness control (ABC).

In a study by Cagnon et al. (1991) on HLC fluoroscopy, the investigators found that the exposure rates from several HLC units ranged from 5.42 to 24 mC/kg/min (21–93 R/min), with an average maximum exposure rate of 12.56 mC/kg/min (48.7 R/min). As Dr. J. Thomas Payne, Director of Medical Physics at Abbott Northwestern Hospital in Minneapolis (also Chairman of the American College of Radiology Commission on Physics), pointed out, "once you start exceeding 40 or 50 R per minute, those are like therapy beams, not diagnostic beams" (Bieze, 1993, p. 69).

GRIDS

While grids improve the contrast of the image in fluoroscopy, the removal of the grid from in front of the image intensifier can reduce the radiation dose by a factor of 2 (Bieze, 1993).

MAGNIFICATION

Magnification of the fluoroscopic image, or more specifically electron optical magnification (Fig. 8-15), is possible with multifield image intensifiers (Seeram, 1985; Bushong, 1993). Magnification degrades the image clarity on the television monitor because there is a decrease in the magnification gain that results in a decrease in the number of photoelectrons striking the output screen of the image intensifier. To keep the brightness level on the television monitor constant, the fluoroscopic mA is increased automatically (Bushong, 1993) and subsequently may double the original dose rate (Wootton, 1993).

LAST IMAGE HOLD

This is a term used to describe fluoroscopic images that can be held in digital storage and subsequently displayed on the television monitor without the need for continuous fluoroscopy. Systems with the last-image-hold feature reduce the dose to the patient by reducing the total fluoroscopic time by 50–80% (Bushberg et al., 1994).

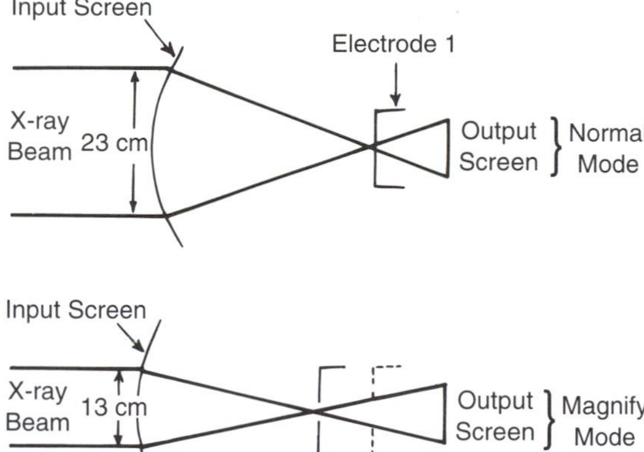

FIGURE 8-15. Electron optical magnification in fluoroscopy. When electrode 2 is at a lower voltage than electrode 1, a wider divergence of the beam results. In addition, the x-ray beam at the input screen must be collimated to a smaller field. [From Seeram, E. (1995). *X-ray imaging equipment: An introduction*. Springfield, IL: Charles C Thomas. Reproduced by permission.]

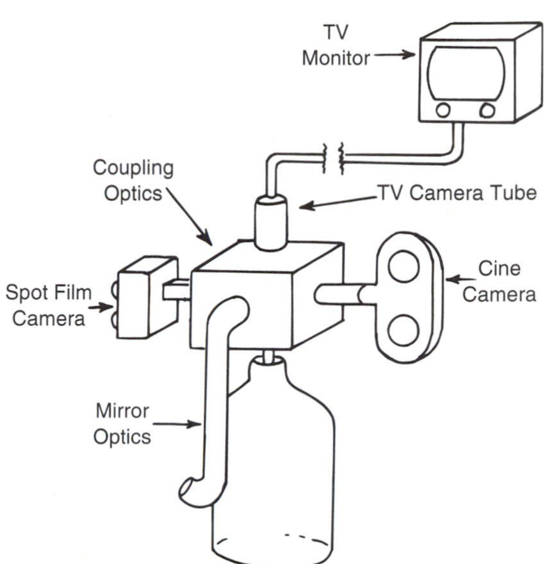

FIGURE 8-16. Two methods of recording the fluoroscopic image with the aid of an image distributor or coupling optics. Shown here are cine fluorography and spot film camera or photospot film recording. [From Bushong, S. (1993). *Radiologic science for technologists* (5th ed.). St. Louis: Mosby–Year Book. Reproduced by permission.]

IMAGE RECORDING TECHNIQUES

Recording fluoroscopic images can be accomplished using several techniques, two of which are illustrated in Figure 8-16. These techniques, *cine fluorography* and *spot film camera recording*, capture the image from the output screen of the image intensifier tube via the coupling optics (image distributor), which directs the light from the output screen to the specific recording device during an examination.

While the photospot camera uses 100-mm cut film or 105-mm roll film with exposures occurring at frame rates of between 6 and 12 frames per second, the cine fluorographic camera uses 35-mm cine film with exposures occurring at frame rates ranging from 30 to 120 frames per second. An important point to note with respect to dose to the patient is that as the framing frequency increases, the radiation dose increases. When compared with cassette-loaded spot films and large-format films in cassettes (which require radiographic exposure technique factors), photospot techniques and cine fluorography reduce the dose by a factor of 5 to 10 (Wootton, 1993).

Finally, videotape can be used to record fluoroscopic images in situations in which high quality recordings are not needed. In this case, there is a dose reduction by a factor of about 5 compared with film-based recording techniques (Wootton, 1993).

C-ARM FLUOROSCOPY

The *C-arm fluoroscopy* machine is used routinely in the operating room and sometimes in cardiology for cardiac pacemaker wire insertions. Apart from several technical factors affecting dose during C-arm fluoroscopy (e.g., fluoroscopic exposure time, fluoroscopic exposure factors, filtration), an important factor influencing the dose is that of the *patient-image intensifier distance* (P-IID). The P-IID should be as short as possible to reduce the dose to the patient, as illustrated in Figure 8-17.

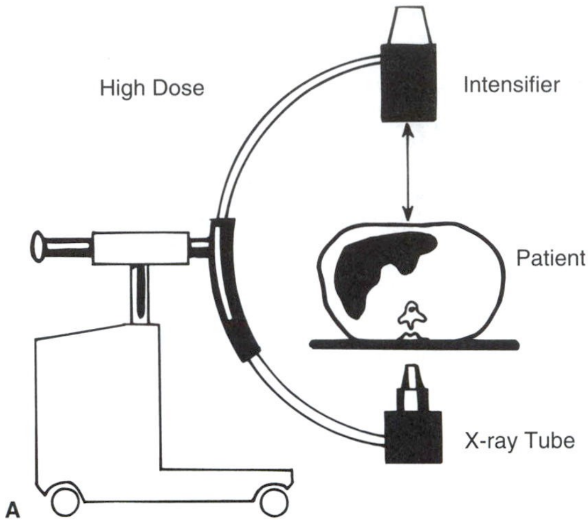

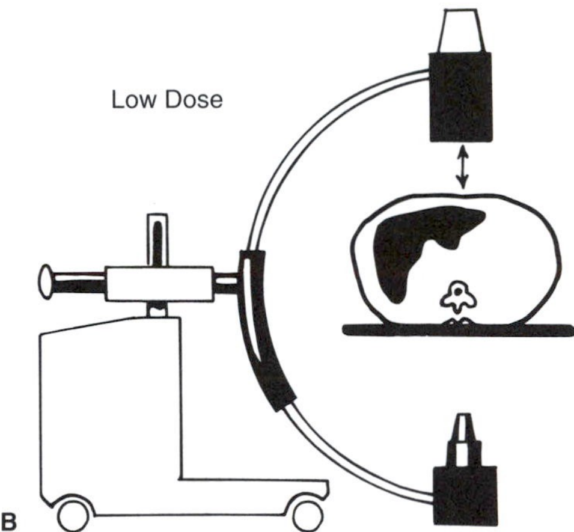

FIGURE 8-17. The P-IID should be as short as possible to minimize the dose to the patient during C-arm fluoroscopy: high dose (A) and low dose (B). [From Wootton, R. (Ed.). *Radiation protection of patients*. Cambridge, England: Cambridge University Press. Reproduced by permission.]

Conduct of the Fluoroscopic Examination

The conduct of the fluoroscopic examination is associated with the three elements shown in Figure 8-14. It involves both the technologist and the radiologist, who must make every effort to ensure that the patient receives the least amount of radiation.

It has been suggested (Bieze, 1993) that during fluoroscopy the radiologist, in an effort to reduce the dose to the patient, should:

1. Collimate the beam to the smallest field sizes.
2. Avoid the use of magnification.
3. Avoid the use of grids during the procedure.
4. Avoid the use of high-level-control fluoroscopy.
5. Use the last-image-hold feature if available.
6. Use intermittent fluoroscopy.
7. Keep track of the cumulative fluoroscopy time.

The technologist, on the other hand, is responsible for the conduct of the radiographic portion of the fluoroscopic examination, apart from performing other tasks such as explaining the examination to the patient, preparation of the contrast medium (barium, for example), assisting the patient during the procedure, assisting the radiologist during fluoroscopy (changing cassettes in the spot film device), and so forth.

In performing the radiographic examination, the technologist should focus attention on the following:

1. Obtain all cassettes for the "overhead" projections before the examination.
2. Set all radiographic exposure techniques prior to final positioning of the patient.
3. Ensure that the positioning is correct, and that the patient understands the breathing instructions.
4. Protect the patient through effective collimation and gonadal shielding when such shielding will not interfere with the information content from the examination.
5. Use the correct SID and beam angulation.
6. Ensure correct placement of markers on the cassette.

The above tasks are representative of a few of the activities that will enhance the conduct of the fluoroscopic examination and will result in unnecessary repeat exposures.

Factors in Computed Tomography

Dose values in CT for different types of examinations are discussed in Chapter 11. While the skin doses in CT are greater than that of selected radiographic examinations, the dose is less than most fluoroscopic examinations (Bushong, 1993; Bushberg et al., 1994). In general, the doses in CT are relatively high (Wootton, 1993; Plaut, 1993). Therefore, the technologist must make every effort to understand those factors affecting dose in an attempt to minimize the dose a patient receives during a CT examination.

The factors affecting dose in CT are those that relate not only to the x-ray beam parameters but also to the image parameters.

X-Ray Beam Parameters

The factors relating to the x-ray beam parameters and those affecting the dose in CT include kVp, mAs, filtration, collimation, the source-to-skin distance, tube motion, and detector efficiency. The first five factors affect dose as described earlier in this chapter. The tube motion refers to the path of the x-ray tube and detectors during data collection. Tube motion specifically affects the distribution of dose in the patient. For those scanners that rotate 360°, the dose is distributed uniformly over the surface of the patient (Seeram, 1994).

Detector efficiency refers to the ability of the CT detector to capture as many photons from the beam that is transmitted through the patient (detection efficiency) and convert those photons (conversion efficiency) into a usable signal (electrical signal). Detectors with high detection efficiency, such as cadmium tungstate detectors, require less dose in forming the CT image (Seeram, 1994) than do gas-ionization detectors, which have lower conversion efficiencies.

Image Parameters

The image parameters affecting dose in CT include signal-to-noise ratio (SNR), which determines the contrast resolution of the image; spatial resolution (e); and slice thickness (h). A simple algebraic expression that relates dose (D) to these three image parameters is as follows:

$$D = K\left[\frac{SNR^2}{e^3 h}\right]$$

where K is a constant.

This relationship implies the following:

1. The dose is directly proportional to the square of the SNR (contrast resolution). To improve the contrast resolution by a factor of 2 will require an increase in the dose by a factor of 4.
2. The dose is inversely proportional to the cube of the spatial resolution. This means that to improve the spatial resolution by a factor of 2 will require an increase in the dose by a factor of 8.
3. The dose is inversely proportional to the slice thickness. If the slice thickness is decreased by a factor of 2, the dose must be increased by a factor of 2 to maintain the same SNR.

Because one of the goals in conducting a radiological examination is to obtain optimum image quality with a dose as low as is reasonably achievable, the technologist and the radiologist must work together in CT to accomplish this objective. Good communication and understanding between the radiologist and technologist about the nature and conduct (including technical details) of the CT examination are essential ingredients of a successful CT examination.

Factors in Mammography

In Chapter 11, dose in mammography will be discussed in terms of dose parameters (in-air surface exposure, surface dose, midline dose, and the mean glandular dose), measurement of the dose, and dose studies. Radiation dose in mammography is important to the technologist because the female breast is very sensitive to radiation. In addition, various guidelines and recommendations have been issued for diagnostic mammography as well as for screening mammography.

The factors affecting dose in mammography are shown in Figure 8-18 and include exposure technique factors (kVp, mAs), tube target, filtration, focal spot, image receptor type, film processing, breast and lesion composition, thickness and shape, as well as the SID. The influence of these factors on dose is discussed by Dr. Lawrence N. Rothenberg, Ph.D., in Appendix 8-2.

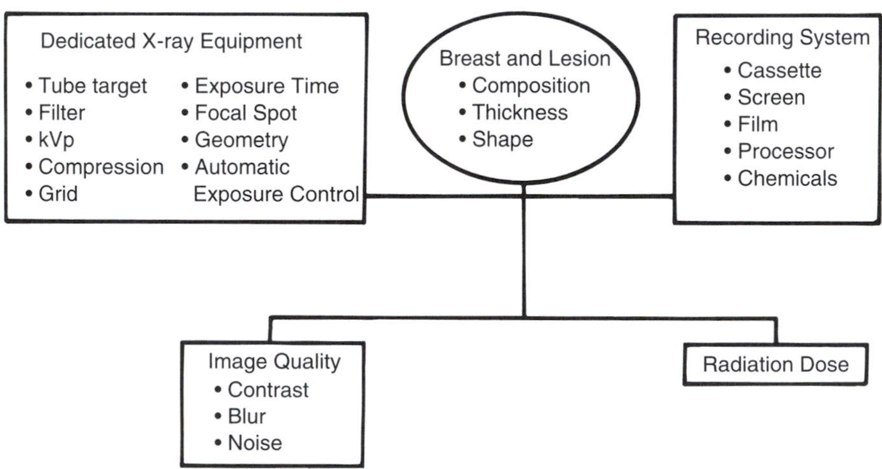

FIGURE 8-18. Factors affecting dose and image quality in mammography. [From Haus, A.G. (1990). Technologic improvements in screen-film mammography. *Radiology, 174*, 628–637. Reproduced by permission.]

REVIEW QUESTIONS

1. The following affect(s) dose in radiography:
   A. Exposure technique factors (kVp and mAs).
   B. The image receptor sensitivity.
   C. Patient positioning and film processing.
   D. All of the above.

2. The components of exposure in fluoroscopy include all of the following except:
   A. Fluoroscopic exposure technique factors (kVp, mA).
   B. Format and type of spot films.
   C. Magnification technique.
   D. Sodium iodide detectors.

3. The components of exposure in CT systems that affect dose to the patient are:
   A. Beam collimation and x-ray tube motion.
   B. Technique factors (kVp, mAs).
   C. Filtration of the beam.
   D. All of the above.

4. The following individuals play a role in determining the dose to a patient except the:
   A. Patient's physician.
   B. Radiology nurse.
   C. X-ray technologist.
   D. Radiologist.

5. The role of the patient's physician in radiation protection of the patient is to:
   A. Provide all clinical data.
   B. Conduct the x-ray examination.
   C. Determine how many views of the patient must be taken.
   D. Shield the patient during an x-ray examination.

6. Who has the responsibility of shielding the patient during an x-ray examination not involving fluoroscopy?
   A. The patient's physician.
   B. The radiologist.
   C. The technologist.
   D. The radiology nurse.

7. What is the central role of the patient during an x-ray examination?
   A. Place the gonadal shield in the proper position.
   B. Select the appropriate film size.
   C. Cooperate with personnel to ensure a successful examination.
   D. Determine the number of views to be taken.

8. Exposure technique factors in radiography include all of the following except:
   A. kVp.
   B. mA.
   C. Exposure time.
   D. Grid.

9. The quality of the radiation beam from the tube is determined by the:
   A. mA.
   B. Exposure time.
   C. kVp.
   D. mAs.

10. The quantity of radiation falling on the patient is affected by the:
    A. mAs.
    B. kVp.
    C. Filtration.
    D. All of the above.

11. Which of the following results in less dose to the patient in a radiographic examination?
    A. High kVp techniques.
    B. Low kVp techniques.
    C. High mAs techniques.
    D. The use of low kVp and high mAs.

12. If the mAs is doubled in radiography, the dose to the patient is:
    A. Doubled.
    B. Increased by a factor of 4.

C. Decreased by a factor of 4.
D. Increased by a factor of 8.

13. Which of the following generators would deliver less dose to the patient for a particular examination?
   A. Single-phase.
   B. Three-phase.
   C. High frequency.
   D. The x-ray generator has no effect on patient dose.

14. Filtration of the x-ray beam is intended to:
   A. Increase the intensity of the beam.
   B. Reduce the dose to the patient.
   C. Increase the quantity of protons falling on the patient.
   D. Decrease the penetrating power of the beam.

15. The field size is:
   A. Determined by the collimation.
   B. Area covered by the beam falling on the patient.
   C. Also referred to as the field of view.
   D. All of the above.

16. Collimation is intended to:
   A. Improve image quality.
   B. Protect the patient from unnecessary radiation.
   C. Decrease scattered radiation.
   D. Shape the primary beam.

17. Collimation reduces the genetically significant dose by:
   A. 65%.
   B. 50%.
   C. 10%.
   D. No relationship exists between collimation and patient dose.

18. The entrance dose to the patient is increased when a ______ source-to-image receptor distance is used.
   A. Long.
   B. Short.

19. The dose to the patient increases:
   A. As patient thickness increases.
   B. As the tissue density increases.
   C. As patient thickness and density decrease.
   D. a and b are correct.

20. Tabletops made of carbon-fiber materials will reduce the absorbed skin dose by:
   A. 50%.
   B. 3–15%.
   C. 20–30%.
   D. 30–50%.

21. Which of the following grid ratios will result in more dose to the patient?
   A. 6:1.
   B. 8:1.
   C. 12:1.
   D. 16:1.

22. Which of the following results in a high patient dose?
   A. Grids with low ratios.
   B. Grids with lower frequencies.
   C. Grids with a high selectivity.
   D. Grids with a low selectivity.

23. The Bucky factor is:
   A. Directly proportional to the patient dose.
   B. Inversely proportional to the patient dose.
   C. Inversely proportional to the square of the patient dose.
   D. Directly proportional to the square of the patient dose.

24. The following may result in an x-ray examination being repeated:
   A. Patient positioning errors.
   B. Exposure technique errors.
   C. Collimation errors.
   D. All of the above.

25. The following will reduce the genetically significant dose:
   A. Avoiding repeat exposures.
   B. Improved exposure techniques.
   C. Education and training.
   D. All of the above.

26. A shield of about 1 mm lead equivalent will reduce the gonadal dose for females by about:
   A. 10%.
   B. 99%.
   C. 90%.
   D. 50%.

27. The gonadal shield is intended to protect the patient's gonads from:
   A. Leakage radiation.
   B. Scattered radiation.
   C. Primary radiation.
   D. All of the above.

28. The thickness of gonadal shields must be at least ________ lead equivalent:
   A. 0.05 mm.
   B. 0.5 mm.
   C. 0.25 mm.
   D. 0.5 cm.

29. The range of mA used in fluoroscopy is:
   A. 100–400 mA.
   B. 1–10 mA.
   C. 1–3 mA.
   D. 5–20 mA.

30. The maximum exposure rate for fluoroscopy according to the FDA is:
   A. 2.58 mC/kg.
   B. 25.8 mC/kg.
   C. 258 mC/kg.
   D. 2.58 C/kg.

31. Which of the following influences the dose in fluoroscopy?
   A. Grids.
   B. Magnification.
   C. Last-image-hold.
   D. All of the above.

32. Which of the following framing frequencies in fluoroscopy will result in the greatest exposure to the patient?
   A. 6 frames per second.
   B. 12 frames per second.
   C. 30 frames per second.
   D. 120 frames per second.

33. The following factors affect dose in C-arm fluoroscopy:
   A. Filtration.
   B. Fluoroscopic technique factors.
   C. Patient-image intensifier distance.
   D. All of the above.

34. The following are x-ray beam parameters in CT except:
   A. Collimation.
   B. Detector efficiency.
   C. kVp and mAs.
   D. Slice thickness.

35. The following are image parameters in CT except:
   A. Signal-to-noise ratio.
   B. Slice thickness.
   C. Spatial resolution.
   D. kVp and mAs.

36. The dose in CT is:
   A. Directly proportional to the square of the signal-to-noise ratio.
   B. Inversely proportional to the cube of the spatial resolution.
   C. Inversely proportional to the slice thickness.
   D. All of the above.

37. To increase the contrast resolution by a factor of 2 in CT requires an increase in dose by a factor of:
   A. 4.
   B. 2.

C. 8.
D. 1.

38. To double the spatial resolution in CT requires an increase in dose by a factor of:
    A. 4.
    B. 2.
    C. 8.
    D. 1.

39. In CT, if the slice thickness is decreased by a factor of 2, the dose must be increased by a factor of:
    A. 2.
    B. 4.
    C. 8.
    D. 1.

40. The following factors affect dose in mammography significantly except:
    A. kVp.
    B. Tube target material.
    C. Focal spot.
    D. Filtration.

REFERENCES

Bieze, J. (1993). Radiation exposure risks haunt interventionalists. *Diagnostic Imaging, 15*, 68–79.

Burns, C.B., & Renner, J.R. (1993). Molybdenum/Al filters perform effectively. *Radiologic Technology, 64*, 216–219.

Bushberg, J.T., Siebert, J.A., Leidholdt, Jr. E.M., & Boone, J.M. (1994). *The essential physics of medical imaging.* Baltimore: Williams & Wilkins.

Bushong, S. (1993). *Radiologic science for technologists* (5th ed.). St. Louis: Mosby–Year Book.

Cagnon, C.H., et al. (1994). Exposure rates in high-level fluoroscopy for image intensification. *Radiology, 178*, 643–646.

Dowd, S.B. (1994). *Practical radiation protection and applied radiobiology.* Philadelphia: W.B. Saunders.

Heriard, J.B., Terry, J.A., & Arnold, A.L. (1993). Achieving dose reduction in lumbar spine radiography. *Radiologic Technology, 65*, 97–103.

International Commission on Radiological Protection. (1993). *Protection of the patient in diagnostic radiology* (ICRP reprint from the Annals of the ICRP). Elmsford, NY: Pergamon Press.

NCRP. (1989). *Exposure of the U.S. population from diagnostic medical radiation* (Report No. 100). Bethesda, MD: National Council on Radiation Protection and Measurements (NCRP).

NCRP. (1990). *Quality assurance in diagnostic imaging* (Report No. 99). Bethesda, MD: National Council on Radiation Protection and Measurements (NCRP).

Pattee, P.L., Johns, P.C., & Chambers, R.J. (1993). Radiation risks to patients from percutaneous transluminal coronary angioplasty. *American Journal of Cardiology, 22*, 1044–1051.

Plaut, S. (1993). *Radiation protection in the x-ray department.* Oxford: Butterworth-Heinemann.

Seeram, E. (1985). *X-ray imaging equipment: An introduction.* Springfield, IL: Charles C Thomas.

Seeram, E. (1994). *Computed tomography. Physical principles, clinical applications, and quality control.* Philadelphia: W.B. Saunders.

Sprawls, P. (1995). *Physical principles of medical imaging* (2nd ed.). Decatur, IL: Perry Sprawls and Associates.

Statkiewicz-Sherer, M.A., Viconti, P., & Ritenour, E.R. (1993). *Radiation protection in medical radiography.* St. Louis: Mosby–Year Book.

Travis, E.L. (1989). *Primer of medical radiobiology* (2nd ed.). Chicago: Mosby–Year Book.

Wolbarst, A.B. (1993). *Physics of radiology.* Norwalk, CT: Appleton & Lange.

Wootton, R. (Ed.). (1993). *Radiation protection of patients.* Cambridge, England: Cambridge University Press.

APPENDIX 8-1

Responsibilities of the Physician, the Radiologist, and the Role of the Technologist (Radiographer). [An extract from ICRP. (1993). ICRP *protection of the patient in diagnostic radiology*. Elmsford, NY: Pergamon Press. Reproduced by permission.]

The decision as to whether an x-ray examination of a patient is justified is sometimes the responsibility of the referring physician and sometimes of the physician who carries out the x-ray examination. In either case, it is imperative that the decision be based upon a correct assessment of the indications for the x-ray examination, the expected diagnostic yield from the x-ray examination and the way in which the results are likely to influence the diagnosis and subsequent medical care of the patient. It is equally important that this assessment be made against a background of adequate knowledge of the physical properties and the biological effects of ionising radiation.

Responsibility of Referring Physician

The referring physician's understanding of the concepts of benefits and risks, as applied to the rapidly changing field of x-ray diagnosis, is often incomplete. The referring physician's chief and proper concern is with the efficacy of the x-ray examination, that is, whether it will contribute to the management of the patient's health problem. However, the referring physician should refrain from making routine requests not based on clinical indications. To achieve the necessary overall clinical judgment the referring physician may need to consult with the radiologist.

The referring physician should provide a clear request describing the patient's problem and indicating the clinical objectives, so that the radiologist can carry out the correct x-ray examination. However, in situations where this information is lacking and if the clinical indications are obvious and the denial of service would place undue hardship on the patient, it is not appropriate to penalise the patient by postponing requested x-ray examinations.

Before prescribing an x-ray examination, the referring physician should be satisfied that the necessary information is not available, either from radiological examinations already done or from any other medical tests or investigations.

Responsibility of Radiologist

To achieve the necessary overall clinical judgment the radiologist may need to consult with the referring physician. This practice is to be encouraged in the interest of obtaining the maximum information at the least radiation risk and economic cost. The radiologist has the responsibility for the control of all aspects of the conduct and extent of x-ray examinations. The radiologist should advise on the appropriateness of proposed x-ray examinations and on the techniques to be used, in the light of the clinical problem presented.

The radiologist should ensure that no person operates x-ray equipment without adequate technical competence, or performs x-ray examinations without adequate knowledge of the physical properties and harmful effects of ionising radiation.

If two or more medical imaging procedures are readily available and give the desired diagnostic information, then the procedure that presents the least overall risk to the patient should be chosen.

The sequence in which x-ray examinations are performed should be determined for each patient. Preferably, the results of each x-ray examination in a proposed sequence should be assessed before the next one is performed, as further x-ray examinations may be unnecessary. On the other hand, the availability and convenience of the patient, as well as the urgency for the clinical information, have to be considered.

Role of Radiographer

The main duty of radiographers is to carry out radiographic examinations under the supervision of a qualified physician, usually a radiologist. The term "radiographer" includes radiological technologist, medical technical assistant, medical radiological technician, or other operator of medical x-ray equipment. Radiographers are in a key position regarding the amount of radiation administered, the optimal use of imaging equipment and the recognition of equipment malfunctions. Education in patient protection should form part of the educational programmes for all radiographers. Each appropriate national body should give due consideration to the content and extent of its programmes for the training and continuing education of radiographers.

APPENDIX 8-2

Factors Affecting Dose in Mammography

The following is an extract from a tutorial paper on *Dose in Mammography* given by Dr. Lawrence Rothenberg, Ph.D., at a meeting of the Radiological Society of North America (RSNA) sponsored by the Association of Physicists in Medicine (AAPM). The paper was published in *Radiographics*, and this extract is reproduced by the kind permission of the RSNA.

Several factors affect dose for a properly exposed mammogram. (Throughout the following discussion, a concurrent change in milliampere seconds may often also be assumed to maintain a properly exposed mammogram or xeromammogram.)

If a longer *exposure time* is necessary to fulfill increased exposure requirements, an extra increase in the overall exposure may be required because of reciprocity law failure. In other words, the required film exposure and its accompanying patient dose will not be determined by a single tube current—exposure time product (mAs); for some screen-film mammography systems, the requirement is greater for a long time—low current product than for a short time—high current product.

At higher *kilovoltages*, with an appropriate reduction in milliampere seconds to maintain the same image density, there will be a reduced dose due to the more penetrating x-ray beam produced but also some loss of subject contrast.

Three-phase and constant-potential x-ray generators will provide a more penetrating beam than single-phase generators, so that as the voltage waveform changes from a high ripple to a constant-potential shape, the dose will be somewhat reduced. Again, some slight loss in contrast may result from a constant potential waveform, compared with that from more varying waveforms.

The effect of changing the *x-ray tube target* from a tungsten to a molybdenum target is that there will be more low-energy photons in the molybdenum spectrum. In a shift from tungsten to molybdenum, the dose will increase, and contrast will be improved.

There may be a choice of *filter type*, such as molybdenum or aluminum filters, with different tube targets. Filters of special metal such as rhodium or of different thicknesses may be used. In general, as the filters are varied to make a beam of higher half-value layer, the dose will be somewhat reduced and so will the contrast. A change of the x-ray tube *focal spot* should produce no effect on dose.

The compression device, which is used for essentially all mammographic exposures, forms part of the overall filtration of the machine, and its thickness and material will affect the half-value layer of the beam. In addition, increased *compression* on the breast will spread the tissue out further and make the compressed breast less attenuating, a characteristic that results in a reduced dose.

Patients with greater *breast thickness* (of the same composition) will require a higher dose. As the *fraction of adipose tissue to glandular tissue* changes toward more adipose tissue as it does in older women, there will be reduced absorption, which will lead to lower required dose.

More *scattered radiation* will be removed as the grid ratio goes up; thus, milliampere seconds must be greatly increased to get a properly exposed image. The transmission factor of the grid will be important in determining how much additional exposure is required when a grid is used. In general, compared with nongrid techniques, the doses are raised by a Bucky factor of 2–3 when a typical low-ratio grid (5:1) is used for mammography. As scattered radiation is reduced by the grid, the dose to the patient must be increased to maintain proper film density.

There are a variety of screen-film *image receptors*, including different speed screens, different speed films, single screens, double screens, single-emulsion films, and double-emulsion films. Whatever changes are made to increase the receptor speed will lead to a reduction in dose.

There are various development chemicals, times of development, and temperatures of the development chemicals for *film processing*. As these are adjusted to increase the speed of development, dose will be reduced.

Adjustments of *distance* can be made on many of the machines, and the source-image distance varies from one unit to another. Newer units tend to have approximately a 65-cm source-image distance.

As the breast is moved up and down for magnification techniques, the overall magnification factor for the image will be changed. An increase in the magnification will lead to increased dose to the patient, since the breast will be relatively closer to the target for the same technique. However, in magnification radiography, the grid may not be needed because scattered radiation is already reduced due to the air gap built into any magnification geometry. In that case, there may be only a small increase, no change, or even a reduction in dose for magnification radiography compared with that resulting from conventional screen-film radiography performed with a grid.

CHAPTER NINE

Methods of Dose Reduction: Guidelines and Recommendations

Learning Objectives

Upon completion of this chapter, the reader should be able to:

1. Identify three reports from which guidelines and recommendations for radiation protection are of importance to technologists.
2. Identify methods of dose reduction.
3. Explain the effect of each of the following on dose reduction: education and training, equipment specifications, personnel practices, and shielding.
4. State the general design and performance recommendations for radiographic equipment.
5. Explain the design and performance recommendations for radiographic equipment with respect to: collimation and beam alignment, filtration, source-to-skin distance, exposure reproducibility, and exposure linearity.
6. State the general design recommendations of mobile radiographic equipment.
7. State the recommendations for fluoroscopic equipment with respect to: direct beam absorber, output radiation intensity, filtration, collimation, source-to-skin distance, exposure switch, cumulative timer, spot film device protective drape, and Bucky slot shielding.
8. State the recommendations for protecting personnel from unnecessary radiation.
9. Explain the recommendations for protecting patients in radiology with respect to: technique selection, filtration, collimation, source-to-skin distance, image receptor sensitivity, immobilization, shielding, and fluoroscopy.
10. Explain the recommendations for radiography in pregnancy with respect to: elective examinations, pregnancy posters, the pregnant technologist and shielding, collimation, and exposure technique.
11. State the general recommendations for quality assurance in diagnostic radiology.

Introduction

Chapter 7 dealt with the concepts of dose limitation, the most important of the principles of radiation protection. This chapter explores the basic ideas relating to the other two principles, justification and optimization, but only in terms of radiation protection guidelines and recommendations.

The principles of justification and optimization govern general methods of dose reduction and essentially relate to medical and technical decisions. Whereas medical decisions are best left to the patient and the patient's physician, the decision to have an x-ray examination is a technical decision in the realm of the radiologist and technologist. Technical decisions center on the choice of the equipment and techniques for carrying out the examination, with the goal of keeping the dose as low as reasonably achievable (ALARA).

Radiation Protection Reports

In Chapters 1 and 7, several radiation protection-related reports of particular interest to the technologist were identified as a basis for further study. Whereas several of these reports deal with general radiation protection topics, others address specifically the guidelines and recommendations for radiation protection in diagnostic radiology. These reports are comprehensive and are prepared by experts in the field of radiation protection. Students should make an effort to consult these protection reports, not only to become aware of them but also to get a glimpse of the wording of the actual statements of the various guidelines and recommendations.

In this chapter, selected guidelines and recommendations for dose reduction will be highlighted from at least the following three reports:

1. Code of Federal Regulations (CFR). Title 21. *Performance standards for ionizing radiation emitting products.* Washington, DC: U.S. Department of Health and Human Services, Food and Drug Administration (FDA). 1992.
2. *Medical x-ray, electron beam and gamma ray protection for energies up to 50 MeV:* Equipment design, performance and use. NCRP Report No. 102. 1989.
3. *Safety code 20A. X-ray equipment in medical diagnosis. Part A: Recommended safety procedures for installation and use.* Radiation Protection Bureau–Health Canada. 1992.

While most countries adopt the current radiation protection practices recommended by the ICRP (1993), others develop their own recommendations in cooperation with the ICRP and other international and national radiation protection organizations (Chapter 7).

REVIEW BOX:
In reviewing recommendations for radiation protection practices, it is important to pay close attention to the use of the words "shall," "should," and "must," whose meanings convey varying degrees of obligation depending on the publications in which they appear. See Chapter 7 for detailed descriptions of accepted usage for these terms.

Methods of Dose Reduction

The factors affecting dose in diagnostic radiology have been identified and discussed in Chapter 8. *Dose reduction* is concerned with the methods and techniques that are intended to vary these factors in an effort to minimize the radiation dose to patients, personnel, and members of the public. These methods and techniques are influenced by the guidelines and recommendations of international (ICRP) and national (NCRP) radiation protection advisory groups and organizations.

Dose reduction can be accomplished in several ways; however, this chapter addresses only those recommendations relating to the following: (1) education and training, (2) equipment design and performance, (3) personnel practices, and (4) shielding.

It is not within the scope of this book to examine the details of all of these; therefore, only the more commonplace elements of each will be presented. Students should consult with their instructors and refer to the radiation protection recommendations specific to their countries and regions for the complete picture.

Education and Training

In Publication 33, the ICRP (1982) stated:

> No person shall operate radiological equipment without adequate technical competence, or perform radiological procedures without adequate knowledge of the physical properties and harmful effects of ionizing radiation (p. 18).

This particular recommendation is supported by national organizations that provide guidelines for the education and training of radiological technologists. In addition, various professional radiologic technology organizations such as the American Society of Radiologic Technologists (ASRT) and the Canadian Association of Medical Radiation Technologists (CAMRT), for example, have a significant role to play in the training and certification of technologists, in an effort to ensure that they meet minimum standards for the clinical practice of radiography. These minimum standards are clearly defined in radiography curricula and allow students to pursue studies in basic physics, instrumentation, anatomy and physiology, patient care, radiographic technique and evaluation, pathology, radiobiology, and radiation protection, after which they write national certification examinations. Successful completion of these examinations indicates that individuals are now capable of working competently in the radiology department.

The education of the radiologic technologist never ceases. The continual introduction of new equipment and techniques into the department provides the radiologic technologist with numerous opportunities to refine and update knowledge. Indeed, the technologist's responsibility for upgrading skills and familiarizing himself or herself with technological innovations is encouraged by the code of ethics of various professional organizations. For example, the ASRT Code of Ethics states that:

> The radiologic technologist continually strives to improve knowledge and skills by participating in educational and professional activities, sharing knowledge with colleagues and investigating new and innovative aspects of professional practice. One means available to improve knowledge and skills is through professional continuing education.

Education and training provide the technologist with the knowledge, skills, and attitudes necessary to reduce the dose to patients, personnel, and members of the public.

Equipment Specifications

All of the x-ray equipment used in diagnostic radiology is designed in accordance with standards set forth in various governmental acts and are intended to optimize image quality and to protect patients and operators from unnecessary radiation exposure. For example, in the United States, the FDA plays a significant role in regulating the manufacture of equipment under the Radiation Control Health and Safety Act of 1968. Additionally, the FDA also establishes performance standards for x-ray equipment. In Canada, on the other hand, equipment specifications must meet the requirements of two acts, the Food and Drugs Act (under Medical Devices Regulations), which addresses the safety and usefulness of equipment, and the Radiation Emitting Devices Act (under the Radiation Emitting Regulations), which deals with design and performance issues for safety. The manufacturer has the responsibility to ensure that the equipment meets the requirements of these regulations.

The topic of dose reduction by equipment design and performance will be elaborated on in the next section of this chapter.

Personnel Practices

Another aspect of dose reduction techniques is related to the manner in which technologists perform x-ray examinations on patients. Such performance is governed by the adherence to the principles of radiation protection including the ALARA philosophy and the guidelines and recommendations of carrying out the examinations. Technologists must always strive to achieve excellence in radiation protection by personally practicing all the safety rules and regulations intended to protect not only the patient but also operators and other personnel, as well as members of the public.

The recommendations for dose reduction by personnel practices will be discussed later in the chapter because they are important elements in a radiation protection program. Additionally, this topic is reflected in the code of ethics of various professional associations. For example, the ASRT Code of Ethics, principle number 7, states that:

> The radiologic technologist utilizes equipment and accessories, employs techniques and procedures, performs services in accordance with an acceptable standard of practice, and demonstrates expertise in limiting the radiation exposure to the patient, self, and other members of the health care team.

By the same token, the CAMRT Code of Ethics requires that each member of the Association shall:

> Conduct all technical procedures with due regard to current radiation safety standards.
>
> Practice only those procedures for which the necessary qualifications are held unless such procedures have been properly delegated by an appropriate medical authority and for which the technologist has received adequate training to an acceptable level of competence.

Shielding

Shielding, which is achieved in one of two ways, is yet another means of reducing the dose of absorbable radiation. Chapter 10 refers to the use of protective barriers (walls) placed between the radiation source (x-ray tube) and the exposed individual. *Specific area shielding*, on the other hand, refers to the use of lead shields to protect radiosensitive organs such as the gonads and breasts (Chapter 8).

Equipment Design and Performance Recommendations

The recommendations and guidelines for equipment specifications *design and performance* are meant to play a significant role in reducing the dose to patients and personnel. These recommendations have been developed for radiographic and fluoroscopic equipment, mammographic and tomographic units, and computed tomographic equipment. It is beyond the scope of this chapter to address all the recommendations; only the more commonplace ones for radiographic and fluoroscopic equipment are reviewed briefly in this section. The student must consult the appropriate documents for further details of the recommendations relevant to his or her country.

Radiographic Equipment: General Recommendations

The general recommendations for equipment design include the use of warning signs, labels, indicator lights and meters; ensuring mechanical stability, exposure control, filtration, indication of exposure; and using technique factors and x-ray tube shielding, to mention but a few. Equipment should be designed so that the operator has a clear view of all warning signs, labels, and meters on the control panel. The location of the focal spot must also be marked on the tube housing. Filtration must be marked on the tube head and the minimum permanent inherent filtration must be indicated. In addition, there are specific requirements for the total permanent filtration, which will be discussed in the next section.

Other general recommendations of importance to the technologist relate to exposure control and x-ray tube shielding. Exposure control refers to the exposure switch and timer, which are used, respectively, to start and stop the exposure to the patient. For radiography and fluoroscopy, the exposure switch must be of a "dead-man" type, which means that the operator must apply continuous pressure to activate the exposure.

For fixed radiographic equipment, the position of the exposure switch is such that the operator must be in the control booth during the exposure. In addition, exposure timers should be accurate to within ±5% of the time selected.

The x-ray tube shielding recommendations are intended to address leakage radiation from the x-ray tube. The NCRP (1989) recommended that the leakage radiation measured at 1 m from the tube not exceed 0.1 centigray (cGy) (0.1 rad) per hour.

Radiographic Equipment: Specific Recommendations

In addition to these general recommendations, there are specific recommendations vital to the practice of radiation protection. They are as follows:

COLLIMATION AND BEAM ALIGNMENT

The FDA, in CFR Title 21 (1992), recommended that for collimation at a source-to-image receptor distance (SID) of 100 cm, the minimum field size must be ≤ 5 cm × 5 cm and the x-ray field size must be aligned to within 2% of the SID at the middle of the image receptor. For systems with automatic collimation or positive beam limitation (PBL), the technologist should not be able to make an exposure if the x-ray field size is greater than the size of the image receptor by >3% of the SID. An override system must be provided to allow the operator to collimate to the size of the image receptor or smaller.

Leakage radiation from the collimator is just as important as leakage from the x-ray tube, and in this regard, the recommendation is that the collimator must offer the same degree of shielding (attenuation) as that of the tube housing.

FILTRATION

Filtration is intended to protect the patient (Chapter 8) and the recommendations are very specific for diagnostic x-ray beams, depending on the kVp used. For example, the required minimum total filtration in the useful beam must be as follows (NCRP, 1989; Health and Welfare Canada, 1992):

1. 0.5 mm aluminum (Al), when the x-ray tube is operated below 50 kVp.
2. 1.5 mm Al, when the tube is operated in between 50 kVp to 70 kVp.
3. 2.5 mm Al, when the tube is operated above 70 kVp.

These filters must be permanently mounted onto the tube housing or collimator.

SOURCE-TO-SKIN DISTANCE (SSD)

The SSD in radiography influences the dose to the patient and, as such, the NCRP (1989) recommended that:

> The SSD *shall not* be less than 30 cm (12 in) and *should not* be less than 38 cm (15 in). Note: For tabletop radiographic procedures, the source-to-film distance (SFD) *should not* be less than 100 cm (40 in). For upright chest radiography, the SFD *should not* be less than 180 cm (72 in) (p. 20).

EXPOSURE REPRODUCIBILITY

When the same exposure technique factors are used repeatedly, the output radiation intensity should be the same for all exposures. This is what is meant by *exposure reproducibility*. To meet the recommendations for reproducibility, the output intensity must not be greater than ±5% of the average intensities of a series of 10 exposures (Bushong, 1993).

EXPOSURE LINEARITY

The combination of different mA and time selections to produce constant mAs values should produce constant output radiation intensities (mR/mAs). This is referred to as *exposure linearity*. For radiographic equipment, the recommendations require that the output intensities for adjacent mA selections not vary by more than 10%.

Mobile Radiographic Equipment

Most of the general design recommendations for fixed radiographic equipment (tube shielding, focal spot location, filtration, collimation, warning signs, indicator lights and meters, exposure timing) apply equally well to mobile radiographic equipment. For example, the recommendation for collimation in mobile radiography is as follows:

> Mobile radiographic equipment *shall be* equipped with adjustable collimators containing light localizers that define the border of the entire field. The difference between the length of each x-ray beam edge and each light-field edge *shall not* be greater than two percent of the source-to-image receptor distance at the image receptor (NCRP, 1989, p. 25).

One specific requirement for mobile radiographic equipment that is fundamentally different from fixed radiographic equipment is that of the exposure switch. The recommendation is such that:

> The exposure switch on mobile radiographic units *shall* be so arranged that the operator can

> stand at least 2 m (6 ft.) from the patient, the x-ray tube and the useful beam (NCRP, 1989, p.25).

Fluoroscopic Equipment

Controlling the factors affecting dose in fluoroscopy (Chapter 8) can significantly reduce the dose to both patients and personnel. Although the design recommendations for fluoroscopic equipment are discussed in detail in CFR Title 21 (FDA, 1992), this subsection highlights only a few important requirements. These include direct beam absorbers, the output radiation intensity, filtration, collimation, source-to-skin distance, exposure switch, cumulative timer, spot film device protective drape, and the Bucky slot shielding.

DIRECT BEAM ABSORBER

All fluoroscopic units must have a *direct beam absorber*, often referred to as a *primary protective barrier*, permanently built into the unit. The purpose of this primary barrier is to limit the exposure during fluoroscopy. If this barrier is removed at any time, the exposure will terminate. In accordance with the FDA's 1992 recommendations, the barrier ensures that the exposure does not exceed 0.002 cGy/hr (2 mrad/hr) at 10 cm from the image receptor.

OUTPUT RADIATION INTENSITY

The *exposure rate* in fluoroscopy should not be <5 cGy/min (5 rad/min) and shall be <10 cGy/min (10 rad/min) unless high-level-control is used. A continuous audible tone shall be heard when high-level-control is used in a fluoroscopic examination (FDA, 1992).

FILTRATION

Because fluoroscopy is usually done at higher than 70 kVp, the total permanent filtration must be at least 2.5 mm Al equivalent.

COLLIMATION

For collimation in fluoroscopy, the NCRP (1989) specifically recommended that:

> An adjustable collimator *shall* be provided to restrict the size of the beam to the area of interest.
>
> 1. The x-ray tube and collimating system *shall* be linked with the image receptor assembly so that the beam is centered on the image receptor assembly. The beam *should* be confined within the useful receptor area at all source-image receptor distances.
>
> 2. For spot film radiography, the shutters *shall* automatically change to the required field size before each exposure (p. 15).

SOURCE-TO-SKIN DISTANCE (SSD)

When the x-ray tube is close to the patient, the skin dose increases and hence a recommended limit has been placed on the SSD. The recommendations are such that the SSD shall not be <30 cm (12 in) for mobile fluoroscopy and must not be <38 cm (15 in) for stationary fluoroscopic equipment.

EXPOSURE SWITCH

As in radiographic equipment, the exposure switch in fluoroscopy, whether it be a foot switch or a switch on the spot film device, must be of the dead-man type.

CUMULATIVE TIMER

The recommendation for such a timer is as follows:

> A cumulative timing device, activated by the fluoroscope exposure switch, *shall* be provided. It *shall* indicate either by an audible or visual signal, or both, obvious to the user, the passage of a predetermined period of irradiation not to exceed five minutes. The signal *should* last at least 15 seconds at which time the timer must be reset manually (NCRP, 1989, p. 15).

SPOT FILM DEVICE PROTECTIVE DRAPE

The distribution of scattered radiation during fluoroscopy is illustrated in Figure 9-1. This can significantly increase the dose to personnel during a fluoroscopic examination. A protective curtain or drape of dimensions not less than 45.7 cm × 45.7 cm (18 in × 18 in) attached to

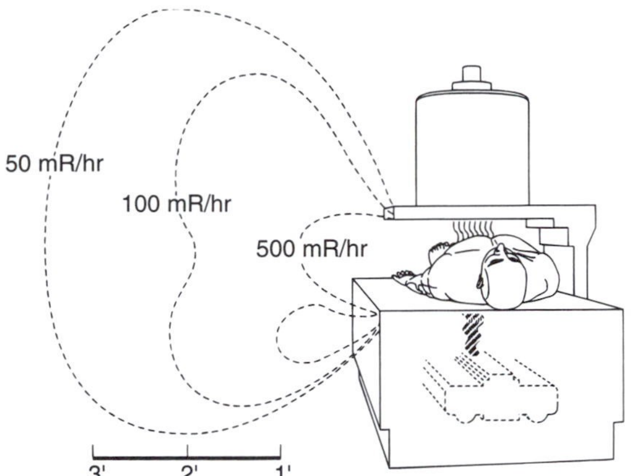

FIGURE 9-1. The distribution of scattered radiation during fluoroscopy without the protective lead curtain mounted on the spot film device. (From Bushong, S. (1993). *Radiologic science for technologists.* 5th ed. Mosby–Year Book. Reproduced by permission.)

the spot film device will minimize the dose to personnel by shielding against radiation scattered above the tabletop. For adequate protection, the drape should have at least 0.25 mm lead equivalent. In Canada, the recommendation requires a lead equivalent of not <0.5 mm at 100 kVp.

There are a few situations (e.g., in a myelogram examination) when it may not be possible to use the lead protective curtain. In these cases, it is recommended that a retractable lead shield with a height of at least 15 cm from the tabletop and a lead equivalent of at least 0.5 mm at 100 kVp be used. This retractable shield must be mounted on the side of the table where the operator stands to use the spot film device during the examination.

BUCKY SLOT SHIELDING

Another aspect of fluoroscopic equipment specifications designed to minimize scattered radiation to personnel during a fluoroscopic procedure is that of the Bucky slot shielding. The shielding must be a part of the equipment and should be of at least 0.25 mm lead equivalent (Fig. 8-1).

Recommendations for Personnel Practices

Personnel practices simply refer to the tasks in carrying out an x-ray examination that has been prescribed by the patient's physician. These practices are intended to protect both patients and personnel from unnecessary radiation. This section addresses the more common recommendations for patient and personnel protection as well as the general guidelines for the reduction of gonadal dose.

Protection of Personnel

In protecting personnel from unnecessary radiation, the goal is to keep exposures below recommended dose limits (Chapter 7) by adhering to the philosophy of ALARA. Accomplishing this goal is guided by several recommendations, not only for operating the equipment but for performing the procedure as well. A few examples are as follows:

PERSONS IN THE X-RAY ROOM

No individual must be present in the x-ray room during the exposure. Those individuals whose presence is required must be protected by some form of shielding (protective aprons and gloves or mobile protective barriers).

DOORS TO X-RAY ROOMS

When rooms are occupied by patients, all doors should be kept closed. Because doors to x-ray rooms are shielded, they offer some degree of protection to individuals outside the room in the vicinity of the doors.

DISTANCE

Personnel must remain as far away as possible from the useful beam. Personnel must not be exposed to the useful beam. During mobile radiography, the operator must stand at least 2 m (6 ft) from the x-ray machine (including the x-ray tube) and the patient. In Canada, the recommended distance is 3 m.

HOLDING PATIENTS

The NCRP (1989) specifically recommended that:

> No person *should* routinely hold patients during diagnostic examinations. When a patient must be held in position for radiography, a mechanical supporting or restraining device *should* be used. If such use of mechanical means is not possible and human support or restraint must be used, the individual holding the patient *should* be chosen so that cumulative doses will be held within acceptable limits. Pregnant women or persons under the age of 18 years *should not* be permitted to hold patients. If a patient must be held by someone, that individual *shall* be protected with appropriate shielding devices such as protective gloves and aprons. Positioning *should* be arranged so that no part of the holder's torso, even if covered by protective clothing, will be struck by the useful beam and so that the holder's body is as far as possible from the useful beam (p. 22, 23).

CONTROL BOOTH

All operators should remain in the control booth during the exposure. They must have an unobstructed view of the patient and be able to communicate without leaving the booth. In procedures in which operators must be at the patient's side, protective clothing must be worn.

WEARING PERSONNEL DOSIMETERS

Personnel dosimeters are often worn at the level of the waist or upper chest level, beside the sternum, during radiographic procedures. In fluoroscopy, when protective aprons are worn, the dosimeter should be worn outside the apron at the level of the collar, a recommendation of the Council of Radiation Control Program Directors (CRCPD). It is interesting to note that in Canada this recommendation states that "the personnel dosimeter *must* be worn under the apron."

In procedures in which the extremities of operators are subject to high exposures, such as in angiography, it is recommended that additional dosimeters be worn on the extremity to monitor these exposures.

PROTECTIVE CLOTHING

Protective clothing in this text refers to aprons, gloves, and thyroid shields. Protective aprons are generally made of lead-impregnated vinyl and worn during fluoroscopic and some radiographic procedures. They are available in varying sizes and shapes and have different lead equivalent thicknesses. In Table 9-1, several characteristics of lead aprons are given. An important characteristic is the percentage attenuation afforded by each of the lead equivalent thicknesses at different kVp values. From Table 9-1, it is clearly apparent that as the lead equiv-

TABLE 9-1. SEVERAL CHARACTERISTICS OF PROTECTIVE LEAD APRONS WORN BY PERSONNEL AND OTHER INDIVIDUALS IN THE RADIOLOGY DEPARTMENT

Equivalent Thickness (mm Pb)	Weight (lb)	X-Ray Attenuation (%) by kVp of Operation		
		50 kVp	75 kVp	100 kVp
0.25	3–10	97	66	51
0.50	6–15	99.9	88	75
1.00	12–25	99.9	99	94

SOURCE: Bushong, S. (1993). *Radiologic science for technologists.* St. Louis: Mosby–Year Book. Reproduced by permission.

alent thickness increases, the percentage attenuation increases for the same kVp value. For example, the percentage attenuation afforded by an apron of 0.5 mm lead equivalent thickness is 75%, whereas it is 94% for an apron of 1 mm lead equivalent thickness at the same kVp (Bushong, 1993).

The NCRP (1989) recommended that:

> Protective aprons of at least 0.5 mm lead equivalent *shall* be worn in the fluoroscopy room by each person (except the patient). People who must move around the room during the procedure *should* wear a wraparound protective garment (p. 18).

Protective gloves are used primarily when it is likely that the hands of operators (and individuals holding patients) will be exposed to the useful beam or that they are in the immediate vicinity of the primary beam. Lead gloves of at least 0.25 mm lead equivalent must be worn to provide some degree of attenuation and thus protect the hand from radiation exposure. In this regard, the NCRP (1989) recommended that:

> The hand of the fluoroscopist *shall* not be placed in the useful beam unless the beam is attenuated by the patient and a protective glove of at least 0.25 mm lead equivalent (p. 18).

The recommendations for protective aprons and gloves in Canada are at least 0.5 mm and 0.25 mm lead equivalent, respectively (Radiation Protection Bureau–Health Canada, 1992).

Thyroid shields are now worn by individuals performing fluoroscopy to protect the neck and thyroid gland from radiation exposure due to scatter. These shields are available commercially and provide attenuation equivalent to at least 0.5 mm of lead.

Protection of Patients

Diagnostic radiology contributes the highest man-made exposure to the population (Chapter 3); therefore, it is absolutely necessary to reduce the dose to patients without compromising the quality of the examination. This goal is also guided by several recommendations and procedures directed to the technologist, radiologist, and the patient's physician (who prescribes the examination) in an effort to minimize patient exposure.

There are several general recommendations to guide technologists and radiologists in carrying out the examination, and they relate to the factors affecting dose discussed in Chapter 8. Examples of these are as follows:

TECHNIQUE SELECTION

Various radiation protection agencies advocate the use of the highest kVp without compromising the quality of the examination because high kVp techniques result in a smaller dose to the patient. In addition, the use of automatic exposure timing is recommended to ensure that exposures and repeat examinations are kept to a minimum.

FILTRATION

Technologists should always ensure that the proper filtration is used and is consistent with the requirements of the particular examination. The total permanent filtration was discussed in Chapter 8. The NCRP (1989) stated that:

> Special care *should* be taken to ensure that adequate and proper filtration is used for all radiographic exposures (p. 23).

COLLIMATION

Collimation is intended to protect the patient by limiting the primary beam to the anatomical area of interest. The recommendation for collimation implies that:

1. The beam must be collimated to the smallest area of interest, consistent with the goals of the x-ray examination.
2. The beam must be collimated to the size of the image receptor or smaller.
3. Evidence of collimation should be seen on the film, that is, the edges of the useful beam

should be visible on the film. This requirement ensures that only the area of interest has been exposed.

Collimation is under the direct control of the technologist (and radiologist, during fluoroscopic procedures), and every effort must be made to ensure correct collimation of the primary beam.

SOURCE-TO-SKIN DISTANCE (SSD)

In carrying out the x-ray examination, the technologist should use the maximum SSD consistent with the requirements of the particular examination. Additionally, the optimum source-to-image receptor distance should be used, based on the requirements of the procedure.

IMAGE RECEPTOR SENSITIVITY

Because the sensitivity of the image receptor affects the dose to the patient, the recommendation for minimizing dose is stated as follows:

> X-ray films, intensifying screens, and other image recording devices *should* be as sensitive as is consistent with the requirements of the examination (NCRP, 1989, p. 22).

The dose to the patient is inversely proportional to the sensitivity of the image receptor. This simply means that if the sensitivity is increased by a factor of 2, the dose will be reduced by 1/2. In other words, going from a 200-speed film-screen system to a 400-speed system will reduce the radiation exposure to the patient by 50%.

IMMOBILIZATION

The use of immobilization is reflected in the recommendation for holding patients stating that restraining devices should be used. In this way, repeat exposures due to patient motion can be avoided.

SHIELDING

Protection of radiosensitive organs by lead shielding is a significant task required of the technologist during an examination. The NCRP (1989), for example, was specific in recommending that eyes and the gonads be shielded from exposure to the useful beam. Specific recommendations for doing so are presented in Appendix A.

> Sensitive body organs (e.g., lens of the eye, gonads) *should* be shielded whenever they are likely to be exposed to the useful beam provided that such shielding does not eliminate useful diagnostic information or proper treatment. Shielding should never be used as a substitute for adequate beam collimation.
>
> *Comment*: Gonadal shielding using at least 0.5 mm lead (usual lead equivalence of aprons) *should* be considered whenever potentially procreative patients are likely to receive direct gonadal radiation in an examination. The lens of the eye *should* be shielded (2 mm lead—usual eye shield thickness) during tomographic procedures that include the eye in the useful beam. Such shielding is unnecessary if the posterior-anterior projection is used. The use of posterior-anterior (PA) projections of the thoracic spine at increased source-to-image distance (SID) *should* be considered in studies of females to reduce the dose to the breasts (p. 8).

FLUOROSCOPY

In carrying out a fluoroscopic examination, both the technologist and the radiologist are responsible for ensuring that the ALARA philosophy is upheld. The recommendations for fluoroscopy will assist personnel in minimizing patient exposure. In Appendix A, 19 NCRP recommendations for personnel performing fluoroscopy are given. The student should note how the terms "shall" and "should" are used in the recommendations.

Recommendations for Radiography in Pregnancy

Carrying out an x-ray examination on pregnant women or women of childbearing age is a topic that demands a great deal of attention because of the increased radiation risks to the embryo or fetus (Chapter 4). The decision to irradiate pregnant patients rests with the patient's physician, usually in consultation with the radiologist. The technologist carries out the examination under the direct guidance of the radiologist.

The general ICRP principles relating to the radiography of women are presented in Appendix B. For radiography of pregnant women, the more common recommendations are centered around the 10-day rule; elective examinations; pregnancy posters, shielding, collimation, and technique factors; as well as the use of diagnostic ultrasound. In addition, there are several concerns regarding the pregnant technologist. Each of these will now be briefly highlighted.

The 10-Day Rule

The goal of the *10-day rule* was to prevent unintentional exposure of the embryo or fetus. The recommendation regarding this was stated by the ICRP in 1970 and implies that if radiography of the abdomen or pelvis on women of childbearing age is needed, then it should be done during the 10 days following the onset of menstruation because it is highly unlikely that a woman might be pregnant during this period. Bushong (1993) pointed out that this rule is "obsolete" in the present-day practice of radiology (in light of the current knowledge of radiobiology); however, if pregnancy is confirmed and an x-ray examination is needed, every effort must be made to reduce the exposure to the embryo or fetus.

Elective Examinations

An *elective examination* is one that is not urgently needed and can be done at a time deemed suitable to the needs and safety of the patient. The NCRP (1989) recommended that "the timeliness of medical needs" be given primary consideration when scheduling elective examinations.

> Ideally, an elective abdominal examination of a woman of childbearing age should be performed during the first few days following the onset of menses to minimize the possibility of irradiation of an embryo. In practice, the timeliness of medical needs should be the primary consideration in deciding the timing of the examination (p. 8).

Pregnancy Posters

To avoid unnecessary radiation exposure of the embryo or fetus, signs or posters that seek to obtain pregnancy information from the patient should be made available. They should appear in areas in the department where they can be clearly seen (reception areas, changing rooms, x-ray rooms) by the female patient who will be undergoing the examination.

The Pregnant Technologist

Bushong (1993) presented an excellent discussion of the issues and concerns surrounding the pregnant technologist. This topic was also discussed by Archer (1994) and Dowd (1994), who pointed out the "posting of notices to employees" and the "legal rights of pregnant radiographers," respectively. The following points are noteworthy:

1. A pregnant technologist should notify the radiology department of her pregnancy so that appropriate plans can be made to monitor her radiation exposure. In addition, the technologist should be counseled during pregnancy while she continues her employment.
2. A pregnant technologist should be provided with a second dosimeter worn under the apron at waist level to monitor fetal exposure for the remainder of the pregnancy (Bushong, 1993).
3. "Under no circumstances should termination or involuntary leave of absence occur" (Bushong, 1993, p. 610).
4. It is not necessary to alter the work schedule of the pregnant technologist because the

dose equivalent limit to the fetus is 5 mSv (500 mrem), a level considered "absolutely safe." Additionally, Bushong (1993) pointed out that workers in fluoroscopy who are protected by lead aprons do not exceed 500 μSv/yr (50 mrem/yr). He further reported that 95% of these workers receive <1 μSv/yr (100 mrem/yr).

Shielding, Collimation, and Exposure Technique

When a medical decision has been made to irradiate a pregnant patient, it is recommended that the technologist: (1) use high kVp techniques, (2) collimate the primary beam effectively and accurately, and (3) place the gonadal shield precisely on the patient so as not to compromise the quality of the examination.

Use of Diagnostic Ultrasound

The ICRP (1993) and other radiation protection organizations recommended that ultrasound be used for the evaluation of fetal maturation and placental localization instead of diagnostic radiography.

Recommendations for Quality Assurance

The basic framework for quality assurance (QA) in radiation protection is discussed in Chapter 13. A QA program is an essential subset of a radiation protection program because it is intended to monitor appropriate activities in a department not only in an effort to reduce costs, but, more importantly, to maintain optimum image quality with minimum radiation dose to patients and personnel. QA encompasses administrative, educational, and preventive maintenance as well as quality control (QC) methods. QC deals specifically with the technical aspects of ensuring optimum image quality with reduced radiation doses.

Depending on their size, radiology departments should have a QA program, in which case QC tests are recommended to be performed on all radiological equipment including photographic, radiographic, fluoroscopic, and special procedures equipment. Whereas some of these tests are performed on a daily basis, it is recommended that others be done monthly, semiannually, and annually. For example, it is recommended that for radiographic equipment, the following tests be performed on an annual basis: filtration; x-ray beam, Bucky, and motion centering; x-ray beam perpendicularity and SID indicator accuracy; visual checks; overload protection; kVp; exposure timers; mR/mAs; linearity; exposure reproducibility; grid alignment and x-ray output waveform (NCRP, 1988), to mention only a few.

For photographic equipment, it is recommended that the following QC tests be done on a daily basis: processor sensitometry, chemicals, fixer, and film washing developer and wash water temperature, water filters, replenishment rate, and processing stand-by limits (NCRP, 1988).

It is not within the scope of this book to discuss the details of these QC tests because this is a topic for a course on QC; however, Chapter 13 presents an overview of the role of quality assurance in radiation protection.

REVIEW QUESTIONS

1. Dose reduction methods and techniques are intended to minimize the radiation dose to:
   - A. Patients.
   - B. Personnel.
   - C. Members of the public.
   - D. All of the above.

2. Which of the following individuals can operate x-ray equipment?
   - A. Radiologic technologists.
   - B. Radiologists.

C. Physicians trained in the physical properties and harmful effects of ionizing radiation.
D. All of the above.

3. For fixed radiographic and fluoroscopic equipment, the exposure switch must:
   A. Be of a "dead-man" type.
   B. Allow the operator to remain in the control booth during the exposure.
   C. Have a cord length of at least 2 m.
   D. A and B are correct.

4. For fixed radiographic equipment, the exposure timer should be accurate to within:
   A. ±0.5% of the time selected.
   B. ±5% of the time selected.
   C. ±25% of the time selected.
   D. ±0.05% of the time selected.

5. The NCRP recommended that the x-ray tube be shielded so that the leakage radiation measured at 1 m from the tube not exceed:
   A. 0.1 centigray (cGy) per hour.
   B. 1 cGy per hour.
   C. 10 cGy per hour.
   D. 0.1 Gy per hour.

6. The FDA recommends that the minimum field size at 100 cm SID must be:
   A. >5 cm × 5 cm.
   B. ≤5 cm × 5 cm.
   C. ≤5 mm × 5 mm.
   D. ≤2% of the area of a cassette of dimensions 8 in × 10 in.

7. The FDA recommended that the x-ray field size must be aligned to within ______ of the SID at the middle of the image receptor.
   A. 5%.
   B. 25%.
   C. 0.2%.
   D. 2%.

8. The required minimum total filtration of the useful beam above 70 kVp is:
   A. 0.5 mm aluminum (Al) equivalent.
   B. 1.5 mm Al equivalent.
   C. 2.5 mm Al equivalent.
   D. 2.5 cm Al equivalent.

9. The NCRP recommended that the source-to-film distance for tabletop radiography should not be:
   A. <38 cm.
   B. <100 cm.
   C. <180 cm.
   D. <40 cm.

10. The recommendations for exposure reproductivity is that the intensity must not be greater than ______ of the average intensities of a series of 10 exposures:
    A. ±10%.
    B. ±1%.
    C. ±2%.
    D. ±5%.

11. For exposure linearity, the recommendations require that the output intensities for adjacent mA stations should not vary by more than:
    A. 10%.
    B. 5%.
    C. 2%.
    D. 1%.

12. The NCRP recommended that the exposure cord length for mobile radiographic units be at least:
    A. 1 m long.
    B. 2.5 m long.
    C. 3 m long.
    D. 2 m long.

13. The total permanent filtration in fluoroscopy must be at least:
    A. 2 mm Al equivalent.
    B. 1.5 mm Al equivalent.
    C. 2.5 mm Al equivalent.
    D. 4.0 mm Al equivalent.

14. In fixed fluoroscopy units, the source-to-skin distance must not be less than:
    A. 30 cm.
    B. 38 mm.
    C. 38 cm.
    D. 30 mm.

15. The protective lead drape hanging from the spot film device should have dimensions of not less than:
    A. 45.7 cm × 45.7 cm.
    B. 45.7 mm × 45.7 mm.
    C. 30 cm × 30 cm.
    D. 50 cm × 50 cm.

16. The drape in Question 15 above should have a lead equivalent of at least:
    A. 5 mm.
    B. 25 mm.
    C. 0.5 mm.
    D. 0.25 mm.

17. The Bucky slot shielding should be at least ________ lead equivalent.
    A. 0.25 mm.
    B. 0.5 mm.
    C. 0.25 cm.
    D. 2 mm.

18. In Canada, the recommended distance for the operator during mobile radiography is:
    A. 1 m from the x-ray machine.
    B. 2 m from the x-ray machine.
    C. 3 m from the x-ray machine.
    D. 10 m from the x-ray machine.

19. The following may be used for patient immobilization except:
    A. Mechanical restraining devices.
    B. A 17-year-old volunteer.
    C. A pregnant mother.
    D. B and C are correct.

20. Which of the following applies with regard to the control booth?
    A. The technologist should remain in the booth during the exposure.
    B. The technologist's view of the patient must be unobstructed.
    C. The technologist can communicate with the patient without leaving the booth.
    D. All of the above.

21. The Council of Radiation Control Program Directors (CRCPD) recommended the following with respect to wearing personnel dosimeters:
    A. They could be worn at the level of the waist during radiography.
    B. They could be worn at the level of the upper chest (beside the sternum) during radiography.
    C. During fluoroscopy, when a lead apron is worn, dosimeters should be worn outside the apron at the level of the collar.
    D. All of the above.

22. According to the NCRP, the lead equivalent for protective aprons worn in fluoroscopy is:
    A. 1 mm.
    B. 0.25 mm.
    C. 0.5 mm.
    D. 2.5 mm.

23. The NCRP's recommendation for protective gloves used in fluoroscopy is:
    A. 1 mm lead equivalent.
    B. 0.25 mm lead equivalent.
    C. 0.5 mm lead equivalent.
    D. 2.5 mm Al equivalent.

24. The NCRP's recommendation for thyroid shields used during fluoroscopy is:
    A. 0.5 mm lead equivalent.
    B. 0.25 mm lead equivalent.
    C. 1 mm lead equivalent.
    D. 2.5 mm Al equivalent.

25. In terms of exposure technique, which of the following will result in less dose to the patient?

A. High mA and low kVp techniques.
B. High mAs and low kVp techniques.
C. High mAs and high kVp techniques.
D. Low mAs and high kVp techniques.

26. Which of the following is true when collimation is used to protect the patient?

A. The beam must be collimated to the smallest area of interest.
B. The beam must be collimated to the size of the image receptor or smaller.
C. Evidence of collimation should be seen on the film.
D. All of the above.

27. Which of the following is intended to protect the patient?

A. Collimation.
B. Filtration.
C. Shielding radiosensitive organs.
D. All of the above.

28. If the sensitivity of the image receptor is doubled, the dose to the patient will be:

A. Reduced by half.
B. Reduced by a factor of 4.
C. Increased by a factor of 2.
D. Increased by a factor of 4.

29. If an examination is done with a 400-speed image receptor rather than a 200-speed system, the dose to the patient will be:

A. Reduced by 100%.
B. Reduced by 50%.
C. Increased by a factor of 2.
D. The dose is not related to image receptor speed.

30. The following should be shielded when they are exposed to the useful beam:

A. Eyes.
B. Gonads.
C. Thyroid.
D. All of the above.

31. The following applies to radiography in pregnancy except:

A. Elective abdominal examinations in women of childbearing age should be performed during the first few days following the onset of menses (NCRP, 1989).
B. Pregnancy posters should be posted in the department.
C. A pregnant mother can hold an infant during a radiographic examination.
D. A pregnant technologist should inform the department of her pregnancy.

32. When a pregnant woman has to undergo a radiographic examination:

A. High kVp techniques should be used.
B. Accurate beam collimation is essential.
C. Gonadal shield must be carefully placed so that it does not interfere with the quality of the examination.
D. All of the above.

REFERENCES

Bushong, S. (1993). *Radiologic Science for Technologists* (5th ed.) St Louis: Mosby–Year Book.

NCRP. (1989). *Medical x-ray, electron beam and gamma ray protection for energies up to 50 MeV: Equipment design, performance, and use.* (Report No. 102). NCRP. Bethesda, MD: National Council on Radiation Protection and Measurements (NCRP).

International Commission on Radiological Protection. (1993). *Summary of the current ICRP principles for protection of the patient in diagnostic radiology.* Elmsford, NY: Pergamon Press.

International Commission on Radiological Protection. (1982). *Protection of the patient in diagnostic radiology.* Elmsford, NY: Pergamon Press.

APPENDIX 9–1

NCRP recommendations for personnel performing Fluoroscopy. [From NCRP. (1989). (Report No. 102). *Medical x-ray, electron beam, and gamma ray protection for energies up to 50 MeV; Equipment, Design, Performance, and Use.* Bethesda, MD: NCRP. Reproduced by permission.]

(a) The useful beam *shall* be limited to the smallest area practicable and consistent with the objectives of the radiological examination or treatment (FDA, 1986).

(b) The tube potential (kilovoltage), filtration and source-skin distance (SSD) employed in fluoroscopic examinations *should* be as large as practical, consistent with the objectives of the study.

(c) Protection of the embryo or fetus during fluoroscopic examination of women known to be pregnant *shall* be given special consideration.

Comment: Ideally, an elective abdominal examination of a woman of childbearing age should be performed during the first few days following the onset of menses to minimize the possibility of irradiation of an embryo. In practice, the timeliness of medical needs should be the primary consideration in deciding the timing of the examination. For a detailed discussion see Report No. 54 (NCRP, 1977b); Report No. 91 (NCRP, 1987) and FDA (1981).

(d) Sensitive body organs (*e.g.*, lens of eye, gonads) *should* be shielded whenever they are likely to be exposed to the useful beam provided that such shielding does not eliminate useful diagnostic information. Shielding should never be used as a substitute for adequate beam collimation. [See Section 2.2(d) comment.]

(e) Fluoroscopy *should not* be used as a substitute for radiography, but should be reserved for the study of dynamics or spatial relationships or for guidance in spot-film recording of critical details.

(f) X-ray films, intensifying screens, and other image recording devices *should* be as sensitive as is consistent with the requirements of the examination. (See Section 4.)

(g) Particular care *should* be taken to align the x-ray beam with the patient and image receptor.

(h) Only persons whose presence is necessary *shall* be in the fluoroscopy room during exposures. All such persons *shall* be protected (*e.g.*, provided with leaded aprons, leaded gloves and/or portable shields).

(i) Special care *should* be taken to insure that adequate and proper filtration is used for all fluoroscopic procedures. [See Section 2.2(k) comment.]

(j) The operator *should* use the maximum SSD consistent with medical requirements of the procedure. For fluoroscopic procedures, distances of less than 30 cm (12 in) *shall not* be used. Distances of less than 38 cm (15 in) *should not* be used.

(k) Radiation source systems and imaging systems, as well as film processors *should* be subjected to appropriate quality assurance programs with documentation, in order to minimize the unproductive application of radiation. [See AAPM (1978a; 1978b) and Report 99 (NCRP, 1988).]

(l) Measurements of fluoroscopic table top or patient entrance kerma rate *shall* be made and documented at least annually. Measurements *shall* also be made of kerma for typical spot film exposures.

Comment: Fluoroscopic kerma rate measurements are especially necessary on apparatus employing imaging devices in which brightness is automatically controlled. Such measurements require the use of an attenuation block in the fluoroscopic beam.

(m) The kerma rate used in fluoroscopy *should* be as low as is consistent with the fluoroscopic requirements and *should not* normally exceed 5 cGy/min (5 rad/min) (measured in air) at the position where the beam enters the patient.

Comment: The fluoroscopist should be aware of the kerma levels associated with the various modes of operation. In procedures where spot film cameras are used and where multiple images are easily obtained, this individual must be fully aware of the manner in which exposures are made and must exercise great care to assure that *only required exposures are made.*

(n) The smallest practical field sizes and the shortest irradiation times *should* be employed. (The option of reducing dose by techniques utilizing high tube potential with low mA and/or single frame techniques using image storage devices *should* be considered where dynamic viewing is not required.)

(o) Medical fluoroscopy *should* be performed only by or under the immediate supervision of physicians properly trained in fluoroscopic procedures.

(p) Protective aprons of at least 0.5 mm lead equivalent *shall* be worn in the fluoroscopy room by each person (except the patient). People who must move around the room during the procedure *should* wear a wraparound protective garment.

(q) The hand of the fluoroscopist *shall not* be placed in the useful beam unless the beam is attenuated by the patient and a protective glove of at least 0.25 mm lead equivalent.

(r) Non-intensified fluoroscopy *shall not* be used.

(s) Where fluoroscopy is performed with under-table intensifier and overhead tube, palpation *shall* be achieved only with mechanical devices.

APPENDIX 9–2

Current ICRP Principles for Radiography of Women. [From ICRP. (1993). *Summary of the current ICRP principles for protection of the patient in diagnostic radiology.* Bethesda, MD: ICRP. Reproduced by permission.]

X-Ray Examinations of Women

Because of the radiation risk to an embryo or fetus, the possibility of pregnancy is one of the factors to be considered in deciding whether to conduct an x-ray examination involving the lower abdomen in a woman of reproductive capacity. During the first 10 days following the onset of a menstrual period, there is no radiation risk to any conceptus, since no conception will have occurred. The radiation risk to a child who has been irradiated *in utero* during the first three weeks after conception is likely to be so small that there need be no special limitation on x-ray examinations required within that time period. Nevertheless, attention should always be paid to details of x-ray examinations that would ensure minimisation of absorbed dose in any embryo or fetus that may be present, whether or not the woman is known to be pregnant.

Irradiation of the pregnant patient, at a time when the pregnancy was unrecognised, often leads to her apprehension, because of concern about possible effects on the fetus. Even though the absorbed doses in the conceptus are generally small, such concern may lead to a suggestion that the pregnancy be terminated. However, on the basis of relative risk increment, it would be exceedingly rare for fetal irradiation from an x-ray examination to justify terminating a pregnancy. When such a concern arises, an estimate of absorbed dose and the associated risk to the fetus, should be made by a qualified expert. With such expert and carefully worded advice, the patient should then be in a position to make her own decision regarding continuation of pregnancy.

X-Ray Examination of Women Who May Be Pregnant

It is prudent to consider as pregnant any woman of reproductive age presenting herself for an x-ray examination at a time when a menstrual period is overdue, or missed, unless there is information that precludes pregnancy (e.g. hysterectomy). In addition, every woman of reproductive age should be asked if she is pregnant. In order to minimise the frequency of unintentional irradiation of the embryo or fetus, advisory notices should be posted at several places within diagnostic x-ray departments (particularly at its reception area) and other areas where diagnostic x-ray equipment is used, other than for dentistry. For example:

IF IT IS POSSIBLE THAT YOU MIGHT BE PREGNANT,

NOTIFY THE PHYSICIAN OR RADIOGRAPHER

BEFORE YOUR X-RAY EXAMINATION

Obstetric Radiography

In many instances, particularly in the evaluation of fetal maturation and placental localisation, ultrasonic examinations are preferable to x-ray examinations. Ultrasonic examinations do not utilise ionising radiation and are reliable. When available, the use of ultrasound greatly reduces the need for x-ray examinations of the gravid uterus.

While radiographic pelvimetry is sometimes of great value, it should be undertaken only on the rare occasion when this is likely to be so and should not be carried out on a routine basis. In particular, the superior–inferior projection for the pelvic inlet, also called the brim view, should not be used in view of the unjustifiably high absorbed doses in the fetus.

Other X-Ray Examinations During Pregnancy

When pregnant women require other x-ray examinations in which the x-ray beam irradiates the fetus directly, special care has to be taken to ascertain that the x-ray examination is indeed indicated at that time and that it should not be delayed until after the pregnancy. Sometimes the radiation risk to the fetus is less than that of not making a necessary diagnosis, so that the x-ray examination should still be done when medical indications are appropriate. In such cases, greater than usual care should be taken to minimise the absorbed dose in the fetus for each irradiation. However, alterations of technique should not reduce unduly the diagnostic value of the x-ray examination.

Radiography of areas remote from the fetus, such as the chest, skull or extremities, can be done safely at any time during pregnancy, if the x-ray equipment is properly shielded and if proper x-ray beam limitation is used.

CHAPTER TEN

PROTECTIVE SHIELDING IN DIAGNOSTIC RADIOLOGY

LEARNING OBJECTIVES

Upon completion of this chapter, the reader should be able to:

1. List two categories of protective shielding in radiology.
2. Explain what is meant by source shielding and structural shielding.
3. Define controlled area and uncontrolled area.
4. Distinguish between primary and secondary protective barriers.
5. Describe the essential features of the control booth in a radiology department.
6. Explain the contribution of each of the following in determining the thickness of protective barriers for diagnostic radiology: dose limits, workload, use factor, distance, energy of the radiation, and attenuation factor.
7. List the materials used in the design of protective barriers for diagnostic radiology.
8. Describe each of the following methods for determining the thickness of protective barriers in diagnostic radiology: half-value

(continued)

layer, shielding requirement tables, and attenuation curves.

9 ■ State the recommended limits for leakage radiation from the x-ray tube.

10 ■ State the shielding requirements for x-ray film.

11 ■ Explain an alternative method of shielding design.

Introduction

While technologists make the best use of time and distance factors in protecting individuals from radiation exposure, "shielding limits personnel exposure by reducing the dose rate" (Turner, 1986). In addition, Martin and Harbison (1979) suggested that shielding is "the preferred method because it results in intrinsically safe working conditions whilst reliance on distance or time of exposure may involve continuous administrative control over workers" (p. 89).

These ideas provide a fundamental rationale for including shielding principles in a radiation protection course for radiologic technologists. This chapter explores two categories of protective shielding: source shielding and structural shielding. In particular, the factors affecting structural shielding requirements are described, and two methods for determining the thickness of primary barriers are highlighted. Finally, the chapter concludes with a brief description of x-ray tube shielding (source shielding) as well as shielding guides for x-ray films.

Categories of Protective Shielding

In Figure 10-1, a typical design of a diagnostic radiology department is shown. The design includes x-ray rooms, offices, waiting rooms, dressing rooms, and so on. While some of these rooms will be occupied by both patients and radiation workers (technologists and radiologists), others will be occupied by patients only (dressing rooms and waiting rooms), and others by radiation workers only (offices, for example). In addition, there may be offices and other facilities (storage rooms, restrooms, children's play areas) adjacent to x-ray rooms.

The walls of a diagnostic x-ray department must be shielded to protect individuals outside x-ray rooms from radiation originating inside x-ray rooms. Additionally, individuals inside x-ray rooms must be protected as well. These considerations have resulted in two types of protective shielding: source shielding and structural shielding.

Source Shielding

Source shielding refers to the lead-lined housing of the x-ray tube, which is designed to offer protection against radiation that leaks through the lead-lined housing. Leakage radiation is discussed later in the chapter.

Structural Shielding

Structural shielding refers to the lead-lined walls of x-ray rooms in the department, which are designed to protect individuals from primary scattered and leakage radiation (Fig. 10-2). Specifically, structural shielding is intended to keep the dose limits (Chapter 7) to individuals within established parameters.

The design of shielding is influenced by several factors, including the areas occupied by various individuals. In this respect, two types of areas have been identified: (1) *controlled areas*—areas routinely occupied by radiation workers who are subject to an occupational dose limit of 1 mSv (100 mrem) per week; (2) *uncontrolled areas*—areas occupied by nonradiation workers (any individuals) who are subject to a dose limit of 0.1 mSv (10 mrem) per week.

For controlled areas, the structural shielding should be such that it reduces the exposure rate (exposure divided by time) outside the area, from primary radiation, to <26 μC/kg per week. For uncontrolled areas, the shielding should reduce the exposure rate outside the area, from leakage and scattered radiation, to 2.6 μC/kg per week.

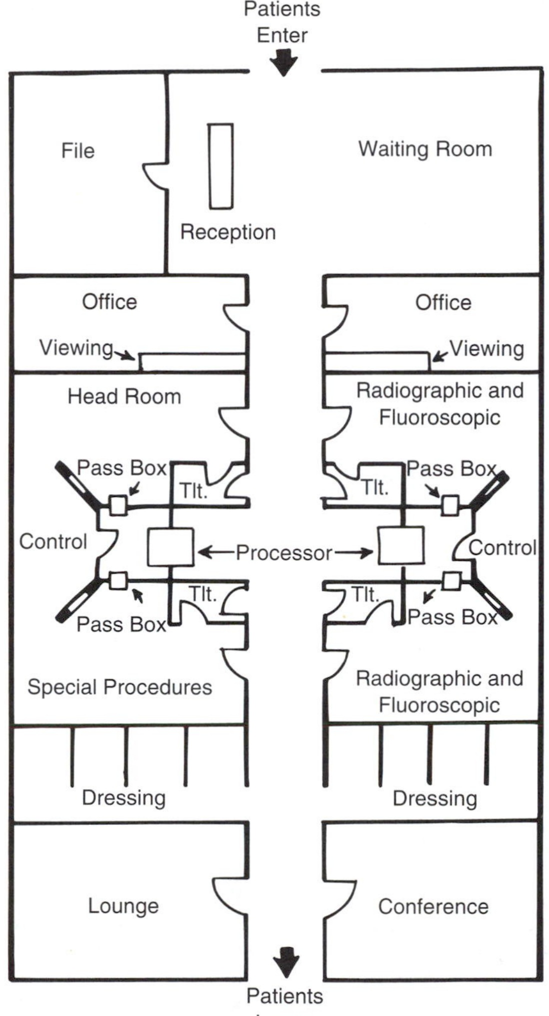

FIGURE 10-1. A basic design of a diagnostic radiology department showing the layout of areas normally occupied by patients and personnel. [From Bushong, S. (1993). *Radiologic science for radiologic technologists* (5th ed.). St. Louis: Mosby-Year Book. Reproduced by permission.]

Protective Barriers

The lead-lined walls of the radiology department are often referred to as *protective barriers* because they are designed to protect individuals located outside x-ray rooms from unnecessary radiation. There are two types of protective barriers: primary barriers and secondary barriers. The basis for such categorization depends on the type of radiation striking the wall.

Primary Protective Barriers

If a wall is struck by primary radiation (the useful beam), it is referred to as a *primary protective barrier.*

Secondary Protective Barriers

A wall that is exposed to secondary radiation (leakage from the x-ray tube and scattered radiation from the patient) is referred to as a *secondary protective barrier.*

These barriers and the type of radiation to which each is exposed are illustrated in Figure 10-3. The following points should be noted about protective barriers (Statkiewicz-Sherer et al., 1993):

1. The direction of the primary beam is perpendicular to the primary protective barrier.
2. The secondary barrier is parallel to the direction of the primary beam.
3. Leakage and scattered radiation can strike both barriers from any direction.
4. Depending on the energy of the primary beam, primary protective barriers are lined with lead of about 1.6 mm (1/16-inch) thick, whereas secondary barriers are usually lined with lead of about 0.8 mm (1/32-inch) thick.
5. The height of protective barriers (from the floor) should be at least 2.1 m (7 ft).
6. Where primary and secondary barriers meet (Fig. 10-3), they should overlap by at least 1.3 cm (0.5 inch), such that the barrier forms a continuous lining.

Control Booth

The *control booth* is an important consideration in the design and structural shielding of an x-ray department for two reasons:

1. It houses the control panel and x-ray exposure switch, which is generally located on

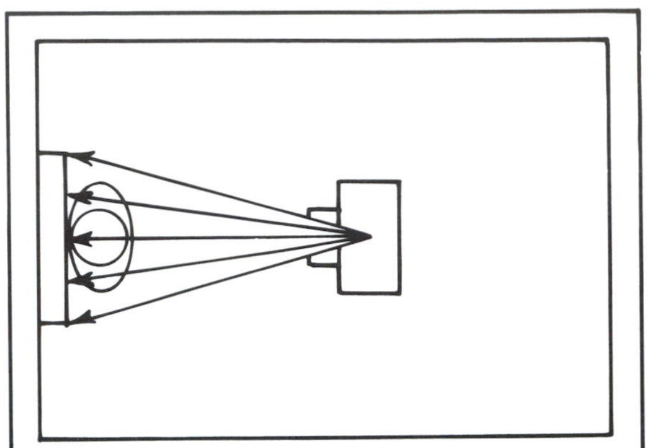

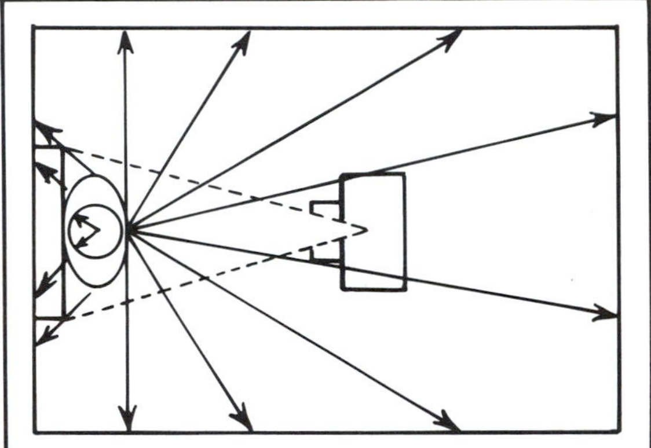

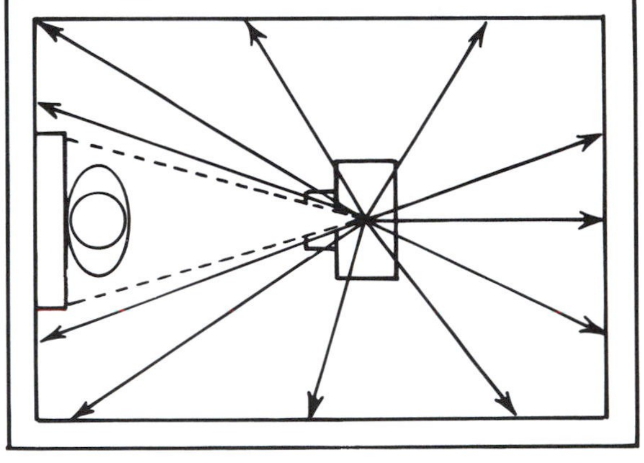

FIGURE 10-2. Structural shielding in an x-ray department depends on several factors, including the type of radiation striking the wall. Here, three types of radiation are illustrated. Primary radiation refers to the useful beam emanating from the target of the x-ray tube, scattered radiation primarily arises from the patient, and leakage radiation emanates from the tube housing. [From Bushberg, J.T., Seibert, J.A., Leidholdt, Jr, E.M., & Boone, J.M. (1994). *The essential physics of medical imaging*. Baltimore: Williams & Wilkins. Reproduced by permission.]

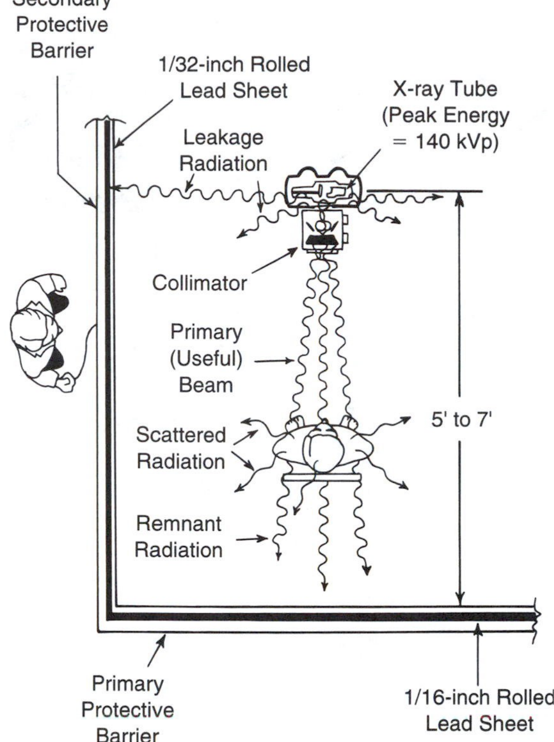

FIGURE 10-3. Two types of protective barriers and the radiation to which each is exposed. The primary barrier provides shielding from primary x-rays, and the secondary barrier provides shielding from both scattered and leakage radiation. [From Statkiewicz-Sherer, M.A., Visconti, P.J., & Ritenour, E.R. (1993). *Radiation protection in medical* radiography (2nd ed.). St. Louis: Mosby-Year Book. Reproduced by permission.]

the control panel (Fig. 10-4). The switch is intentionally positioned within the control booth and designed not to work unless the technologist is actually in the booth during exposures.

2. It serves to protect technologists from scattered and leakage radiation. The walls of the control booth are therefore considered secondary protective barriers.

The location of the control booth in the x-ray room is just as significant as its construction. The Radiation Protection Bureau–Health Canada, for example, recommends:

> (a) Locating the control booth, whenever possible, such that the radiation has to be scattered twice before entering the booth. In installations where the useful beam may be directed towards the booth, the shielding of the booth *must* be that of a primary barrier.
>
> (b) Positioning control booths so that, during an exposure, no one can enter the radiographic room without knowledge of the operator (RPB, 1992, p. 15).

The *viewing window* is a major design feature of the control booth (Fig. 10-5). The window is made of lead glass and is positioned to allow the technologist to observe the patient and equipment during exposures.

The walls and viewing window of the control booth must provide shielding from radiation such that the occupational exposure to personnel is not >1 mSv/wk (100 mrem/wk). The lead glass viewing window usually has a lead equivalency of 1.5 mm (Statkiewicz-Sherer et al., 1993).

Factors Affecting Barrier Thickness

Several factors play a role in determining the thickness of protective barriers for diagnostic installations. These are illustrated in Figure 10-6 and include dose limits, workload, use factor, occupancy factor, distance, energy of the radiation, and the attenuation factor. Each of these are now examined briefly.

Dose Limits

In arriving at the barrier thickness, it is important to know the *occupational dose limits* for controlled and uncontrolled areas. As mentioned earlier in the chapter, the weekly dose limits needed for the calculation are 1 mSv/wk (100 mrem/wk) and 0.1 mSv/wk

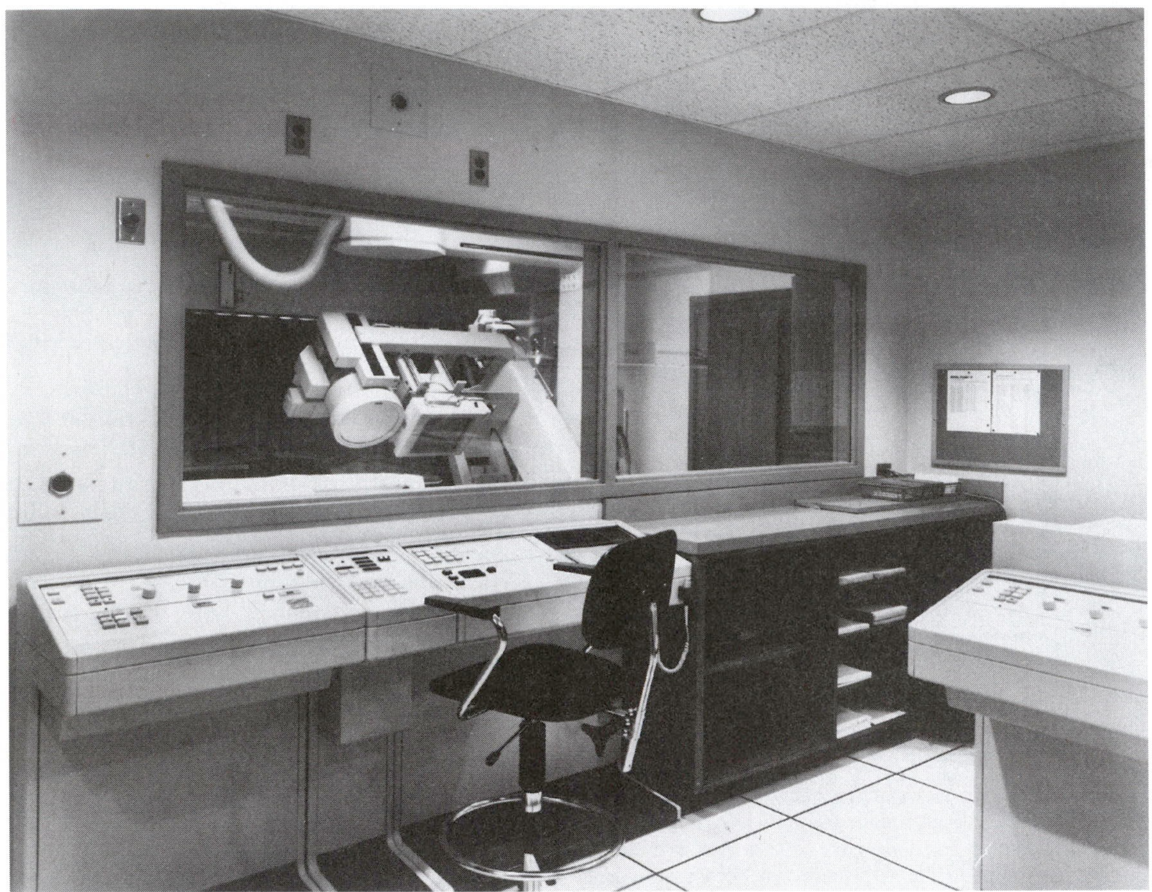

FIGURE 10-4. The control booth of an x-ray room must be shielded to protect operators during the exposure. The control booth also houses the control panel. (Courtesy of Nuclear Associates, Carle Place, NY.)

(10 mrem/wk) for controlled and uncontrolled areas, respectively.

Workload

The *workload factor* (W) refers to the amount of use of the x-ray unit. Specifically, it refers to the time the x-ray tube is energized per week (weekly workload); therefore, it takes into consideration the milliamperage (mA), the kilovoltage (kVp), and the daily patient load.

The workload can be calculated using the following relationship:

$$W = \frac{(\text{mAs/patient}) \times (\text{no. of patients/hr}) \times (\text{no. of hr/week})}{60 \text{ min}} \quad (10\text{-}1)$$

where W = workload in mA-min/wk.

EXAMPLE

A dedicated high voltage (120 kVp) chest room of an x-ray department is designed to handle 40 patients per hour. If the total mAs per patient (2 films, posterior-anterior and a lateral) is about 10, what is the weekly workload for that room?

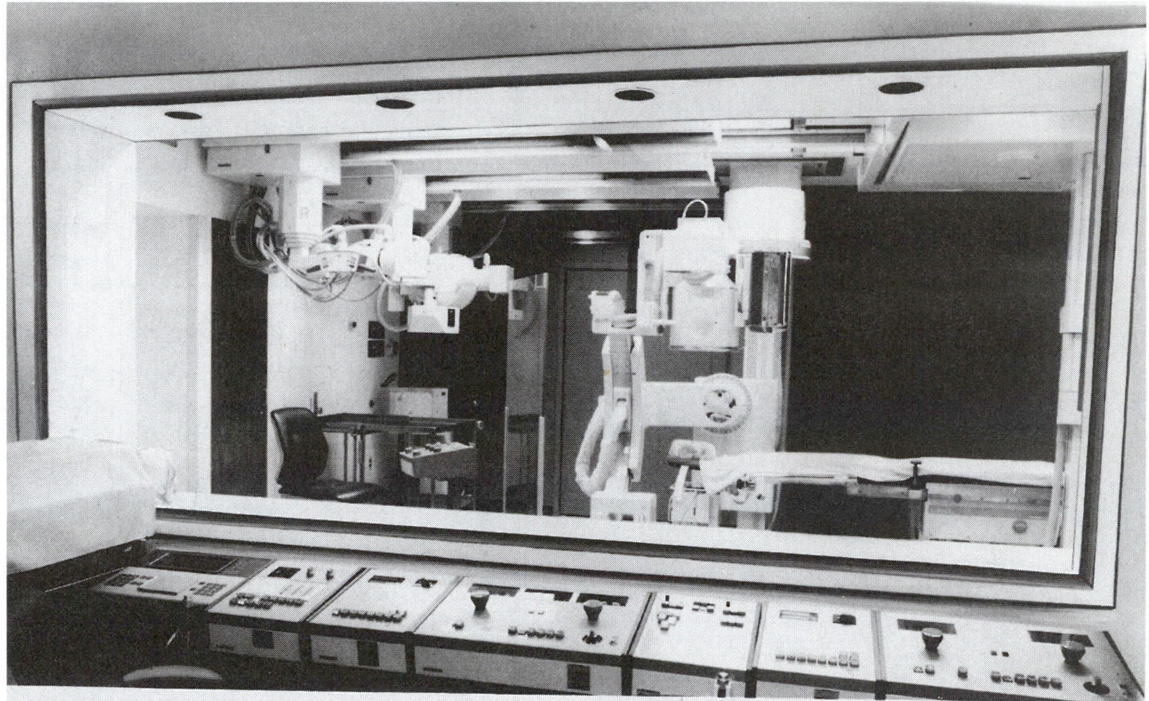

FIGURE 10-5. The viewing window of the control booth is designed in such a way as to allow the technologist to observe both the patient and equipment during the exposure. (Courtesy of Nuclear Associates, Carle Place, NY.)

You may assume that a work week includes 5 days at 8 hours per day.

SOLUTION

Using the relationship

$$W = \frac{(\text{mAs/patient}) \times (\text{no. of patients/hr}) \times (\text{no. of hr/week})}{60 \text{ min}}$$

$$= \frac{10 \times 40 \times 40}{60}$$

$$= \frac{16000}{60}$$

$$= 266.6 \text{ mA-min/wk}$$

$$= 267 \text{ mA-min/wk}$$

Typical weekly workloads for general radiography and other examinations are given in Table 10-1. An important point to note is that as the kVp values increase, workload decreases because fewer mAs are needed. In this particular situation, an increase in shielding may have to be considered because the increased beam penetration is not necessarily offset by the lower workload (Statkiewicz-Sherer et al., 1993).

It is important to note that because of the recently lowered dose limits of the ICRP and NCRP (Chapter 7), shielding calculations using traditional methodologies suggested in NCRP Report No. 49 (1976) may result in "prohibitively and unnecessarily thick barriers" (Simpkin, 1996, p. 578). It is therefore necessary to have accurate information about x-ray tube usage and "accurate models for predicting doses to shielded areas" (Simpkin, 1996, p. 578). In this regard, the study by Simpkin (1996) reports the results of workload and use factors utilized in several modern diagnostic x-ray facilities. The purpose of the study was "to present a sampling of present diagnostic x-ray room usage and

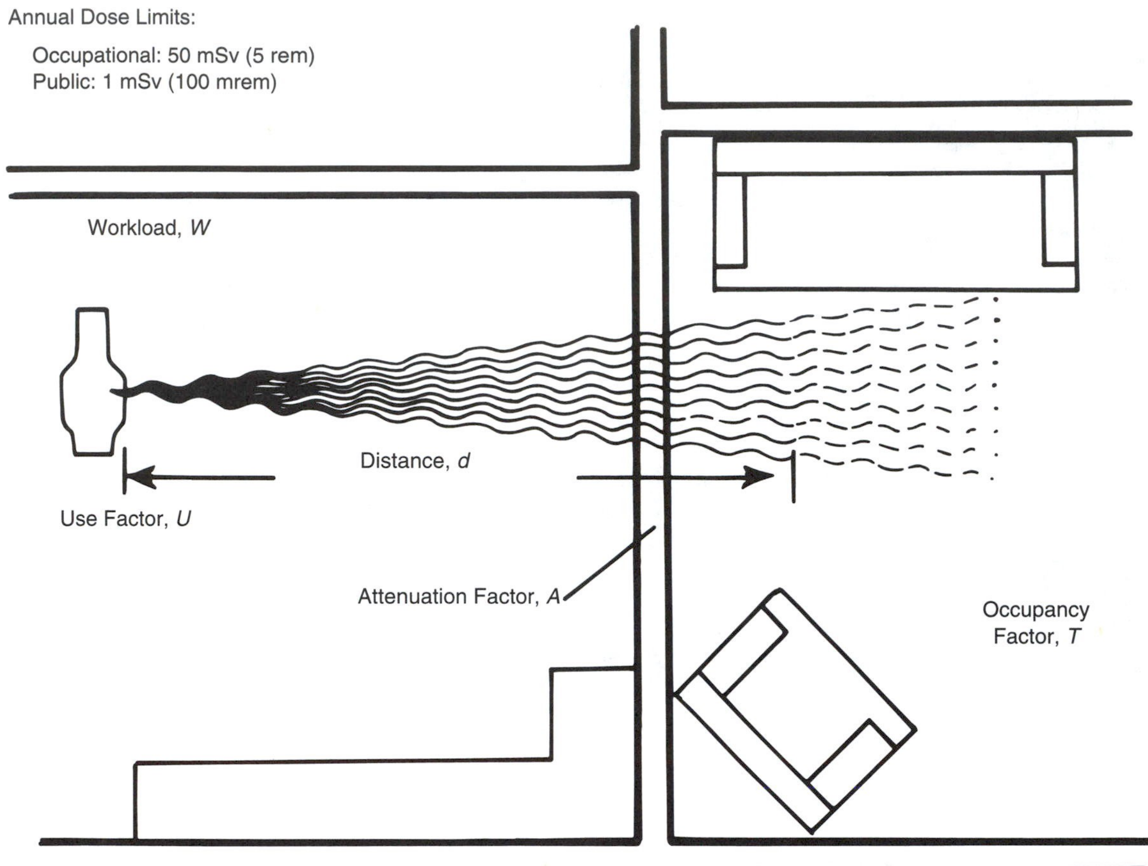

FIGURE 10-6. Factors used in calculating the thickness of protective barriers. [From Wolbarst, A.B. (1995). *Physics of radiology*. Norwalk, CT: Appleton & Lange. Reproduced by permission.]

is offered as a guide when more specific information is unavailable. It is believed that this survey represents the first attempt to measure these fundamentally important parameters" (p. 578).

Use Factor

The *use factor* (U) refers to the amount of time the primary beam is pointed to or directed at any of the walls (barriers) of the x-ray room. For this reason, the use factor is also referred to as the *beam direction factor*.

The use factors for protective barriers are given in Table 10-2. It is important to note that the use factor for the floor is 1 because it is exposed to the primary beam for those examinations done on the x-ray table. For walls occasionally exposed to the primary beam, U is 1/4. On extremely rare occasions when the primary beam is directed toward the ceiling, U is very small and approaches zero. Finally, because all the walls in an x-ray room are exposed to scattered radiation (Fig. 10-2), U for these walls (secondary barriers) is 1.

Occupancy Factor

When designing protective barriers it is important to consider its *occupancy factor* (T) (Fig. 10-6), or the amount of time individuals will

TABLE 10-1. TYPICAL WEEKLY WORKLOADS FOR GENERAL RADIOGRAPHY AND OTHER EXAMINATIONS

	Daily Patient Load	Typical Weekly Workload, [W(mA-min)]		
		≤100 kVp	125 kVp	150 kVp
General radiography	24	1000	400	200
Fluoroscopy with II, including spot films	24	750	300	150

SOURCE: NCRP. (1976). *Structural shielding design and evaluation for medical use of x-rays and gamma rays up to 10 MeV* (Report. No. 49). Bethesda, MD: NCRP. Reproduced by permission.

occupy areas *outside* the x-ray room. These areas fall into three categories according to the NCRP:

1. *Full occupancy*—These are areas occupied by individuals during the course of the workday, such as offices, laboratories, wards, nursing stations, and children's play areas. The occupancy factor for these areas is 1.
2. *Partial occupancy*—These are areas occupied only partially during the full workday, such as washrooms, corridors, elevators, and unattended parking lots (if the department is in close proximity to the lot). The occupancy factor for these areas is 1⁄4.
3. *Occassional occupancy*—These are areas that are occupied only occasionally during the full workday. Waiting rooms, toilets, stairways, unattended elevators, janitor closets, and outside areas for pedestrians or vehicles fall into this category. The occupancy factor for these areas is 1⁄16.

The occupancy factors T = 1, T = 1⁄4, and T = 1⁄16 are for areas occupied by individuals who are not occupationally exposed. For occupationally exposed individuals (e.g., technologists, radiologists, and radiology nurses) who spend most of their workday in a controlled area, the occupancy factor is 1.

Distance

The *distance*, d, in meters, refers to the minimum distance from the x-ray tube to a point on the other side of the barrier that an individual can be, as shown in Figure 10-6. As the distance increases, the exposure rate decreases inversely as the square of the distance (inverse square law). If the distance is large enough, shielding may not be needed (Wolbarst, 1993).

Energy of the Radiation and the Attenuation Factor

The *attenuation factor*, A, of the barrier (Fig. 10-6) depends not only on the barrier material but also on the *energy of the radiation* falling upon it. This energy is actually composed of the

TABLE 10-2. USE FACTORS FOR PRIMARY AND SECONDARY PROTECTIVE BARRIERS

Barrier	Primary Barrier Use Factor (U)	Secondary Barrier Use Factor (U)
Floor	1	1
Wall	1⁄4	1
Ceiling	Very small	1

SOURCE: NCRP. (1976). *Structural shielding design and evaluation for medical x-rays and gamma rays up to 10 MeV* (Report No. 49). Bethesda, MD: NCRP. Reproduced by permission.

different energies of the photons in the beam. The quantity K is introduced to account for these different energies. K is the kerma and represents the kinetic energy transferred to charged particles by uncharged particles per unit mass of the irradiated material. K is related to the attenuated radiation exposure and is expressed in mGy/mA-min at a reference distance of 1 m.

Figure 10-7 shows attenuation curves measured for lead at five different kVp values: 50, 75, 100, 150, and 200. The y-axis (ordinate), drawn as a log scale, gives the value of K in mGy/mA-min at 1 m. The x-axis (abscissa), on the other hand, indicates the thickness of lead needed for the barrier under consideration.

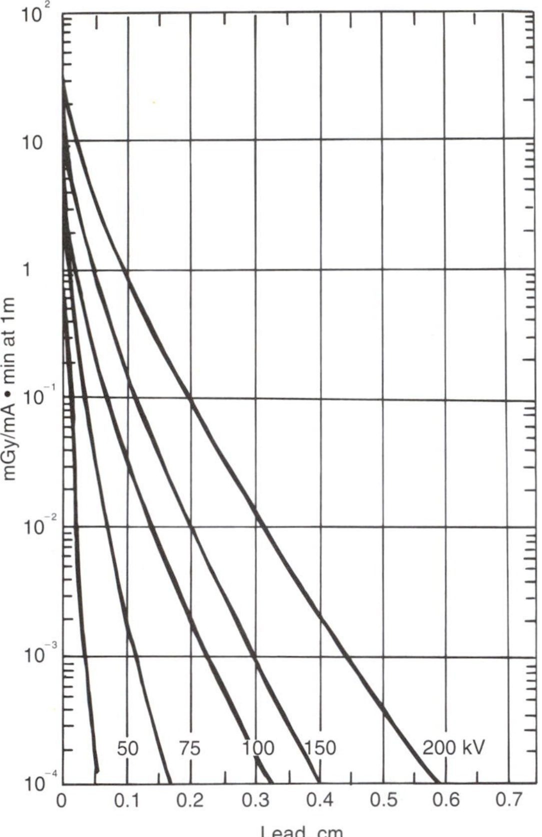

FIGURE 10-7. Attenuation curves measured for lead at five different kV values. The thickness of lead required for protective barriers can be obtained from these curves. [From ICRP. (1982). (Publication No. 33). Protection against ionizing radiation from external sources used in medicine. Elmsford, NY: Pergamon Press. Reproduced by permission.]

Materials for Shielding

The material most commonly used in the design of protective barriers in an x-ray department is lead. Lead is the material of choice because it absorbs radiation efficiently due to its high atomic number and density. While the atomic number for lead is 82, the density of commercially rolled lead is 11.36 g/cm^3.

Another popular choice of shielding material is Clear-Pb (Fig. 10-8), which consists of an acrylic copolymer resin and an organolead salt and contains 30% lead by weight (Nuclear Associates, 1993). Its physical properties (e.g., tensile strength, specific gravity, optical, electrical and electrostatic characteristics) and radiation absorption properties (e.g., linear and mass attenuation coefficients) make Clear-Pb more suitable for use as a shielding material in radiology departments than conventional acrylic lead glass and plate glass.

Clear-Pb is shatter-resistant and is available in large panels (which allow for panoramic viewing, as shown in Fig. 10-9), with a wide range (0.3–2.0 mm) of lead equivalency.

Determining Barrier Thickness

Although technologists are not directly involved in determining the thickness of protective shielding for the radiology department, it is important that they understand how dose limits, workload, and use and occupancy factors are related to barrier computations.

Methods used to determine barrier thickness include half-value layers, shielding requirement tables, and attenuation curves (Curry et al.,

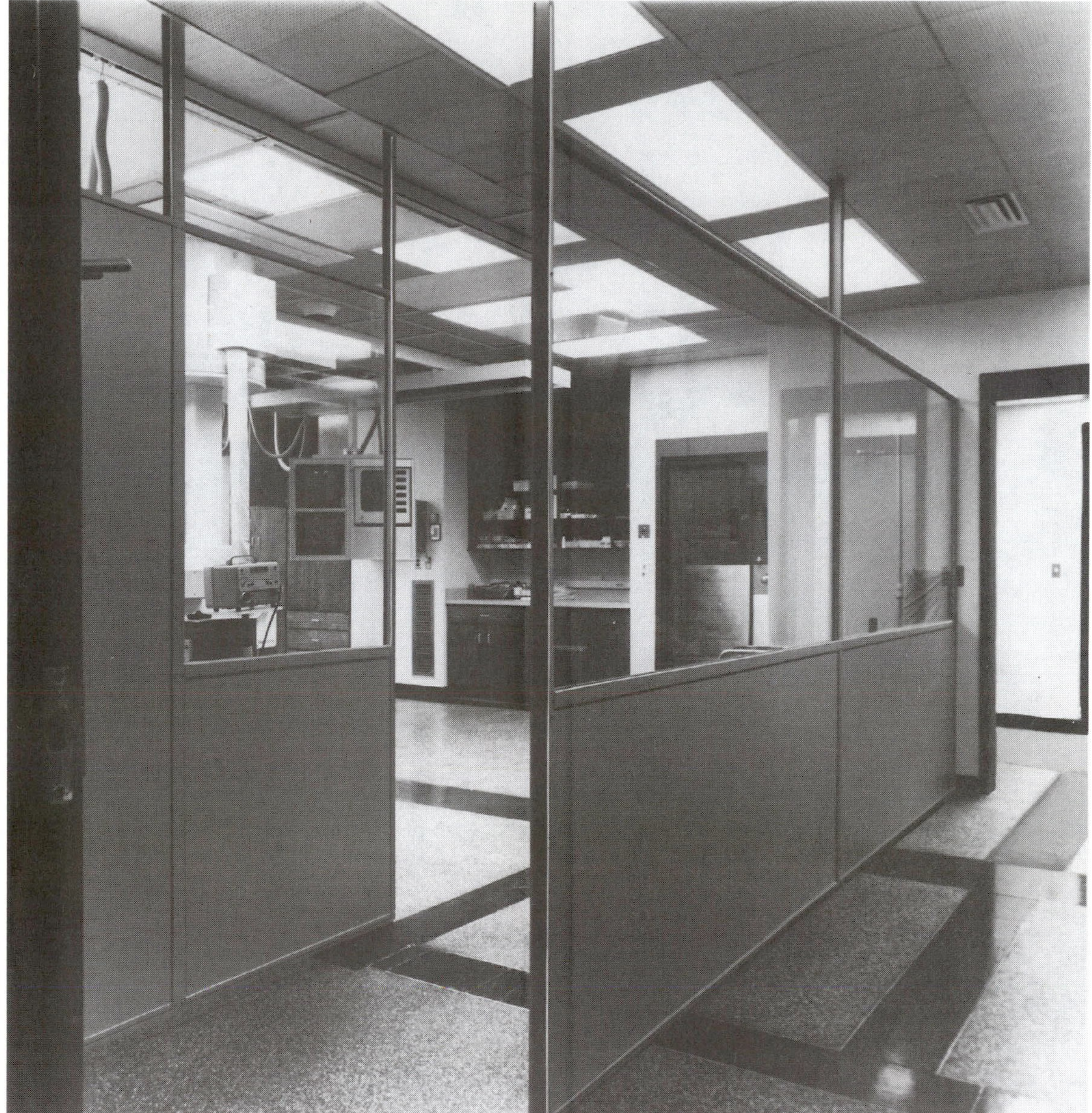

FIGURE 10-8. The use of Clear-Pb for shielding in x-ray departments. (Courtesy of Nuclear Associates, Carle Place, NY.)

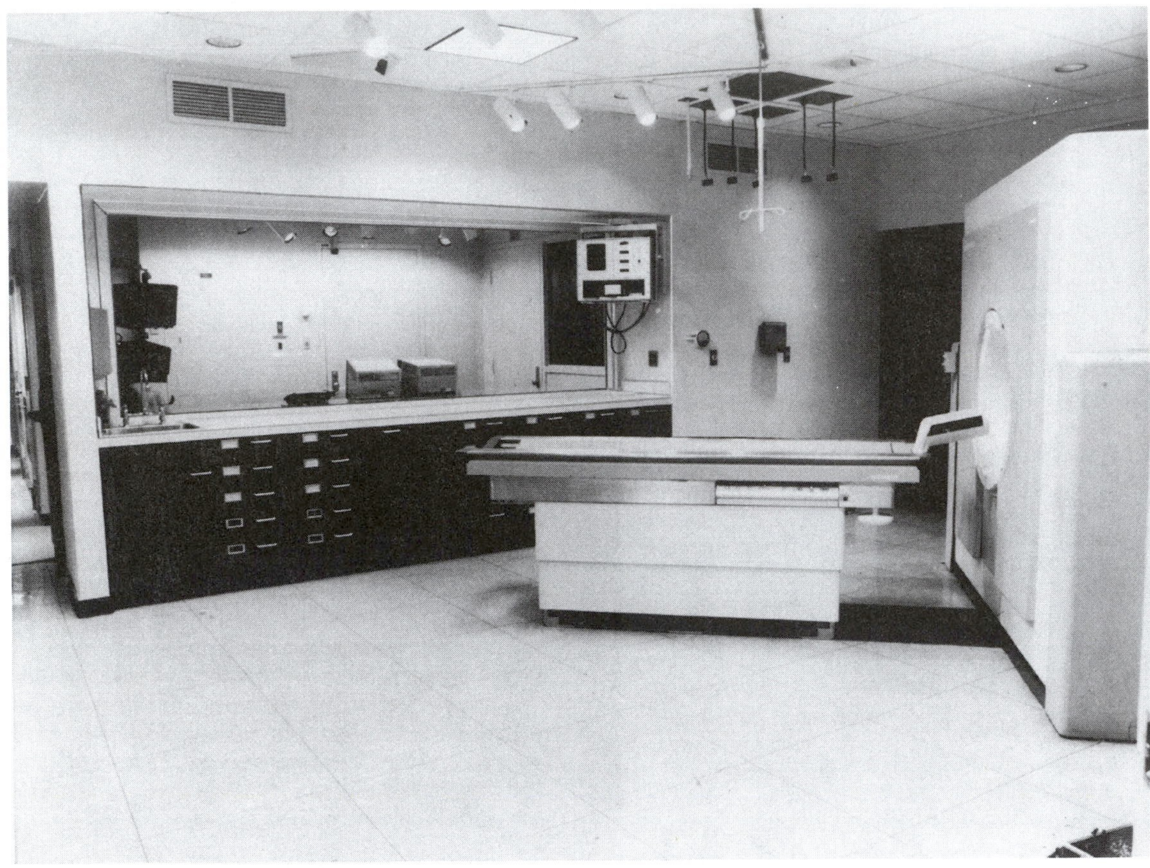

FIGURE 10-9. The use of Clear-Pb in the design of a control booth to provide panoramic viewing. (Courtesy of Nuclear Associates, Carle Place, NY.)

1990). In this section, only primary barrier thickness determination is described because secondary barriers are generally of uniform lead thickness across radiology departments. In addition, only the half-value layer and attenuation curve methods will be described since shielding requirement tables are being revised in accordance with the recently revised dose limits of the ICRP.

Half-Value Layers

The half-value layer (HVL), as discussed in Chapter 2, is that thickness of material that will reduce the radiation intensity to one half its original value. The HVL thicknesses for lead used for shielding at 50, 70, 100, and 125 kVp are 0.06, 0.17, 0.27, and 0.28 mm, respectively (NCRP, 1976).

The fundamental procedure for determining barrier thickness using HVL is as follows:

1. Determine the radiation intensity at some point in the x-ray room.
2. Divide this value of the radiation intensity by 2, several times, until the intensity approaches the recommended level.
3. Multiply the number of times that the intensity was halved by the HVL of the radiation beam.

EXAMPLE

What is the thickness of lead needed for a primary barrier if the radiation intensity at a point in the x-ray room is 10 μC/kg-mAs and the permissible intensity is 0.312 μC/kg-mAs? The HVL of the radiation beam is 0.27 mm lead.

SOLUTION

1. Divide the given radiation intensity of 10 μC/kg-mAs by 2 until the answer is equal to or approaches 0.312 μC/kg-mAs.
   (1) 10 μC/kg-mAs ÷ 2 = 5 μC/kg-mAs.
   (2) 5 μC/kg-mAs ÷ 2 = 2.5 μC/kg-mAs.
   (3) 2.5 μC/kg-mAs ÷ 2 = 1.25 μC/kg-mAs.
   (4) 1.25 μC/kg-mAs ÷ 2 = 0.625 μC/kg-mAs.
   (5) 0.625 μC/kg-mAs ÷ 2 = 0.312 μC/kg-mAs.
2. This results in five HVLs.
3. Multiply the HVL of the beam by 5.
   = 0.27 mm lead × 5
   = 1.35 mm lead

The answer to our original question is that the primary barrier must contain a thickness of 1.35 mm lead.

Shielding Requirement Tables

Another simple method of determining barrier thickness is through the use of precalculated *shielding requirement tables*, where the thickness of the lead needed for shielding can be obtained by looking it up on a table which gives the required thickness, based on the workload, kVp of operation, and the distance in meters of the x-ray tube to the shielded wall.

Attenuation Curves

The use of attenuation curves (shown in Fig. 10-7) to determine barrier thickness involves the use of the formula

$$K = \frac{Pd^2}{WUT} \qquad (10\text{-}2)$$

where K is the exposure per unit workload at unit distance in mGy/mA-min (R/mA-min) at 1 m; P is the maximum permissible air kerma per week for controlled or uncontrolled areas; and d, W, U, and T are as previously defined.

In Figure 10-7, the values of K in mGy/mA-min at 1 m as a function of thickness of lead, in centimeters, are shown for five different kV values. These are the attenuation curves for 50, 75, 100, 150, and 200 kV.

The following example demonstrates not only the use of the above-mentioned formula but also the use of the attenuation curves shown in Figure 10-7.

EXAMPLE

In a general radiographic room, the daily patient load results in an effective workload of 100-mA-min/wk and the tube is operated at 150 kVp. When the x-ray tube is positioned 1 m from the wall that separates the radiographic room from the processing darkroom (keeping in mind that this wall is routinely exposed to the useful beam), what is the thickness of lead needed for this wall?

SOLUTION

In this problem, the values for the various factors are as follows:

P = 1 mGy/wk because the darkroom is a controlled area

d = 1 m

WUT = 100 mA-min/wk

(a) Substitute the above values in the formula

$$K = \frac{Pd^2}{WUT} = \frac{1\ \text{mGy/wk} \times (1)^2}{100\ \text{mA-min/wk}} = \frac{1}{100}$$

$= 0.01$

$= 10^{-2}$ mGy/mA-min

(b) Having calculated K, perform the following steps.

(i) Using Figure 10-7, find the 150 kVp curve.
(ii) On the y-axis, find the value of K equal to 10^{-2} mGy/mA-min at 1 m.
(iii) Trace along the horizontal line until it meets the 150 kVp curve.
(iv) From that point, drop a vertical line to the x-axis to indicate the thickness of lead required.

The answer is 0.2 cm of lead.

Determining the thickness of lead required for secondary barriers, that is, those barriers designed to shield against scattered and leakage radiation, is somewhat more complicated than that of primary barriers. This is due to several influencing factors such as the intensity and energy of the scattered radiation, as well as the size of the field. In addition, certain assumptions have to be taken into consideration as well (Curry et al., 1990).

The factors previously identified and used in calculating primary barrier thickness are all used in calculating secondary barrier thickness except for U. The value of U for secondary barrier calculations is always 1, because scattered radiation is not limited to only one direction, as is the case with the primary beam, but rather is present in all directions.

It is not within the scope of this chapter to explain computations for secondary barrier thickness. This is a task for the health physicist. In general, however, secondary protective barriers for radiology departments have at least 1/32-inch thickness of lead (Statkiewicz-Sherer et al., 1993).

X-Ray Tube Shielding

The housing of the x-ray tube is lined with lead to offer protection from leakage radiation. Leakage radiation is controlled through the guidelines established by various radiation protection agencies such as the ICRP and the NCRP. These guidelines enable manufacturers of x-ray tubes to design the shielding of the tube housing to meet the recommended limits for leakage radiation. For example, in the United States, it is recommended that the limit (measured at 1 m from the x-ray tube) not exceed 0.1 cGy (0.1 rad) in 1 hour (NCRP, 1989). In Canada, it is recommended that the limit not exceed 0.1% of the exposure rate measured at 1 m from the x-ray tube (Radiation Protection Bureau, 1992).

Shielding Guides for Film Storage Areas

The storage rooms for x-ray films must be shielded to prevent exposure from primary and secondary radiation. The shielding computations for these rooms are similar to those previously described with the exception that the storage period of the film must now be taken into consideration.

Barriers must be such that they reduce exposure of film in storage to 0.2 mR, the maximum permissible exposure for the storage life of the film.

The shielding requirements for x-ray film can be obtained from Table 10-3. It can be noted, for example, that for a storage period of 1 month, thicknesses of 3.7 mm lead and 2.8 mm lead are required for a primary barrier ($U = 1/16$) located at 2.1 and 6.1 m, respectively, from the source to the room where the films are stored. For secondary protective barriers ($U = 1$) located 2.1 m and 6.1 m from the x-ray tube and a film storage period of 1 month, the thicknesses of lead needed are 3.0 and 2.2 mm, respectively.

Alternative Method to Shielding Design

So far, the traditional approach to shielding as recommended by the NCRP has been described; however, the NCRP in Report No. 49 pointed out that alternative methods may prove equally

TABLE 10-3. SHIELDING REQUIREMENTS FOR X-RAY FILM

Distance of X-Ray Tube to Stored Film	Barrier Type Thickness of Lead (mm)		Storage Time	
	Primary u = 1/16	Secondary u = 1	Week	Month
2.1 m	3.0	2.4	√	
	3.7	3.0		√
3.0 m	2.7	2.1	√	
	3.4	2.8		√
4.2 m	2.4	1.8	√	
	3.1	2.5		√
6.1 m	2.2	1.5	√	
	2.8	2.2		√

SOURCE: NCRP. (1976). *Structural shielding design and evaluation for medical x-rays and gamma rays up to 10 MeV* (Report No. 49). Bethesda, MD: NCRP.

satisfactory in providing radiation protection. One such method to shielding design was recently described by Dixon (1994).

While in the traditional approach, primary barriers have been described with respect to the floor and walls (in particular) upon which the primary radiation beam falls, and excludes attenuation due to the patient, tabletop, Bucky assembly (grid and cassette holder), and the cassette. Dixon's approach took into consideration the attenuation of the aforementioned materials and he concluded that:

1. For a heavy workload only a small amount of concrete is needed for shielding the floor as a primary barrier.
2. The secondary barrier may be thicker than the primary barrier.
3. Since the actual exposure below the table was found to be very small (0.015 mSv/wk) for a heavy workload of 24 patients per day, "no primary beam shielding would have been required in the floor for these x-ray rooms" (Dixon, 1994).
4. Those who design shielding for x-ray facilities should consult state regulatory requirements before using this approach.

REVIEW QUESTIONS

1. Source shielding refers to:
   A. Lead-lined doors of the x-ray room.
   B. Lead-lined walls of the x-ray room.
   C. Lead-lined housing of the x-ray tube.
   D. Lead-lined floors of the x-ray room.

2. Structural shielding is intended to protect the patient from:
   A. Primary radiation.
   B. Scattered radiation.
   C. Leakage radiation.
   D. All of the above.

3. Structural shielding design is influenced by all of the following except:
   A. Controlled areas.
   B. Uncontrolled areas.
   C. Energy of the radiation.
   D. Thickness of the patient.

4. A controlled area is an area occupied by radiation workers who may experience a dose limit of:
   A. 1 mSv per week.
   B. 0.1 mSv per week.

C. 1 mSv per year.
D. 0.1 mSv per 13 weeks.

5. An area occupied by nurses who are subject to a dose limit of 0.1 mSv per week is called:
   A. A controlled area.
   B. An uncontrolled area.
   C. A restricted area.
   D. A contaminated area.

6. Protective barriers are the:
   A. Lead-lined walls of an x-ray room.
   B. Lead-lined doors of an x-ray room.
   C. Lead-lined walls of the control booth within an x-ray room.
   D. All of the above.

7. A primary barrier is:
   A. A wall exposed to primary radiation.
   B. A wall exposed to secondary radiation.
   C. A wall exposed to leakage radiation.
   D. All of the above.

8. A secondary barrier is one that is exposed to:
   A. Primary radiation.
   B. Scattered radiation from the patient and equipment.
   C. Leakage radiation from the x-ray tube.
   D. b and c are correct.

9. The thickness of the lead lining primary protective barriers is about:
   A. 0.8 mm.
   B. 1.6 mm.
   C. 1.6 cm.
   D. 0.8 cm.

10. The height of protective barriers (from the floor) should be at least:
    A. 2.1 m.
    B. 21 cm.
    C. 1.3 m.
    D. None of the above.

11. Where primary and secondary barriers meet they should overlap by at least:
    A. 1.5 cm.
    B. 1.3 mm.
    C. 1.3 cm.
    D. 13 mm.

12. The lead equivalent thickness of the glass viewing window of the control booth is:
    A. 2.0 mm.
    B. 1.5 mm.
    C. 1.5 cm.
    D. 1.0 cm.

13. Which of the following applies to the control booth?
    A. It should provide shielding such that the occupational exposure is not >1 mSv/wk.
    B. It should be positioned in the x-ray room such that the radiation has to be scattered at least two times before it enters the control booth.
    C. If the useful beam strikes the booth during an exposure, the walls must be that of a primary barrier.
    D. All of the above.

14. The time the x-ray tube is energized per week is referred to as the:
    A. Use factor.
    B. Workload.
    C. Occupancy factor.
    D. mAs.

15. The unit of workload is:
    A. Hours per week.
    B. The roentgen.
    C. Examinations per week.
    D. mA-min per week.

16. As the kVp increases:
    A. Workload increases.
    B. Workload decreases.
    C. Workload and kVp are not related.
    D. The use factor increases.

17. Which of the following refers to the amount of time the primary beam is directed to the walls of an x-ray room?

A. Workload.
B. Use factor.
C. Occupancy factor.
D. Attenuation factor.

18. The use factor for the floor of the x-ray room is:

A. 1.
B. 2.
C. ¼.
D. ½.

19. The radiology department is considered an area of:

A. Occasional occupancy.
B. Partial occupancy.
C. Full occupancy.
D. None of the above.

20. Corridors in an x-ray room fall into the category of:

A. Full occupancy.
B. Partial occupancy.
C. Occasional occupancy.
D. Do not fit into any of the above.

21. The occupancy factor for waiting rooms in an x-ray department is:

A. 1.
B. ½.
C. ¼.
D. 1⁄16.

22. The occupancy factor for washrooms in an x-ray department is:

A. 1.
B. ½.
C. ¼.
D. 1⁄16.

23. For technologists and radiologists who spend most of their workday in a controlled area, the occupancy factor is:

A. 1.
B. ½.
C. ¼.
D. 1⁄16.

24. Which of the following is most commonly used in the design of protective barriers in radiology?

A. Concrete.
B. Lead glass.
C. Lead.
D. Aluminum.

25. The following methods are used to determine barrier thickness except:

A. Half-value layer.
B. Shielding requirement tables.
C. The number of chest x-rays done per week.
D. Attenuation curves.

26. The thickness of material used to reduce the radiation intensity to one half its original value is the:

A. Attenuation factor.
B. Filtration.
C. Barrier factor.
D. Half-value layer.

27. When using attenuation curves to determine barrier thickness, the following formula is applied:

A. $K = Pd^2 \times WUT$
B. $K = Pd^2/WUT$
C. $K = WUT/Pd^2$
D. $K = WUT \times P/d^2$

28. The unit of K in the above formula is:

A. Sieverts per min.
B. mA-min per week.
C. mGy/mA-min.
D. mGy per week.

29. In the United States, the recommended limit for leakage radiation from the x-ray tube is that:

A. The leakage radiation not exceed 0.1 Gy per hour at 1 m from the tube.

B. The leakage radiation not exceed 0.01 Gy per hour at 1 m from the tube.
C. The leakage radiation not exceed 0.1% of the exposure rate measured at 1 m from the x-ray tube.
D. The leakage radiation not exceed 1 cGy per hour at 1 m from the tube.

30. At 4.2 m from the x-ray tube, the thickness of lead required for the primary wall of the film storage cabinet in the radiology department should be:
    A. 2.4 mm if the film storage time is 1 week.
    B. 3.0 mm if the film storage time is 1 week.
    C. 2.8 mm if the film storage time is 1 month.
    D. 2.2 mm if the film storage time is 1 week.

REFERENCES

Curry, T.S., Dowdley, J.E., & Murry, R.C. (1990). *Christensen's physics of diagnostic radiology* (4th ed.). Philadelphia: Lea & Febiger.

Dixon, R.L. (1994). On the primary barrier in diagnostic x-ray shielding. *Medical Physics, 21,* 1785–1793.

Martin, A., & Harbison, S.A. (1979). *An introduction to radiation protection* (2nd ed.). London: John Wiley & Sons.

Martin J. Ratner, Nuclear Associates. (1993). Personal communications. New York: Nuclear Associates.

NCRP. (1976). Structural shielding design and evaluation for medical use of x-rays and gamma rays of energy up to 10 MeV (Report No. 49). NCRP: Bethesda, MD.

NCRP. (1989). *Medical x-ray, electron beam and gamma ray protection for energies up to 50 MeV: Equipment design, performance and use* (Report No. 102). Bethesda, MD: National Council on Radiation Protection and Measurements.

Radiation Protection Bureau. (1992). *Safety code 20A. X-ray equipment in medical diagnosis: Part a: Recommended safety procedures for installation and use.* Ottawa: Health and Welfare Canada.

Simpkin, D.J. (1996). Evaluation of NCRP Report No. 49: Assumptions on workloads and use factors in diagnostic radiology facilities. *Medical Physics, 23,* 577–584.

Statkiewicz-Sherer, M.A., Visconti, P.J., & Ritenour, E.R. (1993). *Radiation protection in medical radiography* (2nd ed.). St. Louis: Mosby-Year Book.

Turner, J.E. (1986). *Atoms, radiation, and radiation protection.* Elmsford, NY: Pergamon Press.

Wolbarst, A.B. (1993). *Physics of radiology.* Norwalk, CT: Appleton & Lange.

CHAPTER ELEVEN

DOSE STUDIES IN RADIOGRAPHY

LEARNING OBJECTIVES

Upon completion of this chapter, the reader should be able to:

1. Define each of the following: entrance skin dose, bone marrow dose, and gonadal dose.
2. List the two most common methods of dose measurement.
3. Identify five major dose studies conducted in the United States.
4. State the major findings of several dose studies in radiography.
5. State the major findings of several dose studies in fluoroscopy.
6. State the major findings of several dose studies in mammography.
7. State the major findings of several dose studies in computed tomography.

Introduction

To address the concept of net benefit and the philosophy of ALARA (see Chapter 5), it is important to have information on the radiation doses from diagnostic radiology. This information can then be used to justify specific practices, assess the risks of radiation exposure to the patient, and identify not only the types of examinations where a decrease in dose is reasonably achievable but also the techniques used to reduce the dose without compromising image quality. Additionally, dose to the patient is measured for a number of other reasons:

1. To compare competitive technologies such as computed tomography and digital fluoroscopy.
2. To assess equipment performance during initial acceptance testing and routine quality control.
3. To comply with recommendations established by international and national radiation protection agencies and provide answers to patient concerns about doses from particular examinations.

This chapter examines various methods of reporting patient dose and subsequently reviews major dose studies in radiography, fluoroscopy, mammography, and computed tomography. Particular emphasis is placed on the results of recent dose studies, rather than their methodologies. In reporting these studies, direct quotation will be used so as not to detract from the original meaning. Finally, the chapter concludes with a general method of determining patient dose from a specific examination.

The overall goal of this chapter is to provide the technologist with further insight into the magnitude of measured doses from various radiological examinations.

Methods of Reporting Patient Dose

The spatial distribution of the dose when a patient is exposed to a beam of x-rays was described in Chapter 3. This distribution leads to doses such as the entrance skin exposure (ESE), entrance skin dose, the average organ dose, the depth dose, the integral dose, and the collective dose. Most dose studies, however, have reported on the entrance skin dose, the bone marrow dose, and the gonadal dose (Bushong, 1993).

Entrance Skin Dose

Even though the *entrance skin exposure* (ESE) is fairly easy to measure, it is the entrance skin dose that is most often reported in dose studies. This dose, which is computed from the ESE, is particularly useful because it takes into consideration the back scatter, or radiation coming back from the floor or wall, depending on the type of examination, that results from the exposure.

The *entrance skin dose* is measured at a point on the skin where the x-ray beam enters the patient (Whalen and Balter, 1984), using a pack of thermoluminescent dosimeters (TLDs) positioned in the middle of the x-ray field. This is illustrated in Figure 11-1.

Bone Marrow Dose

The *bone marrow dose*, or more accurately the *mean active bone marrow dose*, refers to the average dose to the total active bone marrow in both adults and children. This dose is of concern in diagnostic radiology because it can be used as an index of radiation-induced leukemia (Bushong, 1993).

Gonadal Dose

Even though the doses delivered to the gonads are very low, the *gonadal dose* is of importance in diagnostic radiology because of the potential for genetic effects. In this regard, Travis (1989) pointed out that the term *genetically significant dose* (GSD) is used to assess the potential genetic impact of the gonadal dose received by exposed individuals or children in future generations. The assumption is that the GSD would

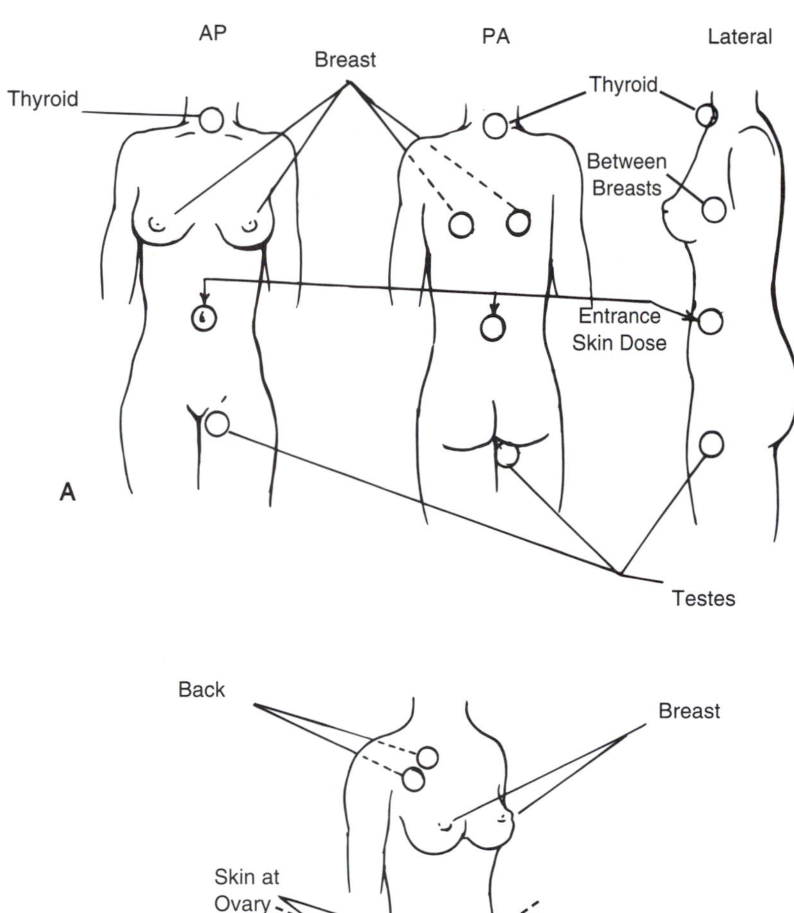

FIGURE 11-1. The arrangement of TLDs on patients during "simple" examinations (A) and "complex" examinations (B). [From Padovani, R., Contento, G., Fabretto, M., Malisan, M.R., Barbina, V., & Gozzi, G. (1987). Patient doses and risks from diagnostic radiology in North-east Italy. *British Journal of Radiology, 60*, 155–165. Reproduced by permission.]

produce the same genetic effect on those receiving it as doses of radiation that are currently administered in medical and/or dental x-rays.

Dose Measurement

One of the critical components of dosimetry studies is the dose measurement technique. The two most common methods used in the majority of studies to measure dose are the ionization chamber method and the TLD method. These dosimeters, particularly TLDs, are small and can be taped onto the patient's skin or inserted into specific sites on a phantom where the dose is to be measured. Because of their energy dependence and variations in sensitivity, TLDs must be carefully calibrated to be used in a dose study. (TLD calibration is beyond the scope of this text and therefore not discussed further.)

Several studies have utilized lithium fluoride (LiF) TLD ribbons and calcium fluoride (CaF_2) as well. Kato et al. (1991) investigated the suitability of magnesium silicate (Mg_2SiO_4) phosphor (MSO TLDs) to measure diagnostic x-ray doses because they are relatively sensitive to low-dose x-rays and are accurate to within a 5% range.

Major Dose Studies

NCRP (1989) identifies and describes five major radiation dose studies dating back several years. This NCRP report focuses attention on assessing the dose to the population from diagnostic x-rays as well as from nuclear medicine and dental radiography. The major studies provided data relating to the types and number of examinations, population demographics, trends, absorbed dose, effective dose equivalent, gonadal and genetically significant doses, films used, dose reduction techniques, and future trends in diagnostic imaging.

The five studies identified in this NCRP report are as follows: the X-Ray Exposure Studies (XES), the Johnson Associates Survey, Radiation Experience Data 1 (RED1), Radiation Experience Data 2 (RED2), and the Nationwide Evaluation of X-Ray Trends (NEXT). Of these, the NEXT study continued to provide data from 1984 to 1987, and these have been published by the Conference of Radiation Control Program Directors (Rueter, 1988; Conway, 1987). Table 11-1 highlights the essential features of each of these studies. Table 11-1 also identifies features of the NEXT study up to 1984. The annual surveys at that time suffered from a few problems such as the lack of standard exposure equivalent phantoms with which to obtain data from automatic exposure timing systems. In 1984, such phantoms were developed and were subsequently used in other annual surveys.

These studies are important to the technologist for several reasons:

1. They have been cited many times in recent dose studies.
2. They provide information on radiation dose trends throughout the decades.
3. They can be used to provide guidance in improving radiation protection practices both in hospitals and private clinics and in meeting new requirements such as those of the Joint Commission on Accreditation of Healthcare Organization (JCAHO). The JCAHO requires that the dose and exposure for each radiographic examination be expressed as a "quantitative value," which can subsequently be used in evaluating a department by comparing these values with a national "average" (Rueter et al., 1990).

The interested reader is referred to the actual NCRP report for the details of data collected from these studies; however, some important findings warrant consideration in this section.

When comparing skin entrance exposures for certain examinations done in 1973 and 1981, the NCRP (1989) pointed out that the results indicate that there may not have been significant changes in "absorbed doses for specific projec-

TABLE 11-1. THE ESSENTIAL FEATURES OF FIVE MAJOR DOSE STUDIES CONDUCTED IN THE UNITED STATES

Study	Essential Features	Year
X-Ray Exposure Studies (XES)	Population-based survey of x-ray examinations individuals had received. Dosimetry data obtained from facility. This study was conducted by the U.S. Public Health Service.	1964, 1970
Johnson Associates Survey	Facility-based survey (hospitals and offices) of the frequency of diagnostic imaging procedures. Study conducted by Johnson Associates.	1973, 1979, 1981
Radiation Experience Data (RED 1)	Hospital-based survey (81 hospitals) of radiological procedures. Done by the Bureau of Radiological Health (BRH), now referred to as the Center for Devices and Radiological Health. Data collected on the number of examinations, age, and sex of patients who received examinations. No dose or patient exposure data were collected.	1980, 1981
Radiation Experience Data (RED 2)	500 hospitals sampled by mail. Trend data such as number of procedures, type and size of hospitals, workloads, contrast media, magnetic resonance imaging procedures, and digital subtraction angiography, as well as geographic location, were collected. Data were extrapolated to the U.S. population.	1982
Nationwide Evaluation of X-Ray Trends (NEXT)	Survey of 40 federal, state, and local health agencies concerning mainly exposure data from several x-ray examinations such as skull, cervical, thoracic, and lumbosacral spines, abdomen, and the retrograde pyelogram. Data on manual techniques obtained on a "standard patient." Doses were calculated for specific organs as a result of exposure received from certain examinations. There was a lack of technical factors for automatic exposure timing systems. Conducted annually in the United States.	1984

SOURCE: Adapted from NCRP. (1989). *Exposure of the U.S. population from diagnostic medical radiation* (Report No. 100). Bethesda, MD: NCRP.

tions in conventional radiography in the United States . . . since 1970" (NCRP, 1989, p. 26).

In addition, the entrance exposure for several diagnostic x-ray examinations have been discussed by the NCRP. These data suggest that radiographic examinations of the lumbar spine, lumbosacral spine, pelvis, and the hip, as well as the intravenous pyelogram and the barium enema, deliver large doses of radiation to patients particularly when compared with low-dose examinations such as those of the chest, skull, and cervical spine.

Finally, the gonadal dose and GSD have been presented by the NCRP. The GSD was ~300 μGy or 0.3 mGy (30 mrad), most of which have been contributed from abdominal, pelvis, and lumbar spine examinations (NCRP, 1989). In addition, the mean active bone marrow dose to adults in 1980 from diagnostic x-rays was 1.15 mGy (115 mrads), a 13% increase from the 1970 estimate. Most of this dose was due to exposures from the barium enema, upper gastrointestinal, and lumbar/lumbosacral spine examinations (NCRP, 1989).

Based on the results of these studies, the NCRP (1989) made the following recommendations:

1. Continuing updates of the frequency of radiological and nuclear medicine examinations are necessary.
2. Uniform expression and methodology for exposure and/or absorbed dose are desirable among the studies reported in the literature.
3. Continuing definition of the influence of new technologies (such as magnetic resonance imaging) upon reduction of the frequency of high-dose examinations would be valuable.
4. Studies on the frequency of new high-dose interventional procedures (such as coronary angioplasty) will be important.
5. Attempts to define the benefit derived from medical radiation, so that possible detriment from these procedures is not discussed out of context, are needed (p. 72).

Two other major dose studies that deserve mention here include one by Shrimpton et al. (1986) and the other by Padovani et al. (1987), who examined patient doses as well as risks from diagnostic x-ray examinations in England and Northeast Italy, respectively. These studies are somewhat similar in their methodology because they both used the following common elements:

1. Frequency survey (number of examinations, age, sex, and so on).
2. Dose measurements on patients undergoing examinations.
3. TLDs used for dose measurements and attached to the patient's skin as illustrated in Figures 11-1A and 11-1B for both "simple" examinations (e.g., chest, abdomen, pelvis, cervical spine, thoracic spine, hip, lumbosacral spine) and "complex" examinations (e.g., barium enema, gastrointestinal series), respectively. This was necessary for the purpose of deriving doses to various radiosensitive organs.

Both of these studies show that the entrance skin doses per radiograph are higher for examinations such as the lumbar spine (22.8 mGy for the lateral projection), thoracic spine (14 mGy for a lateral projection), abdomen (8.43 mGy for the AP projection), and pelvis (6.57 mGy for the AP projection) compared with examinations of the chest and cervical and thoracic spines (0.30 mGy for the AP; 1.31 mGy for the lateral projection; and 16.8 mGy for the lateral projection, respectively). In addition, Padovani et al. (1987) reported an annual GSD of 0.253 mSv to the population and a mean gonadal dose of 0.547 mSv.

Finally, Shrimpton et al. (1986) concluded that their patient exposure results are consistent with those reported in the NEXT surveys done in the United States.

Dose Studies in Radiography

Chapter 1 introduced the basic scheme for patient exposure in radiography as well as several factors affecting the dose delivered to the patient. An important point to remember is that the x-ray beam is fixed during the exposure and is collimated to the anatomy under examination.

Several studies have been done to investigate radiation doses to patients undergoing radiographic examinations, particularly in the area of chest radiography, because this is the most commonly requested x-ray examination. For this reason, few studies of doses to the chest will be examined. It is important to note that the actual units reported in these studies will be cited here and no conversions will be given.

Chest Studies

Faulkner et al. (1986) performed an interesting study to determine whether automatic exposure timing in chest radiography resulted in fewer repeat radiographs and thereby lessened the impact of repeat radiation doses to the patient.

In an overall comparison of the doses due to manual exposures and doses due to automatic exposure timing, the mean anterior dose for automatic timing was 0.03 mGy, which is significantly less than the mean manual dose of 0.06 mGy. The thyroid dose was estimated to vary between 0.06 mGy and 0.12 mGy, while the mean active bone marrow dose was estimated to vary between 0.04 mGy and 0.08 mGy. The study demonstrated that the use of automatic exposure timing resulted in a reduction in patient doses.

In another study, Ewen et al. (1987) investigated the radiation exposure and image quality for several different chest imaging techniques, including photofluorography (now obsolete), conventional high kVp technique, large-screen image intensifier, slot-imaging technique, and the 180-kV technique.

For each of the three most commonplace techniques (conventional high kV, large-screen image intensifier, and slot-imaging), the lung and surface doses were lower for the slot technique and higher for the conventional high kV technique.

Rueter et al. (1990) conducted a dose study to determine the average radiation exposure for chest and two other examinations done in hospitals and private clinics. They measured and calculated the ESE with the goal of providing a "statistically representative national average." The results indicate that whereas the ESE for examinations in the hospital was 4.08×10^{-6} C/kg (15.8 mR), it was 4.05×10^{-6} C/kg (15.7 mR) for private facilities.

Finally, with regard to chest studies, Mayo et al. (1993) measured the skin doses to patients undergoing high resolution computed tomography (HRCT) of the chest to compare it with conventional CT. In HRCT, thin sections (1–2 mm collimation) are scanned in conjunction with a high spatial frequency algorithm. The study compared, in particular, the doses resulting from HRCT with 1.5 mm collimation and either 10-mm or 20-mm intervals, with the dose due to scans of 10-mm contiguous slices by conventional CT.

The researchers found that for the 1.5-mm HRCT, the mean skin dose was 4.4, 2.1, and 36.3 mGy for scans at 10-mm intervals, 20-mm intervals, and conventional 10-mm CT scans at 10-mm intervals, respectively.

The conclusion drawn from the study was that "HRCT scanning at 10- and 20-mm intervals produced 12% and 6%, respectively, of the radiation dose associated with conventional CT. This is considerably less radiation than suggested in earlier studies. Combining HRCT scans at 20 mm intervals with low-dose scans (20 mA, 2-sec scans) would result in an average skin dose comparable with the dose administered with chest radiography" (Mayo et al., 1993, p. 479).

Facial Skeleton Studies

During radiography of the face, critical organs such as the lens of the eye and the thyroid gland are exposed to x-rays. The doses to these organs were measured by Julin and Kraepelien (1984), who used a dedicated head unit (used only for examination of the head) for radiography and a phantom head for absorbed dose measurements using LiF TLD ribbons.

The investigators reported that "the entrance doses to the skin of the head ranged from 0.31 to 2.9 mGy per exposure. The absorbed dose for a full series of sinus exposure averaged 0.33 mGy for the oral mucous membrane, 0.33 mGy for the maxillary sinus mucous membrane, 0.11 mGy for the parotid gland, 0.15 mGy for the submandibular gland, 0.16 mGy for the eye lens and 0.75 mGy for the thyroid gland region. A leaded soft collar adapted to the thyroid region reduced the thyroid doses by more than one order of magnitude, but also reduced the image field" (p. 113).

Dose Studies in Fluoroscopy

The fundamental factors affecting patient dose in fluoroscopy were introduced in Chapter 1 and subsequently described further in Chapter 8. As noted, fluoroscopy is considered a high-dose procedure and contributes the highest collective radiation dose to the population (Padovani et al., 1987).

The literature is replete with studies relating to radiation exposure in fluoroscopy. Most of these studies have examined exposure to personnel (McGuire et al., 1983; Miller et al., 1983; Bush et al., 1985; Boone and Levin, 1991), as well as doses to specific organs (Rowley et al., 1987; Taylor, 1979; McGuire and Dickson, 1986; Suleiman et al., 1991).

Upper Gastrointestinal Studies

Taylor (1979), among others, investigated skin exposures for the barium meal fluoroscopic examination and reported exposures ranging from 0.41 to 23 mC/kg (1.6–90 R). The mean active bone marrow dose from an upper gastrointestinal examination including spot films was investigated by Shleien et al. (1977), who reported a dose of 1950 μGy (195 mrad) in 1964 and 2410 μGy (241 mrad) in 1970.

In a more recent study, Suleiman et al. (1991) investigated tissue doses in the upper gastrointestinal examination. This was a comprehensive study of the doses in a dynamic fluoroscopic environment. Having measured the technical parameters of the fluoroscopy examination and divided up the dynamic aspect of the examination into discrete x-ray fields, the researchers used a computer program to generate tissue dose tables.

The results indicate that for radiation exposures ranging from 2.3 to 7.2 mC/kg (9.1–28 R), the thyroid, lung, active bone marrow, and uterine doses ranged from 0.15 to 3.5 mGy (15–35 mrad), 0.9–4.2 mGy (90–420 mrad), 0.81–5.4 mGy (81–540 mrad), and 0.16–1.0 mGy (16–100 mrad), respectively. These doses compare reasonably well with those of Taylor (1979) and Shleien et al. (1977).

From their study, the investigators made the following important remarks:

> 1. In estimating tissue doses from fluoroscopy examinations, the doses from the radiographic mode as well as the fluoroscopic mode should be included. The radiographic mode constitutes a major contributor to the total tissue dose (pp. 656–657).
> 2. It is obvious that the upper gastrointestinal examination is complex and that how it is conducted may depend on the physician, patient history and technique (single vs double) and equipment used. Careful quantitative analysis of this clinical examination may suggest possible technologic interventions that may result in lower patient doses.
>
> One possible area of intervention is the use of low-dose technology before acquisition of a spot radiograph. In our study, examining physicians routinely used fluoroscopy for positioning several seconds prior to obtaining the spot image. The use of low-dose or freeze-frame technology could significantly reduce the dose to the patient from this portion of the examination (p. 657).

Percutaneous Nephrostomy

Percutaneous nephrostomy has become a commonplace radiologic technique. This procedure involves a good deal of fluoroscopy, either by a multidirectional C-arm fluoroscopic unit in the operating room or by fluoroscopy in the radiology department. During the procedure, a number of personnel can be exposed, such as the radiologist, the technologist, the nurse, the anesthesiologist, and the urologist.

Using a mobile C-arm fluoroscopic unit, as shown in Figure 11-2, Bush et al. (1985) conducted a study to measure the dose to uro-radiological personnel. A pocket dosimeter (quartz-fiber electrometer) was used to measure the dose to the radiologist (Fig. 11-2),

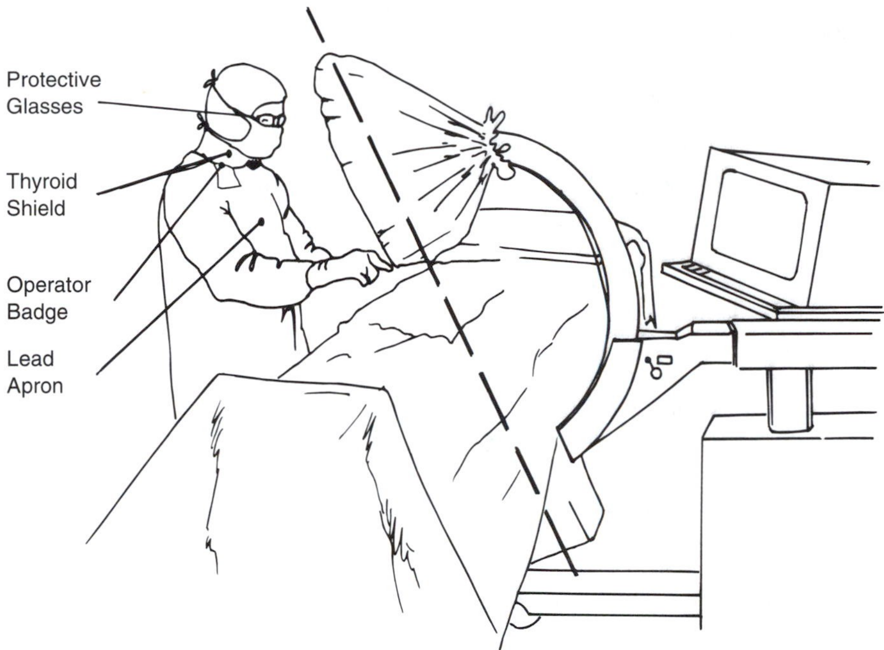

FIGURE 11-2. A radiologist performing percutaneous nephrostomy is exposed to scattered radiation during the procedure. The position of the radiation badge is shown. [From Bush, W.H., Jones, D., & Brannen, G.E. (1985). Radiation dose to personnel during percutaneous renal calculus removal. *American Journal of Roentgenology, 145*, 1261–1264. Reproduced by permission.]

in addition to single-chip TLDs, which were worn as rings on the fourth finger of each hand. Pocket dosimeters were also worn by other personnel.

The authors reported that the average doses to the radiologist's neck and hands were 0.10 mSv (10 mrem) and 0.27 mSv (27 mrem) per case, respectively, for an average of 18 minutes of fluoroscopy time. The average dose to the radiologic technologist during an average fluoroscopy time of 24 minutes was 0.04 mSv (4 mrem) per case. Whereas the average dose to the surgical nurse or assistant and anesthesiologist was 0.04 mSv (4 mrem) and 0.03 mSv (3 mrem) per case, with an average fluoroscopy time of 24 and 25 minutes, respectively, the average dose to the urologist was 0.10 mSv (10 mrem) per case for an average of 8 minutes of fluoroscopy time.

Studies in Angiography

Angiographic studies such as angiocardiography, coronary angiography, and interventional angiography are considered high-dose procedures because they often require long fluoroscopic exposure times for catheter placement and recording the anatomy under investigation.

To date, several dose studies in angiography have been conducted, and these investigations continue even today (Niklason et al., 1993; Boone and Levin, 1991; and Steinbach et al., 1990). The student should refer to these studies for an initial orientation to the nature of angiographic dose studies.

Dose in Mammography

The radiation dose in mammography has been studied by several workers and the results have been published in both NCRP (Report No. 85) *Mammography: A user's guide* (1985) and NCRP (Report No. 100) *Exposure of the U.S. population from diagnostic medical radiation* (1989). Mammography dose studies continue to receive attention because the number of mammography examinations are currently increasing owing to the benefits of screening programs for breast cancer. Recent technical advances have resulted in a significant reduction in the radiation dose to the breast. These advances have proven beneficial not only to the patient but also to the radiologic community as a whole.

First and foremost, the reduction in radiation dose has made protecting sensitive breast tissue from:

1. Cancer induction related to radiologic procedures a more manageable task (ICRP, 1991; NIH No. 85, 1985).
2. It has put compliance with NCRP and JCAHO radiation dose recommendations within the grasp of radiologic personnel everywhere.

Dose Parameters and Measurement

In mammography, dose parameters may include (1) in-air surface exposure, (2) surface dose, (3) the midline dose, and (4) the mean glandular dose (average dose to the glandular tissue of the breast). Although the in-air surface exposure and surface dose are easy to measure, the average glandular dose "provides the best indication of the risk to the patient from a mammographic examination, because it is commonly assumed that the cancer risk is linearly related to the dose and that breast cancer arises in the glandular tissue" (Rothenberg, 1990, p. 740).

Dose measurements in mammography can be made using ionization chambers or TLDs or aluminum filters (for measurements of the half-value layer). However, proper precautions must be taken when using any of these. For example, if TLDs are used, energy and fading corrections are required.

Because it is not possible to measure the average glandular dose directly, it is calculated using known exposure measurements and certain factors referred to as *exposure-to-dose factors* or simply *f-factors*. Specifically, Rothenberg (1990) suggested the basic steps to follow when calculating the average glandular dose:

1. Measure the exposure in-air at the breast entrance surface.
2. Measure the half-value layer of the beam.
3. Determine the average thickness of the compressed breast for the range of patients being examined.
4. Estimate the composition of the breast tissue (the fraction of adipose and glandular tissue).

With these values, the mean glandular dose can be calculated and reported. The actual calculations are usually done by a medical physicist and are beyond the scope of this book.

Dose Studies

Dose studies have been conducted for both xeromammography (currently xeroradiographic systems are not being manufactured) and the more common screen-film mammography.

The NEXT program data published in 1989 reported typical dose values as follows:

1. For screen-film systems, the average value of the mean glandular dose for all examinations, for examinations with grids, and for examinations without grids were 0.93, 1.28, and 0.55 mGy, respectively.
2. For xeromammographic systems, the average value of the mean glandular dose for all examinations, examinations in the positive as well as those in the negative modes were 3.94, 4.08, and 3.40 mGy, respectively (Conway, 1990).

From these values, it is important to note that the dose increases for examinations with grids as well as for xeromammography, which results in significantly higher doses compared with screen-film systems.

For a 4.5-cm-thick compressed breast examined with screen-film mammography, the NCRP (1985) recommended a dose of not >8 mGy for a two-view study using a grid (or <4 mGy for a one-view grid examination), and <1 mGy for a one-view examination without a grid. For xeromammography, the average glandular dose should be <4 mGy.

Recently federal guidelines specify that the maximum dose to a 4.5-cm compressed breast done with a grid in screen-film mammography should be 3 mGy (300 mrad) per view (Federal Register, 1990).

A Canadian Mammography Dose Study

A recent comprehensive dose study in mammography done in Canada is one by Huda et al. (1990). They reported not only the number of mammography examinations done per year in the province of Manitoba, Canada, but also the radiation exposure and the corresponding average glandular dose for a period between 1978 and 1988. The data were collected from three hospitals, three private clinics, and the national breast screening study. They reported an average glandular dose of 1.4 mGy, a value consistent with the findings of other investigators who reported average glandular doses ranging from 1.3 mGy at 25 kVp to 0.8 mGy at 30 kVp (Prado et al., 1988) as well as 1.0 mGy reported by Rueter (1989).

Risk Associated with Mammography

The effective dose equivalent (H_E) can be used to compare the risk of one radiological examination with that of another. Huda et al. (1990) compared the risk of mammography with other radiological examinations by converting the average glandular dose to an H_E value by multiplying it with a weighting factor of 0.15. "The resultant H_E is an estimate of the equivalent whole-body radiation risk, which is taken to include the induction of fatal cancers and serious genetic disorders in the first two generations after the exposure" (Huda et al., 1990, p. 815).

While the average H_E in the Manitoba mammography in 1988 was 0.60 mSv, the H_E values for the chest, skull, abdomen, and lumbar spine from the Shrimpton et al. (1986) study were 0.05, 0.15, 1.4, and 2.2 mSv, respectively.

> The per capita H_E in Manitoba due to mammography was about 14 μSv (1988). This can be compared with the current US average annual per capita H_E of 530 μSv for all types of medical exams using ionizing radiation. These data show that the risk to individual patients undergoing mammography is smaller than that associated with many other diagnostic procedures (Huda et al., 1990, p. 816).

Dose Studies in Computed Tomography

Dose Factors, Descriptors, and Measurement: A Review

The radiation dose in CT is influenced by several factors that were described in Chapter 8. Whereas the x-ray beam parameters include kVp, mAs, filtration, collimation, tube motion, source-to-skin distance, and detection efficiency, the image parameters can be found in the expression:

$$D \propto \frac{1}{\sigma e^3 h} \qquad (11\text{-}1)$$

where D, σ, e, and h are the dose, noise, spatial resolution, and slice thickness, respectively. For this expression, it can be seen that to reduce noise, increase spatial resolution, and decrease slice thickness, the dose must be increased appropriately.

In addition, several methods of describing dose (dose descriptors) were introduced in Chapter 8. These include the single- and multiple-dose profiles (Fig. 11-3), isodose curves, the

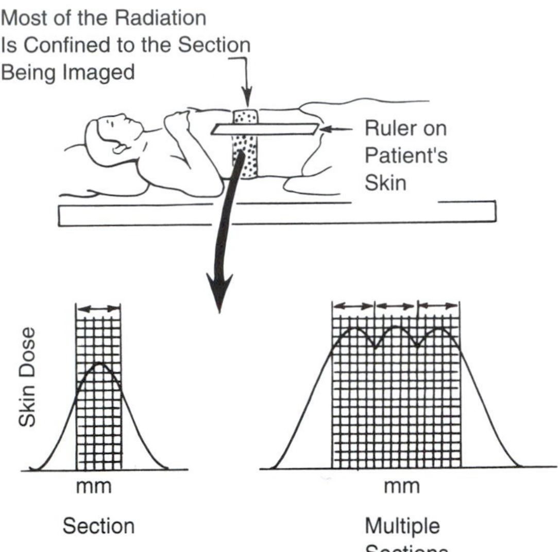

FIGURE 11-3. Single- and multiple-dose profiles showing the distribution of the patient dose for a single section and multiple sections. The ideal dose profiles (cross-hatched areas) cannot be achieved because the x-ray beam is not exactly parallel and blurring occurs due to the focal spot penumbra. [From Whalen, J.P., & Balter, S. (1984). *Radiation risks in medical imaging*. Chicago: Year Book Medical Publishers. Reproduced by permission.]

computed tomography dose index (CTDI), and the multiple scan average dose (MSAD). In review, the CTDI is the average dose at specified locations in a special cylindrical phantom. The CTDI describes the absorbed dose during CT scanning in which a set of contiguous slices (adjacent slices) are being imaged. The MSAD, on the other hand, is the average dose at the center of a series of adjacent scans and is of practical use in the clinical situation. In general, the CTDI is equal to the MSAD.

The Food and Drug Administration (FDA) now requires CT manufacturers to provide dose efficiency information on their scanners using the CTDI. Such information is usually provided in the form of CTDI charts.

The dose in CT can be measured and estimated in a number of ways. These include (1) the use of dose charts, (2) the use of the pencil ionization chamber, and (3) the use of TLDs. One such chart is shown in Table 11-2, together with the phantom used to make the measurements (Fig. 11-4). The pencil ionization chamber is a direct measurement technique and provides information on the MSAD. The TLD method, on the other hand, is the most accurate of the methods described in some detail by Yoshizumi et al. (1989).

Early Studies

The first dose study in CT was reported by Perry and Bridges (1973), who measured radiation doses to the head and gonads from the first CT scanner installed in England. This was followed by a plethora of other dose studies, several of which are cited by Shope et al. (1992), who conducted a comprehensive radiation dose survey of CT scanners from 10 vendors. At that time, patient doses from CT examinations ranged from 0.02 Gy (2 rads) to 0.1 Gy (10 rads) per study for five or more slices (Seeram, 1982).

The dose descriptors in these early studies proved to be inadequate because of the nonuniformity of absorbed doses from CT machines; several factors such as the variety of scan motions, beam geometries, collimation, and operating parameters influenced this nonuniformity (Fearon and Vucich, 1985). Subsequently, other methods of reporting CT doses were developed such as the CTDI and the MSAD.

In 1987, McCrohan et al. published their findings of the average radiation doses from standard CT examinations of the head. Having surveyed 250 CT scanners in a nationwide study, they reported MSAD values to be within 22–68 mGy (2.2–6.8 rads).

Pediatric and Fetal Dose Estimates

Various studies have examined pediatric, fetal, and maternal doses during CT examinations

TABLE 11-2. CTDI DOSE CHART FOR ONE COMMERCIAL CT SCANNER, THE SOMATOM PLUS/PLUS-S, FOR BOTH STANDARD AND SPIRAL CT SCANNING

kV[a] Measurement Point	16 cm Phantom Slice Thickness (mm)					32 cm Phantom Slice Thickness (mm)					Unit
	10	5	3	2	1	10	5	3	2	1	
Standard CT											
80 A	2.2	1.8	1.5	1.3	1.6	0.7	0.5	0.4	0.3	0.4	mGy/100mAs
B–E[c]	2.5	2.4	2.3	2.1	3.2	1.7	1.6	1.6	1.5	2.1	mGy/100mAs
120 A	8.5	6.9	6.0	4.9	6.1	3.4	2.4	1.9	1.5	1.7	mGy/100mAs
B–E	9.2	8.7	8.4	7.7	11.6	6.4	6.0	5.8	5.5	8.1	mGy/100mAs
137 A	11.0	9.0	7.7	6.4	7.9	4.5	3.2	2.5	1.9	2.2	mGy/100mAs
B–E	11.7	11.1	10.8	9.9	14.8	8.3	7.7	7.6	7.1	10.3	mGy/100mAs

	Slice Thickness[c]		Slice Thickness[c]		
	10 mm	5 mm	10 mm	5 mm	
Spiral CT					
120 A	8.5	7.0	3.4	2.4	mGy/100mAs
B–E	9.2	8.7	6.4	6.0	mGy/100mAs

[a] With 0.2 mm Cu filtration.

[b] A, B–E refer to the positions illustrated in Figure 11–4.

[c] Table feed (mm/s) = slice thickness (mm).

SOURCE: Courtesy of Siemens Medical Systems.

because children are especially sensitive to leukemogenesis (Beebe et al., 1978). Fearon and Vucich (1985), for example, have investigated the dose to pediatric patients in routine CT examinations using "typical" technique factors. They reported entrance skin absorbed doses for the chest and abdomen and pediatric head examinations to be 11–24 mGy (1.1–2.4 rads) and 20–34 mGy (2.0–3.4 rads), respectively.

In yet another study, Moore and Shearer (1989) reported fetal and maternal dose estimates for CT pelvimetry using phantom measurements. The results of their study indicate that while the maternal entrance skin dose was ~3.9 mGy (390 mrad), the fetal dose estimate ranged from 1.6 mGy to 2.5 mGy (160–250 mrad) with a resulting dose to the fetus of ~2.3 mGy (0.23 rad).

Patient Doses in CT: A Canadian Study

This is a comprehensive study done to explore several objectives, including the CT radiation doses to patients in the Canadian province of

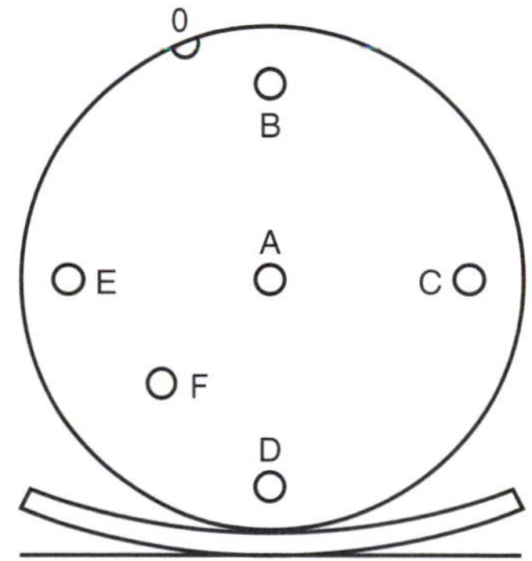

FIGURE 11-4. CT Dose Phantom (BRH) Plexiglas. For doses at positions A, B–E, see Table 11-2.

Manitoba. The study was conducted by Huda et al. (1989), who studied patient doses from 1977 to 1987. Their findings are as follows:

> The annual patient throughput has increased from 4.2 per 10^3 population in 1978 to 18.2 per 10^3 population in 1987. Over the same period, the per capita population dose from CT has increased from 4.2 to 81.0 μSv. This substantial rise has occurred because of an increase in patient throughput, higher radiation doses associated with modern CT scanners with an increasing proportion of (higher dose) body CT studies. The mean patient dose on a second generation (EMI 5005) scanner was about 1.4 mSv, whereas the corresponding doses on third generation scanners operating in Manitoba were 3.9 mSv (GE 9800) and 5.6 mSv (Siemens DRH) (p. 138).

Organ Doses and Effective Dose Equivalents

An exhaustive study on doses in CT was done by Nishizawa et al. (1991), who investigated organ doses (or tissue doses) from 12 new types of CT scanners in Japan. Their goal was not only to calculate the effective dose equivalents using the organ doses but also to evaluate the population doses and radiation risks from CT.

Several tables showing the results of their study are given in their paper, listing not only the characteristics of the scanners used in the study but also the organ or tissue doses for the head, chest, upper abdomen, and lower abdomen CT examinations by type of scanner.

The authors reported the following:

1. Entrance doses in nine scans ranged from 18 to 80 mGy.
2. The mean effective dose equivalent was 0.5 mSv for the head with a range of 0.23–0.7 mSv, 7 mSv for the chest with a range of 4.3–14 mSv, and 3.7 mSv for the upper abdomen with a range of 2.5–7.4 mSv.
3. The mean effective dose equivalent was 3.6 mSv for males and 7.0 mSv for females.
4. In trying to determine an optimum factor for CT examinations, consider image quality as well as the resultant absorbed dose or effective dose equivalent (p. 27).

Head CT Doses: Results of the 1990 NEXT Survey

The NEXT program was introduced earlier in this chapter. The essential feature of this cooperative program between the Conference of Radiation Control Program Directors and the Center for Device and Radiological Health (CDRH) is that it obtains data from a representative sample of facilities across the United States that are performing the particular examination under study.

In 1990, the NEXT program surveyed 48 states and obtained data from a random selection of 252 CT facilities. This was the first study to be conducted in this manner (Conway et al., 1992). The dose descriptor used in the study was the MSAD, for reasons given by Conway et al. (1992).

The results are presented in Table 11–3. The MSAD for most of the CT units ranged from 34 to 55 mGy (3.4–5.5 rad) and doses were found to be as high as 140 mGy (14 rad). Finally, Conway et al. (1992) concluded that "the NEXT 1990 survey provides a reasonable and clinically relevant measure of the dose delivered during CT head procedures. The results reported here provide an indication of the general magnitude of CT doses and are a reasonable basis of comparison that can be used by personnel at CT facilities" (p. 140).

Other CT Dose Studies

Several other studies on doses in CT have been reported in the literature. Of these studies, the ones by Mayo et al. (1995), McCollough et al. (1994), and Mini et al. (1995) should be of interest to radiologic technologists. Mayo and colleagues found that patient dose was reduced by a factor of 3 when 140 mAs was used to image the chest (with acceptable image quality), compared with a 400-mAs technique. In other words, they claim that the dose was reduced from 36 mGy (at 400 mAs) to 12.6 mGy (at 140 mAs).

TABLE 11-3. THE MEAN ORGAN DOSE IN THE THORAX, ABDOMEN, AND PELVIS DURING CT SCANNING

	Dose (mGy) During Localization View			Dose (mGy) During Entire CT Examination		
Organ	Thorax	Abdomen	Pelvis	Thorax	Abdomen	Pelvis
Skin (surface)	0.50	0.79	0.75	22.1	30.3	36.1
Bone marrow	0.05	0.05	0.02	4.7	5.9	11.0
Testes	<0.01	<0.01	0.58	0.03	0.16	8.3
Ovaries	<0.01	0.01	0.25	0.17	1.6	18.9
Uterus	<0.01	0.03	0.31	0.16	1.5	19.3
Bladder	<0.01	0.02	0.30	0.36	1.4	19.7
Colon	<0.01	0.20	0.18	4.2	20.8	20.7
Small intestine	<0.01	0.15	0.38	1.5	15.3	25.8
Kidneys	0.01	0.23	0.03	6.8	24.1	15.8
Liver	0.03	0.30	0.01	13.2	21.3	3.0
Spleen	0.02	0.18	0.01	13.7	21.0	3.2
Pancreas	0.03	0.34	0.01	10.5	15.9	3.6
Stomach	0.03	0.33	0.01	12.2	18.3	2.8
Lung	0.18	0.15	<0.01	17.6	7.0	0.85
Breast	0.38	0.66	<0.01	20.3	4.3	0.52
Esophagus	0.21	0.11	<0.01	13.8	5.1	0.64
Thyroid gland	0.35	0.01	<0.01	5.6	0.28	0.06
Salivary gland	0.02	<0.01	<0.01	1.2	0.10	0.04
Nasal cavities	<0.01	<0.01	<0.01	0.43	0.05	0.03
Brain	<0.01	<0.01	<0.01	0.37	0.05	0.03
Lenses	<0.01	<0.01	<0.01	0.37	0.05	0.03

SOURCE: Mini, R.L., Vock, P., Mury, R., & Schneeberger, P.P. (1996). Radiation exposure of patients who undergo CT of the trunk. *Radiology, 195*, 551–562. Reproduced by permission.

McCullough and co-workers found that the CTDI does not provide a true estimate of the dose delivered by electron beam CT systems. They suggested that the information from their study can be used to convert CTDI data into MSAD data, which provide a more accurate representation of the dose from electron beam CT systems.

Finally, Mini and colleagues investigated the mean organ doses in three regions of the trunk (chest, abdomen, and pelvis) during CT examinations. Their results are shown in Table 11-3. While the skin received 22–36 mGy, the testes and ovaries received 0.03–8 mGy and 0.17–18.9 mGy, respectively. The thyroid and lens of the eye, however, received 5.6–0.06 mGy and 0.37–0.03 mGy, respectively.

Concluding Remarks

In the preceding sections, we reported not only the purpose of various dose studies in radiography, mammography, and CT but also the results of these studies. What we did not describe were the various methods used in the studies. These methodologies are important to the findings of the studies. It was not our goal to examine the methods by which various experiments and measurements were conducted but rather to have an overall appreciation of the magnitude of the doses from various examinations.

For technologists, the studies cited and reported in this chapter can be used:

1. To provide us with an overview of dose trends.
2. To demonstrate that some radiological procedures result in large doses to the patient.
3. To impress upon us that the dose depends on several technical and procedural factors.
4. To suggest ways to minimize the dose to patients and personnel.
5. To help us understand the impact of our own practices on the magnitude of the doses delivered to patients.
6. To provide us with the background needed for our own studies.
7. More importantly, these studies suggest that technologists must observe the fundamental principles of radiation protection not only to reduce doses but to minimize the radiation risks as well.

Elements of a Research Study

Finally, a dose study in radiology is subject to the scientific method, which is governed by the research process. This process consists of several components common to most studies in radiology. These components include an introduction, materials and methods, results, discussion, conclusion, and references. In Appendix 11-1, each component is described briefly with the goal of introducing the student to the nature of research investigations in radiology.

REVIEW QUESTIONS

1. Most dose studies have reported all of the following except:
   A. Depth dose.
   B. Entrance skin dose.
   C. Bone marrow dose.
   D. Gonadal dose.
2. The dose measured at a point on the patient's surface where the x-ray beam enters is the:
   A. Gonadal dose.
   B. Entrance skin dose.
   C. Genetically significant dose.
   D. Integral dose.
3. Which of the following can provide an index of radiation-induced leukemia?
   A. Entrance skin dose.
   B. Genetically significant dose.
   C. Bone marrow dose.
   D. Gonadal dose.
4. Which of the following is most relevant when genetic effects are of concern?
   A. Entrance skin dose.
   B. Bone marrow dose.
   C. Depth dose.
   D. Gonadal dose.
5. Which of the following refers to the population gonadal dose?
   A. Integral dose.
   B. Collective dose.
   C. Genetically significant dose.
   D. Average organ dose.
6. Thermoluminescent dosimeters are used to measure dose because:
   A. They are small.
   B. They can be taped onto the patient's skin.
   C. They can be calibrated for use in a specific dose study.
   D. All of the above.
7. Which of the following TLD materials has been used in dose studies?
   A. Lithium fluoride.
   B. Calcium fluoride.

C. Magnesium silicate.
D. All of the above.

8. Which of the following major dose studies is conducted annually in the United States?
   A. Radiation Experience Data.
   B. X-Ray Exposure Studies.
   C. Nationwide Evaluation of X-Ray Trends.
   D. Johnson Associates Survey.

9. Information on radiation doses from diagnostic radiologic examinations is important to address which of the following?
   A. Justification of a practice.
   B. The philosophy of ALARA.
   C. Evaluate the risks and benefits of radiation exposure.
   D. All of the above.

10. Which of the following is considered a high-dose procedure?
   A. Cardiac angiography.
   B. Barium enema.
   C. Computed tomography.
   D. All of the above.

REFERENCES

Adam, Y., Alberge, S., Castellano, M., Kassab, M., & Escude, B. (1985). Pelvimetry by digital radiography. *Clinical Radiology, 36*, 327.

Beebe, G.W., Kato, H., & Land, C.E. (1978). Studies of the mortality of A-bomb survivors. 6. Mortality and radiation dose, 1950–1974. *Radiation Research, 75*, 138.

Boone, J.M., & Levin, D.C. (1991). Radiation exposure to angiographers under different fluoroscopic imaging conditions. *Radiology, 180*, 861.

Bush, W.H., Jones, D., & Brannen, G.E. (1985). Radiation dose to personnel during percutaneous renal calculus removal. *American Journal of Roentgenology, 145*, 1261.

Bushong, S. (1993). *Radiologic science for technologists* (5th ed.). St. Louis: Mosby-Year Book.

Claussen, C., Kohler, D., Christ, F., Golde, G., & Lockner, B. (1985). Pelvimetry by digital radiography and its dosimetry. *Journal of Perinatal Medicine, 13*, 287.

Conway, B.J. (1987). *Nationwide evaluation of x-ray trends (NEXT): Tabulation and graphical summary of surveys, 1984 through 1987.* Frankfort, KY: Conference of Radiation Control Program Directors.

Conway, B.J., McCrohan, J.L., Rueter, F.G., & Suleiman, O.H. (1990). Mammography in the eighties. *Radiology, 177*, 335.

Conway, B.J., McCrohan, J.L., Antonsen, R.G., et al. (1992). Average radiation dose in standard CT examinations of the head: Results of the 1990 NEXT survey. *Radiology, 135*, 135–140.

Ewen, K., John, V., Lauber-Altmann, I., & Müller, R.D. (1987). Radiation exposure and image quality: A comparison between different chest radiography techniques. *Electromedica, 55*, 18.

Faulkner, K., Gordon, M.D.H., & Miller, J. (1986). A detailed study of radiation dose and radiographic technique during chest radiography. *British Journal of Radiology, 59*, 245.

Fearon, T., & Vucich, J. (1985). Pediatric patient exposures from CT examinations. *American Journal of Roentgenology, 144*, 805.

Federal Register. (1990). *42CFR494(d). 251*, 53525.

Federle, M.P., Cohen, H.A., Rosenwein, M.F., Brant-Zawadski, M.N. (1982). Pelvimetry by digital radiography: A low-dose examination. *Radiology, 143*, 733.

Huda, W., Sandison, G.A., & Lee, T.Y. (1989). Patient doses from computed tomography in Manitoba. *British Journal of Radiology, 62*, 138.

Huda, W., Sourkes, A.M., Bews, J.A., & Kowaluk, R. (1990). Radiation doses due to breast imaging in Manitoba: 1978–1988. *Radiology, 177*, 813.

ICRP. (1991). *Recommendations of the International Commission on Radiological Protection* (Publication No. 60). Elmsford, IL: Pergamon Press.

Julin, P., & Kraepelien, T. (1984). Reduction of absorbed doses in radiography of the facial skeleton. *American Journal of Roentgenology, 143*, 1113.

Kato, K., Antoku, S., Sawada, S., & Russell, W. (1991). Calibration of Mg_2SiO_4 (Tb) thermoluminescent dosimeters for use in determining diagnostic x-ray doses to adult health study participants. *Medical Physics, 18*, 928.

Mayo, J.R., Hartman, T.E., Lee, K.S., et al. (1995). CT of the chest minimal tube current required for good image quality with the least radiation dose. *American Journal of Roentgenology, 164,* 603–607.

Mayo, J.R., Jackson, S.A., & Müller, N.L. (1993). High-resolution CT of the chest: Radiation dose. *American Journal of Roentgenology, 160,* 479.

McCrohan, J.L., Patterson, J.F., Gagne, R.M., & Goldstein, H.A. (1987). Average radiation doses in a standard head examination for 250 CT systems. *Radiology, 163,* 263.

McCullough, C.H., Zink, F.E., & Morin, R.L. (1994). Radiation dosimetry for electron beam CT. *Radiology, 192,* 637–643.

McGuire, E.L., & Dickson, P.A. (1986). Exposure and organ dose estimation in diagnostic radiology. *Medical Physics, 13,* 913.

McGuire, E.L., Baker, M.L., & Vandergrift, J.F. (1983). Evaluation of radiation exposures to personnel in fluoroscopic x-ray facilities. *Health Physics, 45,* 975.

Miller, R.E., & Selink, J.L. (1979). Enteroclysis: The small bowel enema—how to succeed and how to fail. *Gastrointestinal Radiology, 4,* 269–283.

Mini, R.L., Vock, P., Mury, R., & Schneeberger, P.P. (1995). Radiation exposure of patients who undergo CT of the trunk. *Radiology, 195,* 557–562.

Moore, M.M., & Shearer, D.R. (1989). Fetal dose estimates for CT pelvimetry. *Radiology, 171,* 265.

NCRP. (1985). *Mammography: A user's guide* (Report No. 85). Bethesda, MD: National Council on Radiation Protection and Measurements.

NCRP. (1989). *Exposure of the U.S. population from diagnostic medical radiation* (Report No. 100). Bethesda, MD: National Council on Radiation Protection and Measurements.

Niklason, L.T., Marx, M.V., & Chan, H.P. (1993). Interventional radiologists: Radiation doses and risks. *Radiology, 187,* 729.

NIH. (1985). *Report of the National Institutes of Health Ad Hoc Working Group to Develop Radioepidemiological Tables* (Publication No. 85-2748). Rockville, MD: U.S. Department of Health and Human Services.

Nishizawa, K., Maruyama, T., & Takayama, M. (1991). Determinations of organ doses and effective dose equivalents from computed tomographic examination. *British Journal of Radiology, 64,* 20.

Padovani, R., Contento, G., Fabretto, M., Malisan, M.R.; Barbina, V., & Gozzi, G. (1987). Patient dose and risks from diagnostic radiology in North-east Italy. *British Journal of Radiology, 60,* 155.

Perry, B.J., & Bridges, C. (1973). Computerized transverse axial scanning (tomography). III. Radiation dose considerations. *British Journal of Radiology, 46,* 1048.

Prado, K., Rakowski, J., Barragan, F., & Vanek, K. (1988). Breast radiation dose in film/screen mammography. *Health Physics, 55,* 81.

Rothenberg, L.N. (1990). Patient dose in mammography. *Radiographics, 10,* 739.

Rowley, K.A., Hill, S.J., Watkins, R.A., & Moore, B.M. (1987). An investigation into the levels of radiation exposure in diagnostic examinations involving fluoroscopy. *British Journal of Radiology, 60,* 167.

Rueter, F.G. (1988). NEXT 87 Project Preliminary Report. *20th Annual National Conference on Radiation Control.* Frankfort, KY: Conference of Radiation Control Program Directors.

Rueter, F.G. (1989). Mammography in NEXT. *Proceedings of Conference on Radiation Control.* Frankfort, KY. Conference on Radiation Control Program Directors.

Rueter, F.G., Conway, B.J., McCrohan, J.L., & Suleiman, O.H. (1990). Average radiation exposure values for three diagnostic radiographic examinations. *Radiology, 177,* 341.

Seeram, E. (1982). *Computed tomography technology.* Philadelphia: W.B. Saunders.

Shleien, B., Tucker, T.T., & Johnson, D.W. (1977). *The mean active bone marrow dose to the adult population of the United States from diagnostic radiology* [HEW Publication (FDA) No. 77-8013]. Rockville, MD: Department of Health, Education and Welfare.

Shope, T.B., Gagne, R.M., & Johnson, G.C. (1981). A method for describing the doses delivered by transmission x-ray computed tomography. *Medical Physics, 8,* 188.

Shope, T.B., Morgan, T.J., Showalter, C.K., et al. (1982). Radiation dosimetry survey of computed tomography systems from ten manufacturers. *British Journal of Radiology, 55,* 60.

Shrimpton, P.C., Wall, B.F., Jones, D.G., et al. (1986). Doses to patients from routine diagnostic x-ray examinations in England. *British Journal of Radiology, 59,* 749.

Steinbach, W.R., Richter, K., Uhlick F., et al. (1990). Radiation exposure and related risk to patients and operators in angiocardiography and coronary angiography. *Electromedica, 58,* 66.

Suleiman, O.H., Anderson, J., Jones, B., et al. (1991). Tissue doses in the upper gastrointestinal fluoroscopy examination. *Radiology, 178,* 653.

Taylor, K.W. (1979). Exposures to patients from radiological procedures. *Applications of Optical Instrumentation in Medicine* (VII Proceedings SPIE) *173,* 300.

Travis, E. (1989). *Primer of medical radiobiology.* Chicago: Year Book Medical Publishers.

Whalen, J.P., & Balter, S. (1984). *Radiation risks in medical imaging.* Chicago: Year Book Medical Publishers.

Yoshizumi, T.T., Suneja, S.K., & Teal, J.S. (1989). Practical CT dosimetry. *Radiologic Technology, 60,* 505.

APPENDIX 11-1

Elements of a Research Study

In Chapter 11, we examined the results of several research studies investigating the radiation dose to the patient from different radiological examinations. We did not comment on the other elements of the research studies, such as the introduction, the materials and methods, the discussion and the conclusion.

In this appendix, we explain briefly the elements of a research study so that we may have a further understanding of the essential characteristics of each. This will provide us with a fundamental background, should we conduct our own studies.

INTRODUCTION

In this section, the general idea of the study is introduced and, in particular, the nature of the problem to be investigated. This is followed by a review of the literature. Such a review should focus on past research studies that are relevant to the problem. It is important to state explicitly how these past studies are related to the problem to be investigated. Finally, the introduction should indicate the purpose of the study. Variables may be stated, results expected, and why these results are expected.

MATERIALS AND METHODS

This section of the study should provide details of how the study will be conducted. Such details should enable anyone reading the information to be able to replicate the study.

In general, this section should include information on the subjects, equipment, design of the study, and the procedure. Details of the subjects are necessary, especially if they are people. The age, sex, how they were obtained, and the number of subjects per group, together with other relevant characteristics, should be given. A description of the equipment that will be used in the study should be given in some detail and should include brand names and model numbers.

In the procedure subsection, the exact details of how the study will be conducted is mandatory. A step-by-step description of what took place is acceptable. It is here where the scientific method is particularly important. If the study is an experimental one, variables are important, that is, how the independent variables were manipulated and how the dependent variables were measured. In addition, the researcher must also mention how extraneous variables were controlled (such as randomization) and what was done to keep the variables constant during the experiment.

RESULTS

The results should be presented in a brief and comprehensive manner. For example, the results of a study on radiation exposure to the female breast during an upper gastrointestinal tract examination (Homer and Zamenof, 1982) were stated as follows:

> "In these patients, the average skin exposure was 1.1 R (0.28 mC/kg) to the medial half of the right breast and 1.0 R (0.26 mC/kg) to the medial half of the left breast" (p. 498).

In a complicated study design, it may be necessary to use tables and figures to enhance the presentation and interpretation of the results.

DISCUSSION

This is where the results are discussed. First, the purpose of the study and what the expectations were are usually summarized. If the results matched the expectations, the findings are placed within the context of the problem. On the other hand, if the results did not match the expectations, it is important to explain why this occurred.

It is also important to offer criticisms of the study, problems encountered in obtaining the data, and ways to correct the problems. If there are limitations of the study, these should be identified and discussed as well. Implications for practice and suggestions for future research should also be presented in this section.

CONCLUSION

Most researchers have included this section in their reports. It is usually a closing statement that is intended to "wrap up" the research study.

REFERENCES

All references cited in the study must be included and they should conform to the style of the journal in which the study will be published.

Part IV
Magnetic Resonance Imaging

CHAPTER TWELVE

SAFETY ASPECTS OF MAGNETIC RESONANCE IMAGING

LEARNING OBJECTIVES

Upon completion of this chapter, the reader should be able to:

1. State three reasons why MRI safety is of importance to the technologist.
2. List the three fields to which the patient is exposed in MRI.
3. State the units for each of the following: magnetic field strength, switching rates of gradients, frequency of radiowaves, specific absorption rate, and radiofrequency power density.
4. Explain the dose-response model for MRI.
5. Describe the various biological effects of exposure to static magnetic fields, low frequency magnetic fields, and radiowaves.
6. Discuss the physical hazards associated with MRI.
7. Discuss the psychological effects related to MRI.
8. State the guidelines for patient exposure in MRI for each of the following: static magnetic field, gradient magnetic fields, and radiowaves.
9. State the MRI guidelines for occupationally exposed individuals.
10. Describe how the environment is protected from the magnetic field of the MR scanner.
11. Describe how the MR scanner is protected from influences due to the environment.

Introduction

Chapter 2 presented a review of the basic physical principles of magnetic resonance imaging (MRI) and subsequently discussed the biological effects of the exposure fields operating in MRI. This chapter, by contrast, concentrates on the safety aspects of MRI, which have been receiving some attention in the recent radiology literature.

Topics covered range from concerns over both the known and the potential hazards and biological effects associated with exposure to strong magnetic fields and radiowaves as well as safety recommendations.

A Rationale for Protection in MRI

MRI safety measures are based on several major concerns. The patient is exposed to both static and rapidly changing magnetic fields as well as electromagnetic radiation in the form of radiowaves. Exposure to these fields at the levels used in MRI is generally believed to be safe, but the potential for undiscovered biological effects remains. Nevertheless, there are known hazards associated with imaging of patients with implanted electrical conductors or electronic devices, such as pacemakers. Furthermore, ferrous materials in the vicinity of the main magnetic field can become hazardous projectiles. Some patients find placement in the MRI scanning tunnel very confining; therefore, claustrophobia is not uncommon.

Exposure of the Patient in MRI

During an MR examination, the patient is exposed to a strong static external magnetic field, rapidly changing magnetic fields used for spatial localization, and radiowaves.

During the examination the patient is placed in the MR scanner, at which point he or she is exposed to the *strong static external magnetic field*. Exposure to this field causes the patient's protons to align with the field, as illustrated in Figure 12-1.

To produce an image, a set of electrical coils surrounding the patient cause small local variations in the external magnetic field. These coils, called *gradient coils*, slightly change the strength of the magnetic field in a particular direction. For example, the z coils make the external field slightly stronger at one end and slightly weaker at the other along the axis of the bore (hollow section in which the patient lies) of the magnet. The x coils change the field from side to side and the y coils up and down. These gradient fields are used to select the slice that is imaged and to localize information within the slice. Because these gradient fields are switched on and off rapidly, there is potential for producing biological effects from induced currents in the body. A secondary problem with gradient fields is that they create a banging noise when

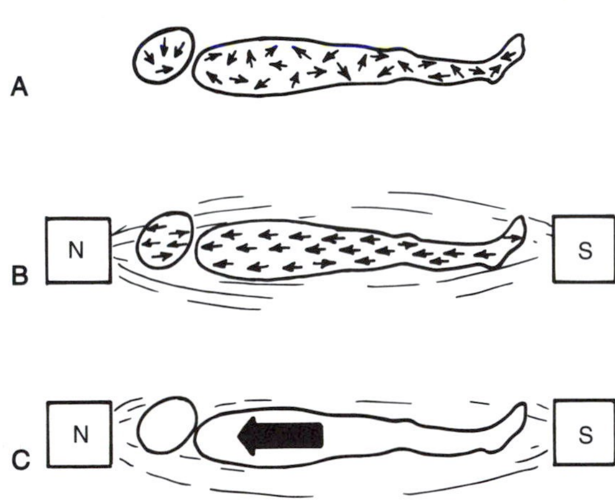

FIGURE 12-1. A patient placed in a strong magnetic field becomes polarized and behaves like a magnet. A: Protons (arrows) are randomly oriented. B: Protons align on parallel and antiparallel with the main magnetic field. Because more protons are parallel with the field, the net magnetization is indicated by the large arrow shown in C. [From Whalen, J.P., & Balter, S. (1984). *Radiation risks in medical imaging*. Chicago: Year Book Medical Publishers. Reproduced by permission.]

they are switched on and off, which may be disturbing to some patients.

During the imaging sequence, the patient is exposed to radiowaves from an antenna (RF coil, as shown in Fig. 12-2) placed either on or around the patient. The absorption of radiowaves is a potential cause of tissue heating (as occurs in a microwave oven).

Exposure Units in MRI

To understand the hazards of exposure to radiowaves and magnetic fields, it is necessary to introduce the units by which they are measured.

The conventional unit of magnetic field strength is the Gauss (G); however, the SI unit is the Tesla (T), where 1 T = 10,000 G. The earth's magnetic field strength is about 0.5 G or 0.00005 T. In MRI the strength of the main magnetic field varies and ranges from 0.1 to 0.3 T for permanent magnet systems, 0.15 to 0.3 T for resistive magnetic systems, and 0.3 to 2.0 T for superconducting magnet systems (Bushong, 1996). Recently, 4.0 T whole-body scanners have been used in several experiments to determine not only practical applications but also human exposure to such strong main magnetic fields (Schenck et al., 1992).

The switching rates of gradients are defined in units of Tesla per second (T/s). The strength of the gradient magnetic fields is small compared with the main magnetic field strength, and is in the order of about 0.01% of the main field strength. For example, in a static main field strength of 1.5 T (15,000 G), the gradient field strength is about 1.5 G or 0.00015 T.

A current of 30 amperes (A) is applied to the gradient coils to produce a change in the magnetic field strength of about 25 microTesla per centimeter (μT/cm). As pointed out by Bushong (1996), a time-varying field (gradient field) of 3 T/s will give rise to a current density of 3 A/cm^2. This is important with respect to biological effects because those cells that conduct electric currents (e.g., nerve cells) may be affected. This, of course, depends on the tissue conductivity and the time of exposure of the patient to the gradient field.

Radiofrequency (RF) radiation (radiowaves) is part of the electromagnetic spectrum and therefore has the properties of electromagnetic radiation. It is often emphasized in the literature that no radiation is used in MRI. This is not totally true. A more accurate statement would be that no ionizing radiation is used.

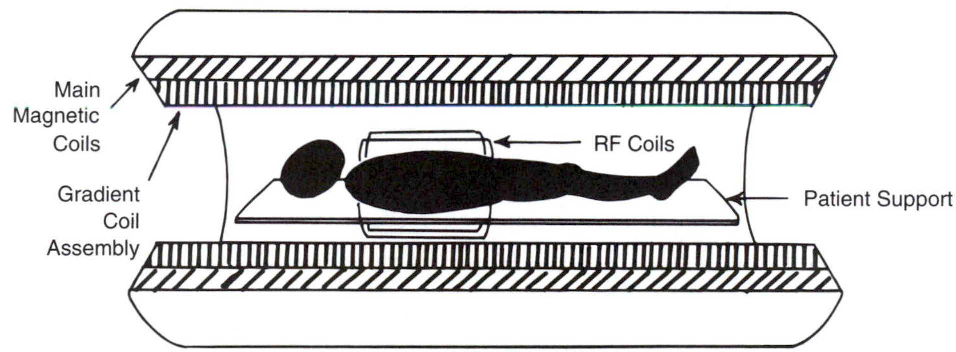

FIGURE 12-2. A patient positioned in an MRI scanner is exposed to a stationary magnetic field produced by the main magnetic coils, as well as a weak changing magnetic field produced by the gradient assembly. In addition, during the examination the patient is also exposed to radiowaves produced by the RF coils. [From Whalen, J.P., & Balter, S. (1984). *Radiation risks in medical imaging*. Chicago: Year Book Medical Publishers. Reproduced by permission.]

REVIEW BOX:
Nonionizing radiation does not lead to the ejection of electrons from their atomic orbits.

In MRI radiowaves are expressed in terms of frequency, or the number of complete cycles per second. The unit of frequency is the *Hertz* (Hz), where 1 Hz = 1 cycle per second. The RF radiation in MRI ranges from ~6.4 Megahertz (MHz) for a 0.15-T system to ~85 MHz for a 2.0-T system. In comparison, the frequency range for AM radio is 530–1640 kHz, and that of FM radio is 88 to 108 MHz.

The hazard to the patient from RF exposure is generally believed to be dependent on the rate and quantity of RF energy absorbed. How much the patient receives is a function of the RF power density [measured in watts per square meter (W/m^2)], as well as the rate at which the patient absorbs the radiation energy [the *specific absorption rate* (SAR)].

The unit of SAR is the watt per kilogram (W/kg). The surface SAR during imaging varies and depends on a number of factors including the size of the object, field frequency, and the field orientation (Persson and Staåhlberg, 1989). The SAR values for imaging with a 1.5-T magnet, for example, vary from 4.4 to 7.1 W/kg for 6 to 10 slices, respectively, when using a spin echo technique. This is a common pulse sequence imaging technique (Brandt, 1984).

Biological Effects of MRI

The second major concern that provides a rationale for protection in MRI is that of biological effects, which were discussed in Chapter 4.

For a perspective on the biological effects of MRI, consider Figure 12-3, which shows a dose–response model for MRI. This model is a nonlinear, threshold dose–response model, where D_T is the threshold dose needed to bring about a biological response. At doses below D_T, no response is observed. "D_T is considerably higher than any of the field intensities employed for clinical MRI examinations. Above D_T, the response to MRI exposure increases slowly at first and then more rapidly until 100% response would be observed" (Bushong, 1996).

Studies of the biological effects of exposure in MRI have been conducted. The general conclusion is that clinical applications of MRI result in no known health hazards, regardless of the field strength of the radiation used (Persson and Staåhlberg, 1989).

The literature is replete with general reviews of biological effects (Budinger, 1985; Saunders, 1984; Tenforde and Budinger, 1985), as well as excellent overviews of the biological effects of static magnetic field exposure (Tenforde et al., 1983; Tenforde, 1985), of changing magnetic fields (Tenforde and Budinger, 1986) and of RF exposure (Elder and Cahill, 1984).

Although it is not within the scope of this chapter to describe these effects, the most significant observations are presented. Figure 12-4 summarizes the most significant observed effects of static magnetic field on growth rates, metabolic rates, genes and reproduction, and cell membranes for animals and plants. Figure 12-5, on the other hand, shows the general effects of static magnetic field exposure on animals and humans.

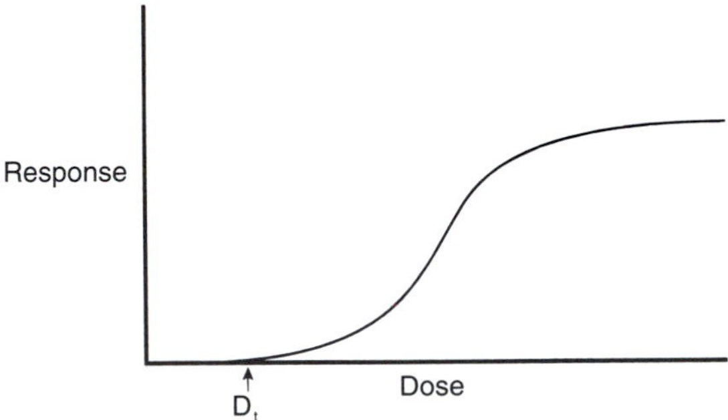

FIGURE 12-3. The dose–response model for MRI. [From Bushong, S. (1996). *Magnetic resonance imaging: Physical and biological principles* (2nd ed.). St. Louis: C.V. Mosby. Reproduced by permission.]

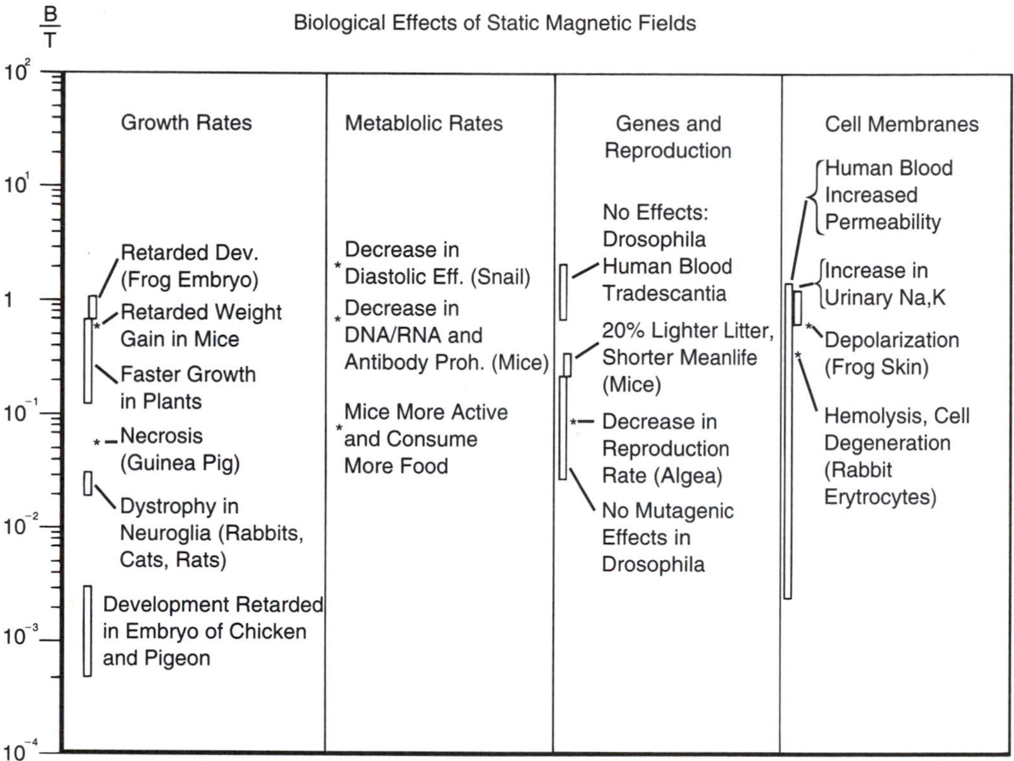

FIGURE 12-4. The most significant observed effects of static magnetic field exposure on various biological systems. [Redrawn with permission from Persson, B.R., & Staåhlberg, F. (1989). *Health and safety of clinical NMR examinations.* Boca Raton, FL: CRC Press.]

The biological effects of extremely low frequency magnetic fields are summarized in Figure 12-6. The effects of time-varying, extremely low frequency magnetic fields, on the other hand, have been studied by several investigators. These reports have been evaluated by Tenforde (1985), who could not arrive at any definitive conclusion regarding biological effects. The common biological effects, however, were those of decreased cellular respiration rate; altered metabolism of carbohydrates, proteins, and nucleic acid; endocrine changes; altered hormonal responses of cells and tissues; decreased cellular growth rate; and developmental effects, among others (Persson and Staåhlberg, 1989).

When a body is exposed to radiowaves at certain levels of SARs, the result is an increase in body temperature (Elder and Cahill, 1984). During MRI the increase in body temperature will depend on RF energy deposition and the rate of heat loss.

According to Athey (1992), a 1-hr exposure at 1 W/kg will result in an increase of ~1°C. This rule of thumb can be alternatively restated so that the same increase can be predicted if the total energy over the duration of exposure is 60 W·min/kg. It is important to note that Athey (1992) was talking about an SAR averaged over 1 kg. In actuality, the nonuniform deposition of RF can result in hot spots or local hyperthermia.

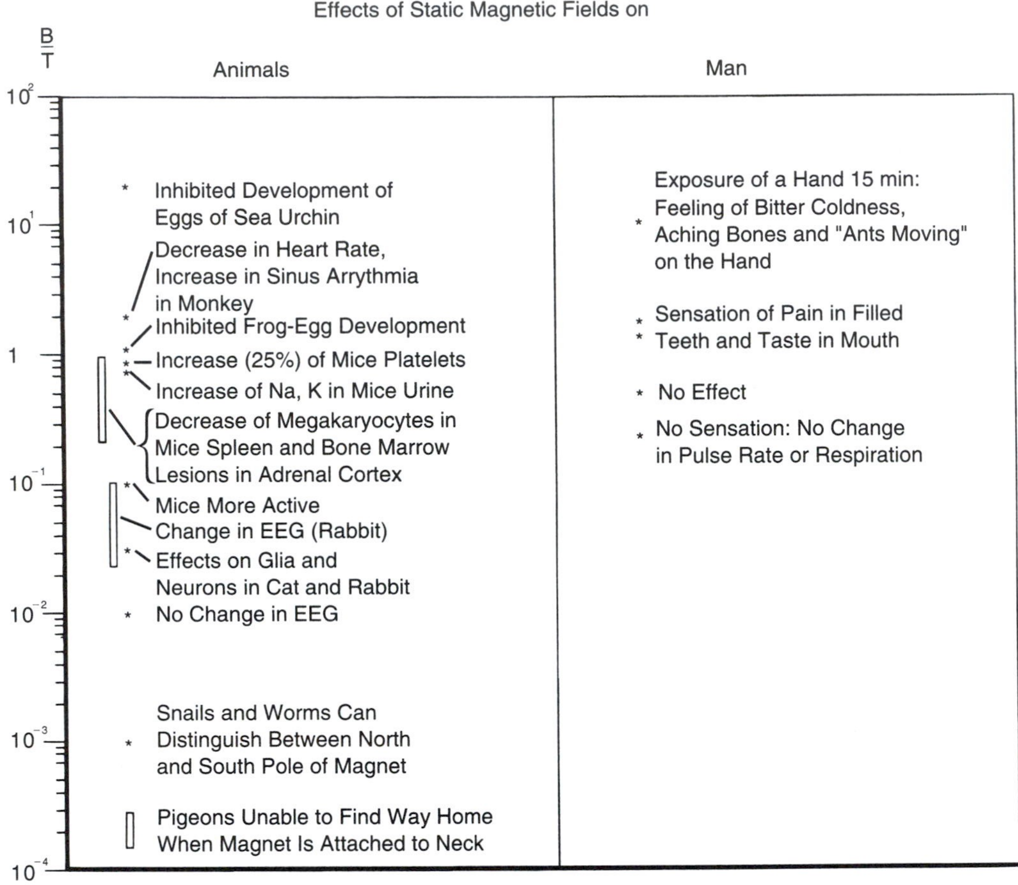

FIGURE 12-5. The most significant observed effects of static magnetic field exposure on animals and humans. [Redrawn with permission from Persson, B.R., & Staåhlberg, F. (1989). *Health and safety of clinical NMR examinations*. Boca Raton, FL: CRC Press.]

Several studies have been conducted to investigate the effects of RF deposition in biological systems at different SAR levels. Although the details of these studies are not important to this text, the general results are summarized in Table 12-1. A number of important points should be noted:

1. The table shows a wide range of SAR levels, from a high of (100 W/kg) to a low of (0.4 W/kg).
2. Below 10 W/kg, some studies have reported effects while others have found no effects.
3. At SAR levels of ≤0.4 W/kg, effects are unlikely and there is no significant change in the health of the organism.

Physical Hazards Associated with MRI

The physical hazards associated with MR scanners are caused by the magnetic fields, the gradient coils, and the nature of superconducting MRI scanners.

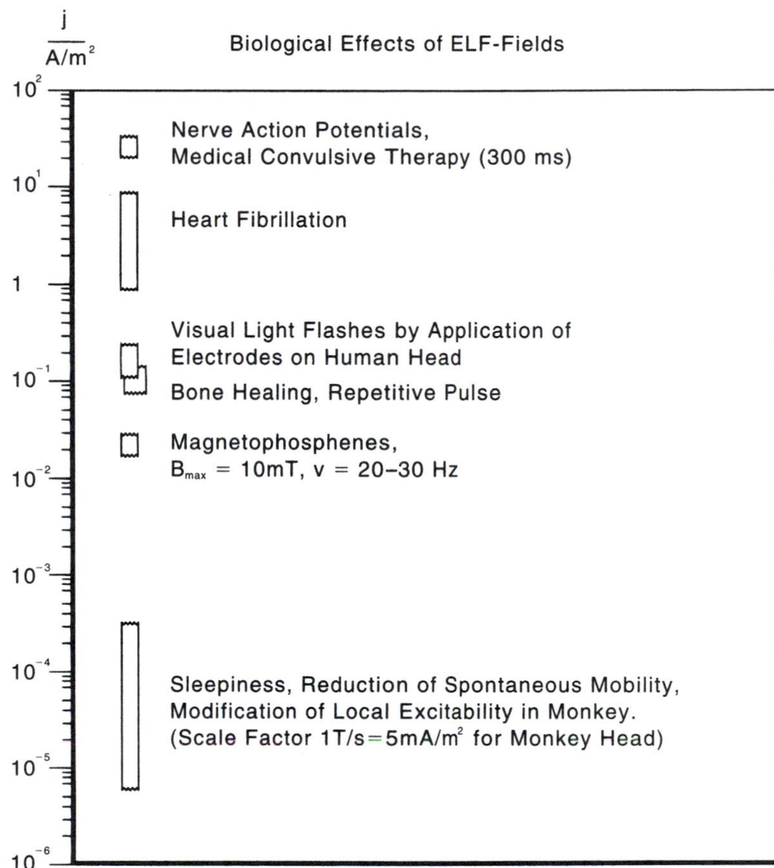

FIGURE 12-6. The biological effects of extremely low frequency magnetic fields. [Redrawn with permission from Persson, B.R., & Staåhlberg, F. (1989). *Health and safety of clinical NMR examinations.* Boca Raton, FL: CRC Press.]

The hazards associated with the main magnetic field in MRI arise from the "forces exerted on ferromagnetic objects that are either within, on, or distant from the patient and health practitioners who are exposed to the static magnetic field" (Kanal et al., 1990, p. 594).

One important consideration is that of the projectile, or missile, effect. This refers to the attraction of ferromagnetic objects distant to the MR magnet by the main magnetic field. Because this is a very strong field, the attraction is so great that it causes the object to accelerate toward the magnet. The speed at which the object travels depends on its size; the smaller it is, the faster it moves. This effect turns a simple object into a dangerous projectile, which can seriously harm any patient or health professional who may be in the path of the speeding object.

The objects reported to have been exposed to the external field or attracted to the MR magnet are listed in Table 12-2. The force of attraction is stronger for ferromagnetic objects than for paramagnetic objects, which are weakly attracted, and diamagnetic objects, which are minimally affected (Shellock, 1992).

Metallic implants or foreign bodies also pose problems for patients undergoing MRI examinations because they can either be moved or dislodged during the procedure. To prevent these types of accidents, patients are routinely screened before the MRI examination (Shellock and Kanal (1994)).

TABLE 12-1. THE EFFECTS OF RF DEPOSITION IN BIOLOGICAL SYSTEMS AT DIFFERENT SAR LEVELS

SAR (W/kg)	Type of Biological Effect Expected or Reported
100	Increased embryonic and fetal resorptions, birth defects, postnatal weight decrements, and reduced survival upon reirradiation of the offspring of mice exposed during pregnancy
50 (45)	No mutation in bacteria
	No enzyme effects
	No change in lymphocyte transformation
	Increased K^+ efflux and Na^+ influx
	Intact mammalian systems are affected
	Increased response of the immune system
	No effects on postnatal survival, adult body weight, or longevity
10	—
<6	Gray area: "effects" with inconsistent results (90% of "effects" involve behavioral, hematological, or immunological elements, CNS structure and/or function, or hormone levels)
1.4	Core temperature <0.5°C
0.8–0.3	Onset of thermoregulatory response at 25% of resting metabolic rate (RMR)
0.4	SAR not likely to be associated with "effects"
<0.4	No significant change in health status

SOURCE: Persson, B.R., & Staåhlberg, F. (1989). *Health and safety of clinical NMR examinations.* Boca Raton, FL: CRC Press. Reproduced with permission.

In addition to problems caused by the main magnetic field, there are those created by time-varying magnetic fields. A major problem is that of the induction of electric currents in devices that are electrical conductors. Electric currents can also be induced when the patient is moved into and out of the bore of the magnet (this occurs when a conductor moves in a stationary magnetic field). Changing magnetic fields can also cause heating of ferromagnetic implants; however, a number of studies have concluded that for the field strengths used in MRI, such heating does not pose a problem (Buchli et al., 1988; Goldman et al., 1989; Hurwitz et al., 1989).

Changing magnetic fields (as well as RF exposure) may induce an electric current in cardiac pacemaker wires and thus cause fibrillation, burns, or other serious problems (Edelman et al., 1990; Kanal and Shellock, 1990) such as movement of the pacemaker, changes in the programming, and/or switch closure (Hayes et al., 1987; Persson and Staåhlberg, 1989).

Another major physical hazard is the acoustic noise produced by the gradient coils during an MR examination. The noise is in the form of loud sounds (banging), which arise from switching the gradient coils on and off. When current flows through the coils (located in the main field), they experience a force, which causes them to vibrate. It is this motion or vibration that generates the loud sounds. Because the noise may be disturbing to some patients, the use of earplugs on all patients has been encouraged to alleviate this problem.

The final physical hazard to be dealt with in this chapter relates to superconducting MR scan-

TABLE 12-2. VARIOUS OBJECTS EXPOSED TO THE EXTERNAL MAGNETIC FIELD OR ATTRACTED TO THE MR MAGNET

Metal fan	Pacemaker	Tile roller	Magnet
Tile cutter	Vacuum cleaner	Identification badge	Pen, pencil, paper clip
Buffing machine	Hearing aid	Calculator	Nail clipper
Pulse oximeter	"Sand" bag	Pole for intravenous solution bag	Insulin infusion pump
Shrapnel	Jewelry	Hairpin	Gurney
Wheelchair	Forklift tines	Oxygen tank	Tools
Knife	Scissors	Prosthetic limb	Clipboard
Cigarette lighter	Mop	Chest tube stand	Key
Stethoscope	Film magazine	Bucket	Watch
Pager	Steel tipped/heeled shoes	MR table parts	
Assorted prosthetic devices and surgical implants			

SOURCE: Kanal, E., Shellock, F.G., & Talagala, L. (1990). Safety considerations in MR imaging. *Radiology, 176*, 593–606. Reproduced by permission.

ners. In superconducting systems, liquid helium is used to maintain the superconductivity of the magnetic coils. If for some reason this superconductivity is not maintained, the magnet will become resistive and heat will be given off. This heat will result in a conversion of the liquid helium into the gaseous state. This is referred to as *quenching*. The gas may escape into the MR scanning room and displace the oxygen, thus leading to problems such as asphyxiation and possible frostbite (Kanal et al., 1990).

Psychological Effects Related to MR Examinations

Psychological effects before and during MR examinations have been studied by a number of workers, including Flaherty and Hoskinson (1989), Quirk et al. (1989), and Fishbain et al. (1988). These effects include claustrophobia, anxiety, panic disorders, and emotional distress. There are several factors affecting these psychological reactions and, as pointed out by Quirk et al. (1989), they include the small space in which the patient is positioned when placed in the bore of the magnet, the acoustic noise generated by the gradient coils, the length of the examination, and the climatic conditions within the bore of the magnet.

To alleviate these problems, several methods have been suggested, such as explaining the details of the examination to the patient prior to scanning. The technologist should explain clearly the length of the examination, the small space in which the patient will be positioned, the acoustic noise, and the ambient conditions in the bore of the magnet. In addition, an individual may be encouraged to stay with the patient during the examination. This is important because patients must be observed while scanning is in progress and in between sets of image acquisition.

In some institutions, MR scanners are equipped with a mirror system in the bore of the magnet to allow the patient to see not only the technologist but also the room surroundings.

Pregnancy Considerations in MRI

Pregnancy is a major concern in MRI because of the potential risks to the fetus, especially during the first trimester.

The literature on pregnancy considerations in MRI is sparse for patients and technologists. However, guidelines for the prudent use of MRI in pregnancy have been issued by both the United States Food and Drug Administration (FDA) and the National Radiological Protection Board (NRPB) of Great Britain. While the FDA requires labeling of the MR equipment to indicate that the safety of imaging the fetus "has not been established" (FDA, 1982), the NRPB's guideline is written to suggest excluding pregnant women during the first trimester (NRPB, 1984).

Exposure Guidelines

Exposure guidelines for the prudent use of MRI in medicine have been issued in several countries, including the United States, Canada, Great Britain, and Germany. In 1982, the FDA issued its first set of guidelines, which were subsequently revised in 1988.

Exposure guidelines can be discussed in terms of patient exposure and occupational exposure.

Guidelines for Patient Exposure

The current FDA guidelines (Athey, 1992) are as follows:

1. *Static magnetic field*—For whole-body exposure, 2.0 T is recommended, whereas for extremities 5.0 T is the limit.
2. *Gradient magnetic fields*—For frequencies below 1 kHz, the limit is 20 T/s for pulses longer than 0.12 msec. If the pulses are shorter and the frequencies are higher, then higher values are allowed.
3. *Radiofrequency (RF) fields*—The guidelines are such that there are two options:
   a. The whole-body SAR limit is 0.4 W/kg, which is the same as the limit recommended by the American National Standard Institute (ANSI); the SAR limit to 1 g of tissue is 8.0 W/kg or 3.2 W/kg averaged over the head.
   b. The temperature increase does not exceed 38°C for the head, 39°C for the trunk, and 40°C for the extremities.

In Canada, the guidelines are as follows, as stated by the Environmental Health Directorate (1987):

1. 2.0 T for static magnetic fields.
2. 3 T/s for changing magnetic fields.
3. SAR limit of <1 W/kg >15 min exposure and an SAR limit of <2 W/kg <15 min exposure in 25% of body weight.

With the advent of 4.0-T MR scanners, several of which are undergoing clinical testing in the United States (Schenck et al., 1992), there are concerns about revision of the guidelines. These systems result in higher frequencies for RF fields and greater RF power deposition. In addition, the interest in fast imaging techniques means that the changing magnetic fields due to the gradient coils will be higher. The question is as follows: Will these concerns have implications for future guidelines? Athey (1992) pointed out that "the FDA guidance value was chosen to include a safety factor of about three with respect to the theoretical threshold. The actual safety factor now appears to be closer to two; thus to avoid peripheral nerve stimulation, it will probably not be possible to relax the guidelines very much, if at all" (p. 252).

Occupational Exposure

Guidelines for occupationally exposed individuals have been established by the International Radiation Protection Association (IRPA, 1984). For these individuals, the limits are based on SAR levels for whole-body exposure of 0.4 W/kg. The power density (W/m^2) limit for individual occupational exposure to a frequency range of 10–400 MHz, for example, is 10 W/m^2.

In Canada, the guidance on exposures to operators is such that they:

> Should not be continuously exposed to a magnetic flux density exceeding 0.01 T during the working day. Exposures to higher flux densities are permitted for short-time durations (about 10 minutes per hour); their number and duration should be minimized (Environmental Health Directorate, 1987, p. 15).

Other Safety Considerations

There are several other safety considerations in MRI that warrant special attention. These include protection of the environment from effects due to the MR scanner and protection of the MR scanner from environmental factors.

Protecting the Environment

The MR scanner should be installed in a location where the effects on the environment from the magnetic field that extends beyond the MR scanner are negligible. This stray magnetic field is referred to as the *fringe field*.

The fringe field decreases in strength as one moves away from the MR scanner. This variation in fringe field strength tends to have detrimental effects on various equipment and objects. The types of equipment and objects that should be excluded from the fringe field are shown in Figure 12-7.

It is also important for the public to be aware of the presence of the fringe field, and in this regard it is recommended that warning signs be posted in appropriate areas in the department. Several warning signs are shown in Figure 12-8.

Protecting the MR Scanner

There are several reasons why the MR scanner must be protected from environmental influences stemming from the presence of ferromagnetic objects and equipment near to or within the fringe field.

1. Ferromagnetic objects can be attracted to the MR scanner due to the strong attractive force of the main magnetic field. This can result in the "missile" or projectile effect, as discussed previously.
2. Ferromagnetic objects may degrade the field uniformity in the bore of the magnet. Such uniformity is essential for good image qual-

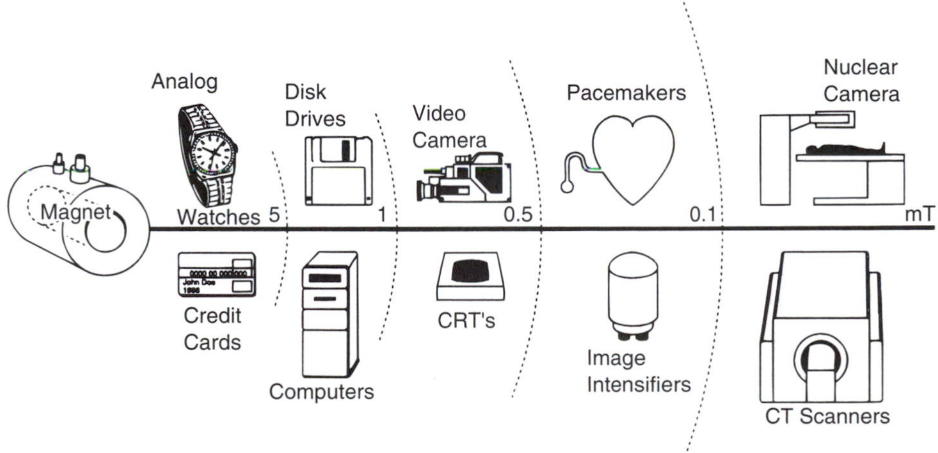

FIGURE 12-7. The equipment and objects that should be excluded from the fringe field in MRI. [From Bushong, S. (1996). *Magnetic resonance imaging: Physical and biological principles* (2nd ed.). St. Louis: C.V. Mosby. Reproduced by permission.]

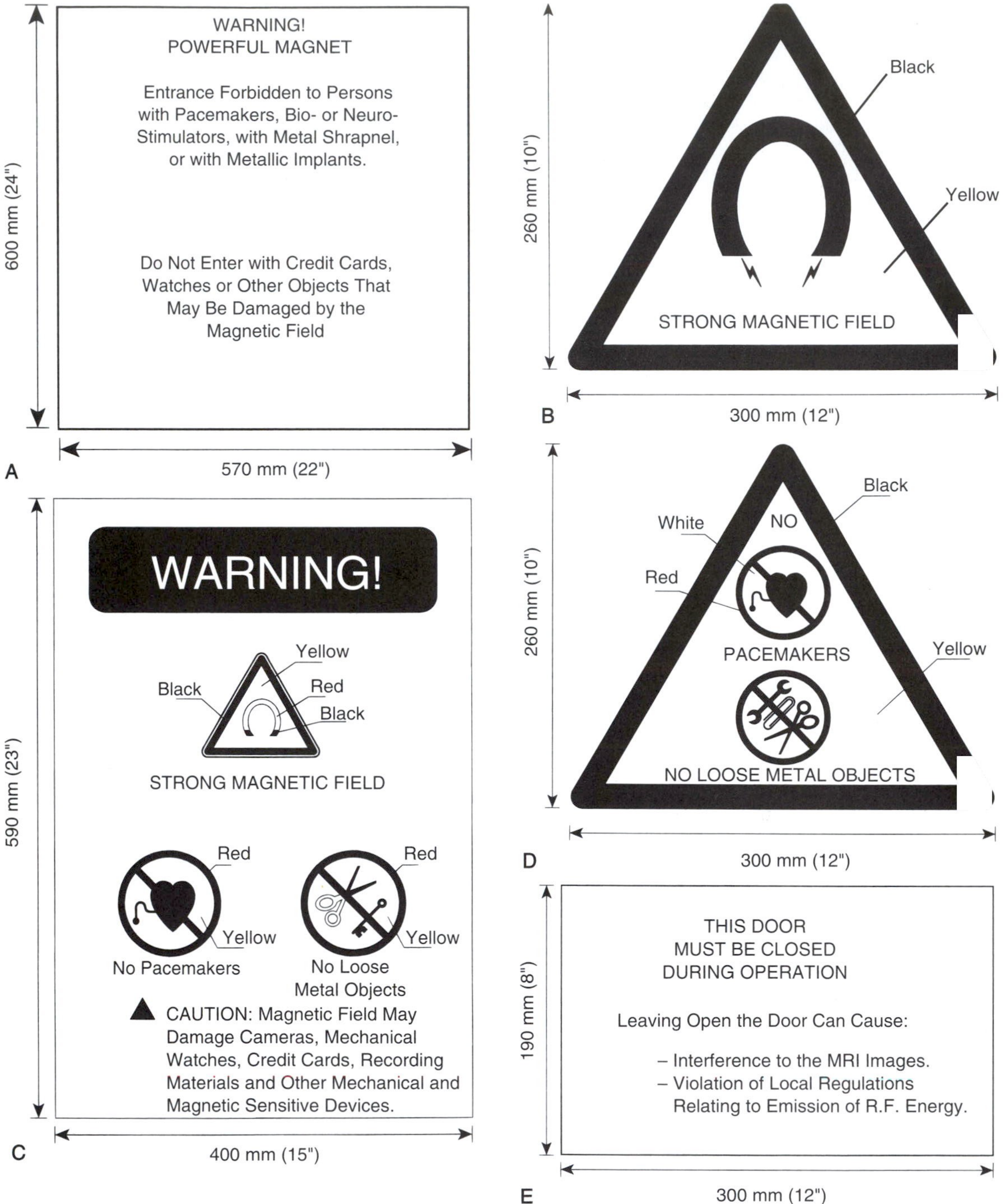

FIGURE 12-8. A–E. Examples of warning signs to be posted in a department with an MR scanner. (Courtesy of Elscint Ltd., Ontario, Canada.)

ity. In this regard, Figure 12-9 shows several objects that should remain outside the fringe magnetic fields.

3. The MR scanner must be shielded from external RF waves such as those from broadcast radio because the MRI operates at 1–100 MHz RF range. Protecting the scanner is accomplished by:
   a. Lining the walls of the MR scanner room with copper or aluminum mesh to absorb any external RF waves. The operator's viewing window is also shielded from external RF radiation.
   b. Shielding the magnet by one of the three schemes shown in Figure 12-10.
4. Last, but certainly not least, is the presence of a metal detector through which patients and personnel must pass before they get close to the MR scanner; however, metal detectors may not be sensitive enough to detect all metallic objects.

MRI is an exciting imaging modality that has opened up new avenues and challenges for technologists. Already, MRI has become commonplace in diagnostic imaging, and experts believe that MRI may even become a routine procedure in radiology departments. Therefore, the technologist must make every effort to understand not only how MRI works but also the biological effects associated with exposure to magnetic fields and radiowaves in MRI. The safety aspects and the guidelines for the prudent use of this marvelous technique must also be studied and rigorously observed.

This chapter provided a small but meaningful step in that direction.

REVIEW QUESTIONS

1. Which of the following major concerns provides a rationale for protection in MRI?
   A. The patient is exposed to magnetic fields and radiowaves.
   B. There are potential biological effects of the fields in MRI.

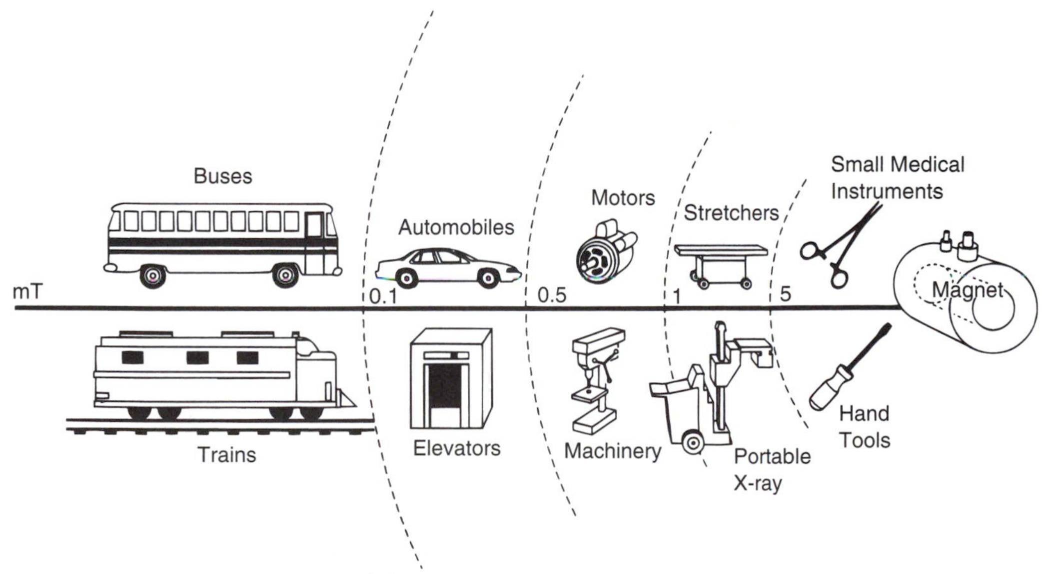

FIGURE 12-9. Several objects that should remain outside the fringe field in MRI. [From Bushong, S. (1996). *Magnetic resonance imaging: Physical and biological principles* (2nd ed.). St. Louis: C.V. Mosby. Reproduced by permission.]

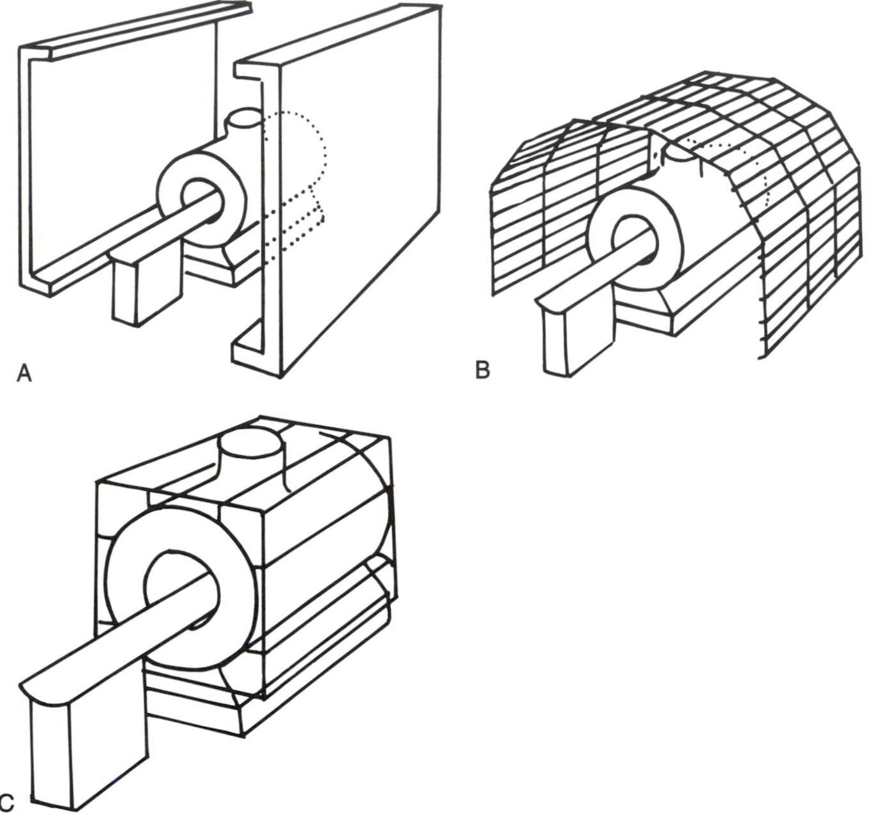

FIGURE 12-10. Three schemes used to shield the MR scanner. A: Parallel plates. B: Cylindrical cage or magnetic dome. C: Integrated self-contained shield or flux return yoke. [From Einstein, S.G., & Hilal, S.K. (1985). In H.Y. Kressel (Ed.), *Magnetic Resonance Annual 1985*. New York: Raven Press. Reproduced by permission.]

   C. There are associated physical hazards and psychological effects associated with MRI.
   D. All of the above.

2. During an MRI examination, the patient is exposed to:
   A. A strong static magnetic field.
   B. Rapidly changing magnetic fields.
   C. Radiowaves.
   D. All of the above.

3. The SI unit for magnetic field strength is the:
   A. Tesla.
   B. Gauss.
   C. Tesla per second.
   D. Watts per kilogram.

4. One Tesla is equal to:
   A. 1000 G.
   B. 10,000 G.
   C. 100 G.
   D. 100,000 G.

5. The switching rates of gradients used in MRI are defined in units of:
   A. Gauss.
   B. Tesla.

C. Tesla per second.
D. All of the above.

6. The unit of frequency is the:

A. Cycle.
B. Angstrom.
C. Watts per kilogram.
D. Hertz.

7. The unit of RF power density is:

A. Watts.
B. Watts per kilogram.
C. Watts per square meter.
D. Coulombs per kilogram.

8. The unit of specific absorption rate is:

A. Watts per kilogram.
B. Watts per meter squared.
C. Coulombs per kilogram.
D. None of the above is correct.

9. The dose–response model for MRI is the:

A. Linear, threshold model.
B. Supralinear, nonthreshold model.
C. Nonlinear, threshold model.
D. Linear quadratic threshold model.

10. One of the biological effects of exposure to radiowaves at certain levels of SARs is:

A. Tissue heating.
B. Cavitation.
C. Microstreaming.
D. Chromosome breakage.

11. The physical hazards associated with MRI stem from:

A. The main magnetic field.
B. Gradient magnetic fields.
C. Quenching.
D. All of the above.

12. The following are physical hazards in MRI except:

A. Claustrophobia.
B. Projectile or missile effect.
C. Induction of electric currents in electrical conductors.
D. Acoustic noise caused by gradient switching.

13. A quench in MRI will result in all of the following except:

A. Permanent damage to the magnet.
B. Loss of superconductivity of the coil for the main magnetic field.
C. The magnet becomes resistive and heat is released.
D. The liquid helium can evaporate very quickly.

14. The following have been classified as psychological effects that may be experienced by some patients during an MR examination, except:

A. Claustrophobia.
B. Anxiety.
C. Panic.
D. Acoustic noise.

15. The FDA guidelines for the use of MRI in pregnancy require that:

A. Pregnant patients can be imaged during the first trimester.
B. The equipment be labeled to indicate that the safety of imaging the fetus has not been established.
C. Pregnant patients cannot be imaged during the first trimester.
D. The equipment be labeled to indicate that MRI is safe and that a pregnant patient should not be concerned about possible risk.

16. The FDA guidelines for patient exposure to the static magnetic field in MRI is:

A. 2.0 T for whole-body exposure.
B. 4.0 T for whole-body exposure.
C. 20 T for whole-body exposure.
D. 5 T for whole-body exposure.

17. The FDA limit for exposure of the patient to gradient magnetic fields is:
    A. 2.0 T/s for frequencies >1 kHz and pulses <0.12 msec.
    B. 20 T/s for frequencies <1 kHz and pulses >0.12 msec.
    C. 20 T/s for frequencies >1 kHz and pulses >0.12 msec.
    D. 20 T/s for frequencies <1 kHz and pulses >2 msec.

18. The FDA whole-body SAR limit for patient exposure in MRI is:
    A. 4 W/kg.
    B. 40 W/kg.
    C. 0.4 W/kg.
    D. 0.4 W/m^2.

19. The IRPA whole-body SAR limit for MRI workers is:
    A. 4 W/kg.
    B. 40 W/kg.
    C. 0.4 W/kg.
    D. 10 W/m^2.

20. The MR scanner is protected from influences due to the environment because:
    A. The walls of the scanner room are shielded with lead.
    B. The walls of the scanner room are lined with copper or aluminum mesh.
    C. The magnet may be shielded with parallel plates or a cylindrical cage or an integrated self-contained shield.
    D. b and c are correct.

REFERENCES

Athey, T.W. (1992). Current FDA guidance for MR patient exposure and considerations for the future. *Annals of the New York Academy of Sciences, 649*, 242.

Brandt, G. (1984). Tissue heating by radiofrequency magnetic fields magnetic resonance imaging. *Proceedings of the Third Annual Meeting of the Society of Magnetic Resonance in Medicine.* Berkeley, California: Berkeley Society of Magnetic Resonance in Medicine.

Buchli, R., Boesiger, P., & Meier, D. (1988). Heating effects of metallic implants by MRI examinations. *Magnetic Resonance in Medicine, 7*, 255.

Budinger, T.G. (1985). Health effects of in vivo nuclear magnetic resonance. *IEEE Engineering in Medicine and Biology Magazine, 1*, 31.

Bushong, S. (1996). *Magnetic resonance imaging: Physical and biological principles* (2nd ed.). St. Louis: C.V. Mosby.

Edelman, R.R., Shellock, F.G., & Ahladis, J. (1990). Practical MRI for the technologist. In R.R. Edelman & J. Hesselink (Eds.), *Clinical Magnetic Resonance Imaging.* Philadelphia: W.B. Saunders.

Elder, J.A., & Cahill, D.F. (Eds.). (1984). *Biological effects of radiofrequency radiation* (Report No. EPA-600/8-83-026F). North Carolina: U.S. Environmental Protection Agency.

Environmental Health Directorate. (1987). *Guidelines on exposure to electromagnetic fields from magnetic resonance clinical systems.* Ottawa: Environmental Health Directorate.

FDA. (1982). *Guidelines for evaluating electromagnetic risk for trials of clinical NMR systems.* Bethesda, MD: Bureau of Radiological Health Report.

Fishbain, D.A., Goldberg, M., Labbe, E., et al. (1988). Long term claustrophobia following magnetic resonance imaging. *American Journal of Psychiatry, 145*, 1038.

Flaherty, T.A., & Hoskinson, K. (1989). Emotional distress during magnetic resonance imaging. *New England Journal of Medicine, 320*, 467.

Goldman, A.M., Grossman, W.E., & Friedlander, P.C. (1989). Reduction of sound levels with antinoise in MR imaging. *Radiology, 173*, 549.

Hayes, D.L., Holmes, D.R., & Gray, J.E. (1987). Effect of a 1.5 Tesla nuclear magnetic resonance imaging scanner on implanted permanent pacemakers. *Journal of the American College of Cardiology, 10*, 782.

Hurtwitz, R., Lane, S.R., & Bell, R.A. (1989). Acoustic analysis of gradient coil noise in MR imaging. *Radiology, 173*, 545.

IRPA. (1984). Interim guidelines on limit of exposure to radiofrequency electromagnetic fields in the frequency range from 100 kHz to 300 GHz. *Health Physics, 46*, 975.

Kanal, E., & Shellock, F.G. (1990). Burns associated with clinical MR examinations. *Radiology, 175*, 585.

Kanal, E., Shellock, F.G., & Talagala, L. (1990). Safety considerations in MR imaging. *Radiology, 176*, 593–606.

NRPB. (1984). Ad hoc advisory group on NMR clinical imaging: Revised guidance on acceptable limits of exposure during nuclear magnetic resonance clinical imaging. *British Journal of Radiology, 56*, 974.

Persson, B.R., & Staåhlberg, F. (1989). *Health and safety of clinical NMR examinations.* Boca Raton, FL: CRC Press.

Quirk, M.E., Letendre, A.J., Ciottone, R.A. (1989). Anxiety in patients undergoing MR imaging. *Radiology, 170*, 463.

Saunders, R.D., & Smith, H. (1984). Safety aspects of NMR clinical imaging. *British Medical Bulletin, 40*, 148–154.

Schenck, J.F., et al. (1992). Human exposure to 4.0 Tesla magnetic fields in a whole-body scanner. *Medical Physics, 19*, 1089.

Shellock, F.G., & Kanal, E. (1994). Magnetic resonance imaging bioeffects, safety and patient management. New York: Raven Press.

Tenforde, T.S. (1985). Biological effects of stationary magnetic fields. In M. Gandolfo & S.M. Michaelson (Eds.), *Biological Effects and Dosimetry of Non-Ionizing Radiation: Static and ELF Electromagnetic Fields.* Elmsford, NY: Plenum Press.

Tenforde, T.S. (1986). Interaction of time-varying ELF magnetic fields with living matter. In C. Polk & E. Postow (Eds.), *Biological Effects of Electromagnetic Fields.* Boca Raton, FL: CRC Press.

Tenforde, T.S., & Budinger, T.F. (1986). Biological effects of physical safety aspects of NMR imaging in vivo spectroscopy. In: *NMR in Medicine*: The Instrumentation and Clinical Applications. S.R. Thomas & R.L. Dickson (Eds.). New York: American Institute of Physics.

Tenforde, T.S., et al. (1983). Cardiovascular alterations in Macaca monkeys exposed to stationary magnetic fields: Experimental observations and theoretical analysis. *Bioelectromagnetics, 4*, 1.

Part V
Radiation Protection Through Quality Control

CHAPTER THIRTEEN

RADIATION PROTECTION THROUGH QUALITY CONTROL

LEARNING OBJECTIVES

Upon completion of this chapter, the reader should be able to:

1 ■ Define quality assurance (QA) and quality control (QC).

2 ■ State the goals of a QA program for diagnostic radiology.

3 ■ Trace the history of QA in radiology.

4 ■ Define the term "dose optimization" and describe briefly the components of dose optimization in radiology.

5 ■ Discuss the concepts of QC leading to dose optimization.

6 ■ Explain what is meant by the term "tolerance limit" in QC.

7 ■ Cite examples of exposure reduction as a consequence of a QC program.

8 ■ Identify one NCRP report on QA for diagnostic radiology.

Introduction

The concepts of *quality assurance (QA)* and, more specifically, *quality control (QC)* have become increasingly important in radiation protection of the patient. Other concepts such as total quality management (TQM) and continuous quality improvement (CQI) were explained in Chapter 1.

This chapter identifies and describes the essential features of QC in diagnostic radiology, with the goal of emphasizing the role of QC in radiation protection of the patient. More specifically, this chapter defines both QA and QC, traces the development of QC, states the goals of a QC program, and describes the concepts leading to dose reduction. These concepts relate to responsibilities, principles, test procedures, and parameters for QC monitoring. It is not within the scope of this chapter to describe QC tests and how to conduct and interpret them; these topics are best described in texts that are devoted to comprehensive treatment of quality control.

Definitions

The idea and concepts of QA and QC can be traced back to the early 1970s. Several definitions of these concepts emerged in 1973, and were updated in 1979 and in the 1980s to reflect advancements in knowledge and technology. In 1988, the National Council on Radiation Protection and Measurements (NCRP) offered their version of the definitions.

Quality Assurance (QA)

According to the NCRP (1988), QA

> . . . is a comprehensive concept that comprises all of the management practices instituted by the imaging physician to ensure that: (1) every imaging procedure is necessary and appropriate to the clinical problem at hand; (2) the images generated contain information critical to the solution of that problem; (3) the recorded information is correctly interpreted and made available in a timely fashion to the patient's physician; and (4) the examination results in the lowest possible radiation exposure, cost and inconvenience to the patient consistent with objective (2) (p. 1).

The objectives inherent in this definition identify several individuals who play significant roles in establishing a successful QA program. While objective 1 implicates the patient's physician in the initial decision-making process, objective 2 assigns the responsibility for making decisions about image quality to both the radiologist and technologist. Objective 3, on the other hand, narrows its focus to the radiologist, who is assumed to possess a reliable degree of competency in image interpretation. Finally, objective 4 is really what a QA program is all about, that is, dose reduction, image quality standards, and cost.

Overall, QA is a management concept that includes administrative, educational, and technical measures to ensure that image quality standards are met, dose is kept to a minimum and consistent with image quality, and the cost of establishing and maintaining the program is low and reasonable. QA ensures efficient utilization of the resources in the department.

Quality Control (QC)

QC deals with technical measures. The NCRP (1988) defined QC as:

> . . . a series of distinct technical procedures which ensure the production of a satisfactory product. Its aim is to provide quality that is not only satisfactory and diagnostic but also dependable and economic (p. 4).

QC, then, is the component of the QA program that deals with techniques for measuring imaging quality as well as testing and maintaining the integrity of the components of the x-ray system. In other words, QC deals with the equipment. It includes several concepts leading to dose reduction, and it is effective in ensuring radiation protection of the patient.

Goals of QA and QC

The overall goals of a QA program are usually discussed in terms of primary and secondary goals. While the primary goal is to facilitate accurate diagnosis, the secondary goals are to:

1. Reduce the radiation exposure to the patient (ICRP, 1982).
2. Reduce the radiation risk to the patient.
3. Ensure patient comfort and privacy.
4. Ensure communication. In this regard, films should be correctly identified and labeled, and accurate reports should be sent to the patient's physician as quickly as possible.
5. Keep the cost to the consumer as low as possible but should in no way compromise diagnosis.

To accomplish these goals, those who are responsible for the integrity of the QA program, as well as those who participate in conducting QC procedures, must understand the factors affecting image quality because these factors influence the ability to make an accurate diagnosis. In addition, individuals must also understand the factors that play a role in minimizing the radiation exposure to the patient, thus subsequently reducing the radiation risks to the patient. (See Chapters 1 and 4 for an expanded discussion of these issues.)

In summary, both education and training in QC procedures are mandatory if the QA program is to be successful in achieving these goals.

QA: Historical Perspectives

The idea of QA may be traced back to a project of the National Institute for Occupational Safety and Health (NIOSH) in 1970. In this project, the chest x-rays of coal miners were deemed to be of poor quality due to overexposure, underexposure, and poor processing technique (Felson et al., 1973). These factors resulted in a high reject rate (rate at which unacceptable films are discarded).

Later, other studies, such as those by Trout et al. (1973), Burnett et al. (1975), Beideman et al. (1976), and Hall (1977), reported significant reject rates in various facilities. The major cause of the rejection was attributed to poor equipment performance. In yet another study, Showalter et al. (1977) found that 50% of the exposure variation for PA chest projections may be due to equipment malfunction as well. These studies provided data to show that poor performance was a major cause of poor image quality, which in turn resulted in unnecessary radiation to the patient who had to be reexposed to radiation to obtain films of diagnostic quality.

In 1979, the Bureau of Radiological Health (BRH), now called the Center for Devices and Radiological Health (CDRH), a division of the Food and Drug Administration (FDA) of the United States Department of Health, Education and Welfare (USHEW) supported and encouraged the development of QA programs in radiology departments. The CDRH took an educational approach (as opposed to a regulatory one) and promoted QA as a voluntary activity, to be established by individual radiology facilities. In addition, the Joint Commission on Accreditation of Healthcare Organizations (JCAHO) has completely endorsed the goals of the CDRH with respect to QA programs.

The CDRH goals focused on ways to ensure that radiological equipment performance was effective because a number of studies, such as those done by Barnes et al. (1976) and Burkhart (1980), showed that routine QA programs could make a difference. Around this same period, several other groups such as DuPont, Agfa-Gavert, Eastman Kodak Company, Radiation Measurements Incorporated (RMI), and the American College of Radiology (ACR) expressed an interest in QA and began presenting workshops on how to establish a QA program. QA is now commonplace in most radiology departments, and already several reports have indicated the dose reduction benefit as well as other benefits, all attributed to QA programs (NCRP, 1989).

Dose Optimization

To gain a perspective on the role of QA in radiation protection, it is important that we understand *dose optimization.* This term refers to the use of the lowest possible radiation dose in an examination without compromising the image quality required for accurate interpretation (Philips, 1993). Dose optimization is an integral part of QA because its components not only affect the integrity of the program but maintain it as well.

Components

The components of dose optimization are broadly illustrated in Figure 13-1. These include education and training, technical factors, and personnel practices.

Education and training have been discussed in the literature (Bushong, 1993; Carlton and Adler, 1992; NCRP, 1988; Seeram, 1985; Gray and Stears, 1984; Gray et al., 1983; McLemore, 1981; Carlton, 1980). It is important that all personnel in the department including technologists, radiologists, physicists, biomedical engineers, and related individuals be trained in the technical aspects of radiology. This includes QA education.

Recently, we have seen the evolution of the QC technologist, an individual who has received special training in QC procedures. In this regard, Gray and Stears (1984) pointed out that the technologist spends a substantial amount of time pursuing both formal and informal courses of study designed to improve on-the-job proficiency. Approximately 8% of the formal education time of the technologists interviewed was dedicated to the Mayo Radiologic Technologist School; the remainder of the time was spent on in-service education and presentations within and outside of the Mayo Clinic. Thus, the "nonformal education" of these technologists was obtained via hands-on experience within the department.

Today, we see an increasing number of QC technologists, as well as QC courses, which have become commonplace in radiologic technology programs.

Technical factors relevant to the role of QA and QC in radiation protection are those factors that affect patient exposure, many of which also affect image quality. These factors also play a role in dose optimization, because, as dose is minimized by changing one factor, image quality is subsequently decreased. Therefore, a balance must be maintained between dose and image quality.

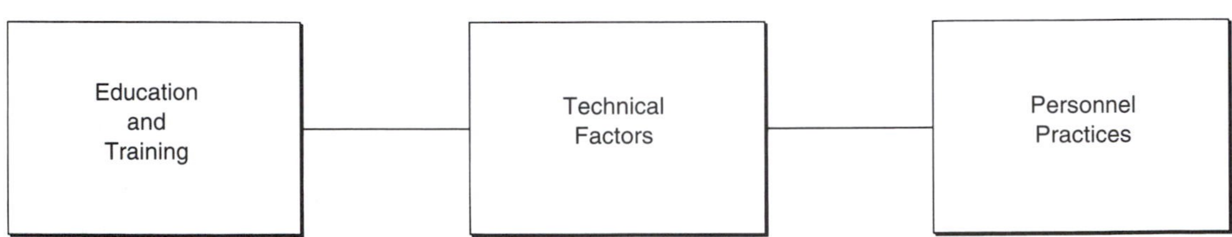

FIGURE 13-1. The components of dose optimization, a concept relevant to QA and radiation protection.

Technical factors were discussed in the previous chapters. It is not within the scope of this chapter to elaborate on these factors. However, the major factors include kVp, mA, time, waveform, filtration, collimation, image receptor sensitivity, grids, tabletop, and distance.

As noted, these are factors related to the equipment. QC is thus concerned with monitoring these factors to ensure that patient exposures are within acceptable limits and that the patient is not subject to unnecessary radiation doses.

The final component of dose optimization is that of personnel practices, which refers to activities performed by individuals in the course of their daily work. These activities are wide and varied and range from patient scheduling, patient reception, patient preparation, patient examination, and film processing to image quality control, image interpretation, report preparation, report distribution, and file room operation (NCRP, 1988).

For the technologist, it is mandatory that duties be performed in a meticulous manner, with the goal of radiation protection as a primary consideration within the framework of a QA program. The technologist must ensure that the examination is conducted accurately, the patient is protected, and the image quality is acceptable for accurate interpretation by the radiologist.

QC Concepts Leading to Dose Optimization

There are several concepts of a QA/QC program leading to dose optimization. These include responsibilities, principles of QC, QC test procedures, and parameters for QC monitoring. Each of these is now described because they represent the backbone of QA programs.

Responsibilities

For a QA program to be successful, it is important that responsibilities be defined so that individuals understand the nature of the tasks associated with a particular responsibility. A QA scheme illustrating responsibilities and interaction among different individuals is shown in Figure 13-2.

In this scheme, the radiologist in charge of the department assumes the primary responsibility for the entire program, as identified by the FDA, the CDRH, and the JCAHO. In most cases, however, this responsibility is assigned to the radiological physicist, biomedical engineer, or the technologist.

The responsibility for QA is a group effort. Everyone in the department should play a role, no matter how small, to maintain the integrity and ensure the success of the program. Because physicists are trained at a higher level than technologists, they play major roles in developing tools and tests for QC and teach others how to conduct these tests and interpret the results. The engineer's role relates to repair and calibration of the equipment (Seeram, 1985).

Principles of QC

The principles of QC are related to three major steps: (1) acceptance testing, in which equipment is tested to verify that it functions according to the specifications provided by the manufacturer, (2) routine performance evaluation, and (3) error correction (Bushong, 1993).

Conducting the performance evaluation tests requires the use of a definite set of rules for solving a problem, an algorithm, to ensure accurate and reliable measurements. An example of a generalized algorithm is shown in Figure 13-3. There are at least three major items that warrant further consideration. These are the test procedure, image quality standards, and performance criteria or tolerance limit.

The *test procedure* informs the QC technologist about the steps that should be taken when performing performance evaluations. These steps should be clear and precise and should be based on a format that is easy to follow. One such format may be as follows:

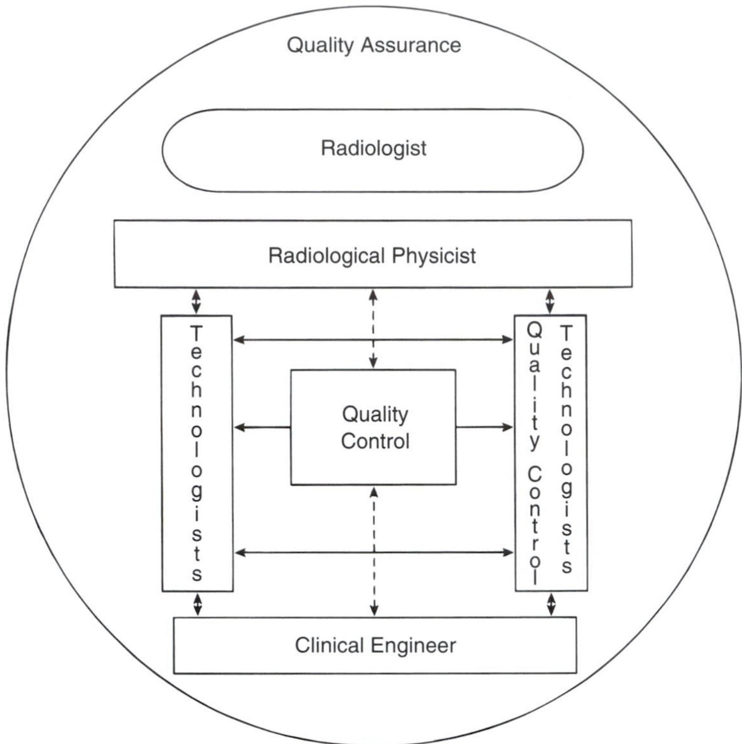

FIGURE 13-2. A QA scheme showing responsibilities and interaction among individuals in a radiology department. [From Seeram, E. (1985). *X-ray equipment: An introduction*. Springfield, IL: Charles C Thomas. Reproduced by permission.]

1. The name and purpose of the test.
2. The equipment needed to perform the test.
3. How often the test should be conducted, in other words, the testing frequency.
4. Equipment setup and measurements to be recorded.
5. Documentation of the test results.
6. Interpretation of the results.
7. Measures to correct unsatisfactory results (Seeram, 1985).

Image quality standards, however, must be established by the department. These standards are usually based on both subjective and objective criteria. Whereas subjective standards are based on the feelings and opinions of radiology workers, objective standards are based on the results of scientific research. In QA programs, objective standards should prevail.

Standards should have "certain defined limits," which are alternatively defined as performance criteria or tolerance limits. Equipment performance is deemed acceptable when the results of a test fall within these limits. In this case, the patient is not subjected to unnecessary exposures due to faulty equipment.

The principles of QC involve other considerations that affect the integrity of the program. These include preventive and corrective maintenance measures, record keeping, and the development of a QA policy and procedural manual, which should contain information on pertinent items listed in Table 13-1.

Elements and Variables for QC Monitoring

There are several elements in the imaging chains for radiography, fluoroscopy, mammography, computed tomography, and digital systems,

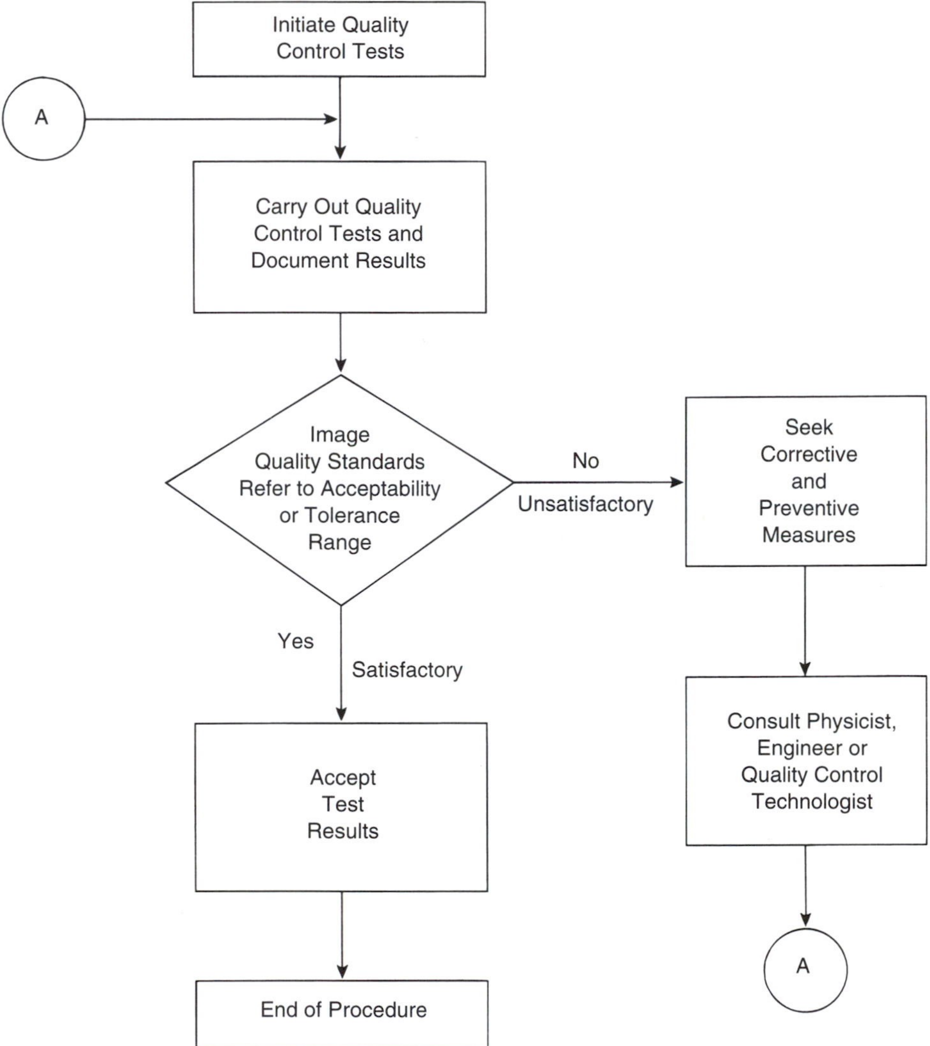

FIGURE 13-3. A flow chart illustrating the fundamental principles of QC. [From Seeram, E. (1985). *X-ray equipment: An introduction.* Springfield, IL: Charles C Thomas. Reproduced by permission.]

> . . . each of which is subject to variability or change with time. . . . Each element in the imaging chain can drift such that the image quality may be degraded. Consequently, to ensure optimum image quality with minimal radiation exposure to the patient and staff and to do so in a cost effective manner, it is essential to measure and control all of the appropriate variables. . . . (NCRP, 1988, p. 61).

It is not within the scope of this chapter to list all of the elements or to describe how the variables are tested (these are covered in QC courses). It is important, however, to identify those elements common to several of the imaging systems and to give examples of the tolerance limits for a few representative variables.

TABLE 13-1. PERTINENT ITEMS THAT MAY BE INCLUDED IN A QA MANUAL TO ENSURE A SUCCESSFUL PROGRAM

Introduction
Objectives of the QA program
Individual responsibility protocol
Parameters to be monitored
Frequency of testing
Image quality standards
Test equipment available
Description of each test procedure
Photographs and/or diagrams illustrating the equipment setup procedure
Record-keeping protocol
Protocol for reporting problems
References
Additional educative materials including audiovisual aids
An appendix that includes all data recording forms

SOURCE: From Seeram, E. (1985). *X-ray imaging equipment: An introduction.* Springfield, IL: Charles C Thomas. Reproduced by permission.

Common elements for radiography, fluoroscopy, mammography, and some digital imaging systems include, for example, x-ray generators, x-ray tubes, collimators, filtration, grids, cassettes, screens, films, and processing.

Generator variables include kVp, exposure time, output waveforms, exposure per unit of tube current and time [$\mu C \cdot kg^{-1}$(mR)/mAs], linearity, exposure reproducibility, and automatic exposure control (NCRP, 1988).

The variables for x-ray tubes and collimators are filtration, alignment of the light field and the radiation field defined by the collimator, focal spot size, off-focus radiation, and several others. Because filtration and collimation are intended to protect the patient, they are considered extremely important. The thickness of the filter depends on the kVp used. Specifically, if the operating range of kVp is 50–70, the minimum half-value layer (HVL) in Al ranges from 1.2 to 1.5 mm. Above 70 kVp, the filtration increases and ranges from 2.1 to 3.8 mm Al for operating voltages ranging from 71 to 140 kVp, respectively (NCRP, 1988).

The variables for grids and image receptors (cassettes, screens, and films) are also important because they play a major role in determining the amount of radiation needed to produce an acceptable image. While the variables for grids (subject to QC) are grid uniformity and grid alignment, variables for image receptors are several, the three most common being screen-film contact, screen-film-cassette speed matching, and screen cleanliness (NCRP, 1988).

Exceeding the Tolerance Limit

Each of the QC tests for the different variables has an associated tolerance limit, previously derived by various radiologic and physics groups through scientific research. The results of QC tests are matched against the tolerance limit, which can be expressed qualitatively (pass-fail or no significant areas of poor contact seen) or quantitatively (± 0.05 or $\pm 3\%$ or ≤ 1.3 $mC \cdot kg^{-1}$/min). The tolerance limit usually has a $\pm$ value.

If the results of the QC test fall within the tolerance limit, the test is considered acceptable. If, however, the results exceed the tolerance limit, the test indicates that equipment performance is unacceptable.

Consider Figure 13-4, which conceptualizes the notion of tolerance limit and the consequences of exceeding the $\pm$ values that define the limit. For example, in the case of the QC test of the kVp variable, the tolerance limit is ± 2 kVp for the 60–100-kVp range. Suppose, however, that the test was done at 70 kVp. Then we would accept 68–72 kVp. Any value >72 or <68 would render the test result unacceptable and would suggest the need for repairs and/or calibration.

In addition, if the results of those factors affecting dose fall beyond the positive value of the tolerance limit, this would imply that the pa-

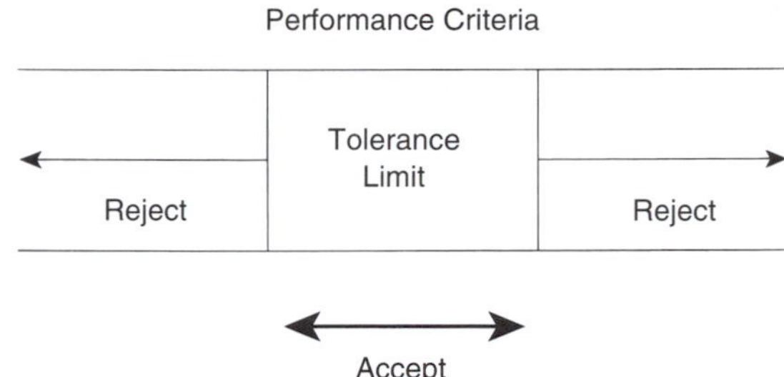

FIGURE 13-4. The concept of tolerance limit in QC. If the results of the QC test exceeded this limit, the performance criteria would not have been met, subsequently indicating that the equipment be repaired or calibrated to give the proper results.

tient will receive unnecessary radiation. However, if the results of the factors that influence image quality fall below the negative value of the tolerance limit, image quality is deemed unacceptable. QC ensures minimum radiation exposure to the patient without compromising image quality. The tolerance limits for several essential QC tests are listed in Table 13-2.

Exposure Reduction as a Consequence of QC

There is no doubt that an effective QA/QC program results in dose reduction as well as dose optimization (NCRP, 1988; Phillips, 1993). This is well documented in the literature.

In 1980, *Imaging Management* reported that retake rates at Cerritos Garden General Hospital in California were reduced from 17% to 5% in just 2 months after a QA program was implemented. Additionally, another hospital, Kennestone Hospital in Georgia, lowered their repeat rate from 5.3% to 4.2%. In 1981, Meeks reported that Chippenham Hospital in Virginia reduced its retake rate from 10–15% to about 3% as a result of QA efforts.

Later, in 1984, Gray and Stears reported low rejection rates on the order of 1.8% for mammography, 8.6% for pediatric radiography, 3.1% for outpatients, and an overall rate of 5.2% as a result of their quantitative QC program, which was based on objective evaluation measures.

TABLE 13-2. TOLERANCE LIMITS FOR SEVERAL ESSENTIAL QC TESTS

Test	Tolerance Limit	Frequency
Light field and x-ray field alignment	±2% of source-to-image distance (SID)	Semiannually
Automatic collimation	±3% of SID	Semiannually
kVp	±5%; less over limited range, e.g., ±2 kVp for 60–100 kVp	Annually
Exposure times	For three phase generator: ±5%	Annually
mR/mAs	±10%	Annually
Linearity	±10% over clinical range	Annually
Exposure reproducibility	±5%	Annually
Sensor panel function of phototimers	±10%	Semiannually
Grid alignment	Density of 1.0 ± 0.10	Annually
Screen-film contact	No significant areas of poor contact	Annually
Maximum fluoroscopic exposure rate	$\leq$1.3 mC·kg^{-1}/min for manual $\leq$2.6 mC·kg^{-1}/min for automatic systems	Semiannually

SOURCE: National Council on Radiation Protection and Measurements. (1988). *Quality assurance for diagnostic imaging equipment* (Report No. 99). Bethesda, MD: NCRP.

Cohen (1985) reported that as an optimizing procedure, QA in diagnostic radiology will lead to a reduction of 50% of the mean whole-body dose equivalent from 1.0 mGy (100 mrad) to 0.5 mGy (50 mrad) per year.

Finally, as a result of knowledge of QC coupled with the understanding of the factors affecting radiation dose to the patient, the technologist is in a much better position to make significant contributions to dose reduction and dose optimization in radiology.

NCRP Report No. 99

As QA programs evolve, we shall see the appearance of more and more information on this topic. Currently, an excellent report is that of the National Council on Radiation Protection and Measurements (NCRP) Report No. 99. This report is extensive and covers a wide range of topics including:

1. General concepts of quality assurance and quality control.
2. Quality assurance—personnel performance and keeping records.
3. Establishment of a quality control program.
4. Procedures, objectives, and policies.
5. Photographic quality control.
6. Quality control in radiography, fluoroscopy, conventional tomography, mobile radiography, mammography, special procedures, computed tomography, digital imaging, magnetic resonance imaging, video systems, and computers.
7. Summary of quality control tests.

The overall goals of the report are to "encourage the establishment of practical and comprehensive quality assurance programs in medical imaging facilities and to provide guidance for developing and implementing such programs" (NCRP, 1988, p. 1).

The technologist will find this report an extremely useful resource in all aspects of QA.

REVIEW QUESTIONS

1. Quality assurance (QA) deals with:
   A. Cost savings.
   B. The use of the smallest dose to produce the best image quality.
   C. Optimum image quality to facilitate diagnostic interpretation of the film.
   D. All of the above.

2. QA is a management concept that includes:
   A. Administrative measures.
   B. Educational measures.
   C. Technical measures.
   D. All of the above.

3. QC deals specifically with:
   A. Technical procedures (tests) to ensure that the best possible image quality is obtained.
   B. Administrative measures.
   C. People.
   D. All of the above.

4. Which of the following is not a goal of QC?
   A. Reduction of patient dose.
   B. Reduction of radiation risk to the patient.
   C. Ensure patient comfort and safety.
   D. Identify technologists with poor radiation protection skills.

5. The history of QA may be traced back to the 1970s through a project of the:
   A. NIOSH.
   B. CDRH.
   C. JCAHO.
   D. DuPont Company.

6. Which of the following refers to dose optimization?
   A. Uses of the smallest film size and minimum number of films to save money.
   B. Use of the clinical information about the patient to determine the number of x-rays to perform.

C. Use of the smallest possible radiation dose to provide an accurate diagnosis.
D. All of the above.

7. The following are components of dose optimization except:
   A. Education and training.
   B. Technical factors.
   C. Administrative costs of the QA program.
   D. Personnel practices.

8. The principles of QC are based on all of the following except:
   A. Acceptance testing.
   B. Routine performance evaluation.
   C. Error correction.
   D. Cost of the imaging equipment.

9. The results of a QC test are deemed acceptable when:
   A. The results fall within the tolerance limits of the test.
   B. The results exceed the tolerance limit of the test.
   C. The results fall within certain defined limits called performance criteria.
   D. a and c are correct.

10. Which of the following should be subject to QC monitoring to ensure radiation protection of the patient?
   A. Radiographic systems.
   B. Fluoroscopic systems.
   C. Computed tomography and mammography systems.
   D. All of the above.

REFERENCES

Barnes, G.T., Nelson, R.E., & Witten, D.M. (1976). A comprehensive quality assurance program: A report of four years' experience at the University of Alabama in Birmingham. Application of Optical Instrumentation in Medicine. V. *Proceedings of the Society of Photo-Optical Instrumentation Engineers, 96*, 19.

Beideman, R.W., Johnson, O.N., & Alcox, R.W. (1976). A study to develop a rating system and evaluate dental radiographs submitted by a third-party carrier. *Journal of the American Dental Association, 93*, 1010.

Burkhart, R.L. (1980). *Quality assurance programs for diagnostic radiology* [HEW Publication (FDA) 80-8110]. Washington, DC: U.S. Department of Health, Education and Welfare.

Burnett, B.M., Mazzaferro, R.J., & Church, W.W. (1975). *A study of retakes in the radiology department in two large hospitals.* (FDA No. 76-8016). Washington, DC: FDA.

Bushong, S. (1993). *Radiologic science for technologists* (5th ed.). St. Louis: C.V. Mosby.

Carlton, R. (1980). Establishing a total quality assurance program in diagnostic radiology. *Radiologic Technology, 52*, 23.

Carlton, R., & Adler, A. (1992). *Principles of radiographic imaging.* Albany, NY: Delmar Publishers.

Cohen, N. (1985). Quality assurance as an optimizing procedure in diagnostic radiology. *British Journal of Radiology, 18* (Suppl. 1), 134.

Felson, B., Morgan, W.K.C., & Bristol, L.J. (1973). Observations on the results of multiple readings of chest films in coal miners pneumoconiosis. *Radiology, 109*, 50.

Gray, J.E., & Stears, J. (1984). Quality control in diagnostic radiology at Mayo Clinic. *Applied Radiology, 2*, 89.

Gray, J.E., Winkler, N.T., Stears, J., & Frank, E.D. (1983). *Quality control in diagnostic imaging.* Rockville, MD: Aspen Publishers Inc.

Hall, C.L. (1977). Economic analysis of a quality control program. Application of Optical Instrumentation in Medicine. VI. *Proceedings of the Society of Photo-Optical Instrumentation Engineers, 127*, 271.

ICRP. (1982). *Protection of the patient in diagnostic radiology* (Publication No. 34). Elmsford, NY: Pergamon Press.

McLemore, J.M. (1981). *Quality assurance in diagnostic radiology.* Chicago: Year Book Medical Publishers.

Meeks L.E. II (1981). Quality control program cuts costs and reduces patient exposure. *Radiology/Nuclear Medicine Magazine, Vol. 1*, 26.

National Council on Radiation Protection and Measurements. (1988). *Quality assurance for diag-*

nostic imaging equipment (Report No. 99). Bethesda, MD: NCRP.

National Council on Radiation Protection and Measurements. (1989). *Medical x-ray, electron beam and gamma ray protection for energies up to 50 MeV: Equipment design, performance and use* (Report No. 102). Bethesda, MD: NCRP.

(1980). *Imaging management: A sense of direction.* Wilmington, DE: DuPont.

Philips, B. (1993). *Personal communication.* Radiation Protection Service, Health and Welfare British Columbia, Canada.

Seeram, E. (1985). *X-ray imaging equipment: An introduction.* Springfield, IL: Charles C Thomas.

Showalter, C.K., Bunge, R.E., Gross, R.E., & Seville, M.E. (1977). An analysis of film/screen combinations and patient exposures from nationwide evaluation of x-ray trends (NEXT). Application of Optical Instrumentation in Medicine. VI. *Proceedings of the Society of Photo-Optical Instrumentation Engineers, 127,* 136.

Trout, E.D., Jacobson, G., Moore, R.T., & Shoub, E.P. (1973). Analysis of the rejection rate of chest radiographs obtained during the coal mine black lung program. *Radiology, 109,* 25.

Answers to Review Questions

CHAPTER 1

1. D
2. C
3. D
4. A
5. C
6. D
7. D
8. A
9. B
10. C
11. A
12. B
13. A
14. A
15. D
16. B
17. A
18. A
19. C
20. C
21. B
22. C
23. D
24. B
25. A

CHAPTER 2

1. A
2. C
3. A
4. A
5. D
6. A
7. B
8. B
9. D
10. C
11. A
12. B
13. A
14. A
15. D
16. A
17. B
18. A
19. A
20. A
21. B
22. A
23. D
24. C
25. D
26. D
27. B
28. A
29. D
30. C
31. A
32. D
33. B
34. A
35. A

CHAPTER 3

1. D
2. A
3. D
4. B
5. B
6. D
7. D
8. A
9. B
10. A
11. B
12. C
13. A
14. A
15. A
16. B
17. C
18. A
19. C
20. C
21. D
22. B
23. C
24. A
25. D
26. D
27. B
28. D
29. B
30. D

CHAPTER 4

1. D
2. A
3. D
4. B
5. C
6. A
7. D
8. D
9. B
10. B
11. A
12. A
13. D
14. D
15. C
16. C
17. B
18. C
19. D
20. A
21. D
22. B
23. D
24. D
25. C
26. C
27. C
28. B
29. A
30. D
31. C
32. D
33. C
34. D
35. D
36. D
37. C
38. C
39. D
40. D
41. C
42. A

CHAPTER 5

1. A
2. D
3. C
4. D
5. A
6. D
7. D
8. A
9. B
10. B
11. B

12. C
13. A
14. D
15. B
16. D
17. B
18. C
19. A
20. D
21. C
22. D
23. B
24. C
25. C
26. C
27. D
28. D
29. D
30. D

CHAPTER 6

1. D
2. A
3. A
4. D
5. C
6. B
7. C
8. D
9. A
10. C
11. A
12. D
13. D
14. A
15. B

CHAPTER 7

1. A
2. B
3. B
4. D
5. C
6. D
7. C
8. C
9. D
10. D
11. D
12. B
13. A
14. A
15. D
16. B
17. D
18. D
19. B
20. C
21. C
22. B
23. A
24. D
25. C
26. A
27. D
28. B
29. D
30. A
31. A
32. C
33. C

CHAPTER 8

1. D
2. D
3. D
4. B
5. A
6. C
7. C
8. D
9. C
10. D
11. A
12. A
13. C
14. B
15. D
16. B
17. A
18. B
19. D
20. B
21. D
22. C
23. A
24. D
25. D
26. D
27. C
28. B
29. C
30. A
31. D
32. D
33. D
34. D
35. D
36. D
37. A
38. C
39. A
40. C

CHAPTER 9

1. D
2. D
3. D
4. B
5. A
6. B
7. D
8. C
9. B
10. D
11. D
12. D
13. C
14. C
15. A
16. D
17. A
18. C
19. D
20. D
21. D
22. C
23. B
24. A
25. D
26. D
27. D
28. A
29. B
30. D
31. C
32. D

CHAPTER 10

1. C
2. D
3. D
4. A
5. B
6. D
7. A
8. D
9. B
10. A
11. C
12. B
13. D
14. B
15. D
16. B
17. B
18. A
19. C
20. B
21. D
22. C
23. A
24. C
25. C
26. D
27. B
28. C
29. A
30. A

CHAPTER 11

1. A
2. B
3. C
4. D
5. C
6. D
7. D
8. C
9. D
10. D

CHAPTER 12

1. D
2. D
3. A
4. B

5. C
6. D
7. C
8. A
9. C
10. A
11. D
12. A
13. A
14. D
15. B
16. A
17. B
18. C
19. C
20. D

CHAPTER 13

1. D
2. D
3. D
4. d
5. a
6. c
7. c
8. d
9. d
10. d

Glossary

Absorbed dose (3): The amount of energy absorbed per unit mass of the exposed tissue.

Algorithm (13): A set of rules for solving a problem employed to conduct performance evaluation tests. These algorithms incorporate three components: the test procedure, image quality standards, and performance criteria (tolerance limit).

As low as reasonably achievable (ALARA) (3): Optimization can be said to occur if a positive net benefit is achieved at a dose that is as low as reasonably achievable.

Atom (2): The building block of the universe. It is made up of a dense nucleus surrounded by electrons.

Atomic mass (2): Actual mass of the atom.

Attenuation (2): The reduction of radiation that occurs as it passes through matter.

Attenuation factor (10): This property of a barrier material (A) is determined by the properties of the barrier material as well as by the energy of the radiation falling upon it.

Average dose to the patient (3): The average dose received by all the tissue within the defined area of the x-ray beam.

Average organ dose (3): The average radiation energy absorbed by a particular organ.

Backscatter (11): Radiation scattered from walls or floors or the Bucky mechanism back to the film. Backscatter causes film fogging.

Base units (3): One of the two classes of units used by the SI system. Base units for the physical quantities length, mass, and time are, respectively, the meter (m), kilogram (kg), and seconds (s).

Bone marrow dose (11): Radiation dose to the bone marrow.

Bremsstrahlung radiation: German for "braking," this term refers to the radiation produced when a high-speed electron is decelerated in an interaction with the charged nuclei of target atoms.

Bucky factor (B) (8): The ratio of the incident total radiation striking the grid to the total radiation transmitted through the grid.

Cardinal principles of radiation protection (1): These principles, which incorporate the concepts of time, shielding, and distance, are intended to reduce the radiation exposure an individual may receive. The principles are as follows: (1) keep exposure time as short as possible, (2) place a protective shield between the source of radiation and vulnerable areas of the exposed patients that should not absorb any scattered radiation, and (3) keep the distance between the source of radiation and the exposed individual as great as possible.

C-arm fluoroscopy (8): A procedure that is routinely used in operating rooms and in pacemaker wire insertions.

Characteristic x-rays (2): When high-speed electrons interact with inner shell electrons of target atoms to cause ionization, characteristic radiation results.

Cine fluorography (8): The use of 35-mm cine film with exposures occurring at a rate of between 30 and 120 frames per second to capture the image from fluoroscopic examination.

Classical scattering (2): The absorption of a low-energy photon by the entire atom with which it interacts excites the atom. It quickly releases a photon whose energy equals that of the incident photon.

Collimation (3, 7): The act of collimating. In this process the radiation beam is limited to the anatomy of interest.

Compton scattering (2): Also referred to as inelastic or nonclassical scattering, this photon–electron interaction predominates in x-ray imaging. In Compton scattering, the incident photon has enough energy to eject the electrons from the outer shell of the atom, which results in the ionization of the atom.

Computed tomography dose index (CTDI) (11): This is the average dose at specified locations in a special cylindrical phantom; it describes the absorbed dose during CT scanning in which adjacent slices are being imaged.

Contact shields (8): Lead shields that rest directly on the patient to protect tissues or organs (gonads) from radiation.

Continuous x-ray spectrum (2): This spectrum shows that the energies of Brems radiation range from zero to some maximum.

Control booth (10): The room that houses the control panel and protects the radiologic technologists from scattered and leakage radiation. The x-ray exposure switch is located in the control panel and is designed to require the technologist's presence to control exposure to the patient. This ensures that the technologist will be in the control booth, and thus protected from exposure.

Cosmic radiation (3): This type of radiation includes radiations of different energies, including solar and galactic radiation.

Coulomb per kilogram (3): The Roentgen produces 2.58×10^{-4} coulomb of ionization per kilogram (C/kg).

Cumulative timer (8): Every fluoroscopic unit is equipped with this device, which keeps track of fluoroscopic exposure time. It automatically notifies the radiologist when each 5-minute time period has elapsed, at which point it interrupts the production of x-rays.

Depth dose (3): The absorbed dose measured at some point below the skin surface.

Deterministic effects (1): The severity of these effects increases as the dose increases. There is a threshold for these effects, which were formerly known as nonstochastic effects.

Direct action (2): One of two classes of radiation interaction that lead to biological responses in living things. Direct action is characterized by the excitation or ionization of biological macromolecule, such as DNA, which leaves it in a chemically unstable state.

Direct beam absorber (9): Also referred to as a primary protective barrier, this built-in barrier in all fluoroscopic units limits the exposure during fluoroscopy. If the barrier is removed, the exposure will terminate.

Discrete emission spectrum (2): This continuum shows that characteristic x-rays are emitted only at specific photon energies.

Distance (10): The minimum distance from the x-ray tube to a point on the other side of the barrier that an individual can be. As the distance, d, increases, the exposure rate increases inversely as the square of the distance.

Division delay (4): The interruption of the progression of cells through the cell cycle.

Dose equivalent (3): The quantity (H) that is used to define the differences in biological effectiveness between radiations of different types and energies.

Dose equivalent limit (7): Part of a more comprehensive system of radiation protection that relates to dose limitations.

Dose limit (1): Numerical standards that represent a range of "safe" radiation amounts (sometimes called occupational dose limits).

Dose limitation (5): Restricting the dose to a certain amount during a period of time.

Dose reduction (9): The methods and techniques by which radiation doses are minimized to patients, personnel, and members of the public. The dose reduction practices covered in this text include education and training, equipment design and performance, personnel practices, and shielding.

Dose–risk relationship (1) (dose–response model) **(1):** The relationship between the size of the radiation dose and its associated risk of injury (biological response) to the exposed individual.

Earth radiation (3): This type of radiation occurs naturally in the air, soil, and rocks. Additionally, radionuclides are found in food and drink, and the human body gives off its own endogenous radiation.

Effective dose (3): Previously known as the effective dose equivalent, this quantity (E) is defined as the total of the weighted equivalent doses in all the body's tissues and organs. Mathematically, it is expressed as:

$$E = \sum_{T} W_T \cdot H_T$$

Elective examination (9): One that is not urgently needed and can, therefore, be done at a time that is deemed suitable to the needs and safety of the patient.

Electromagnetic radiation (2): Consisting of an electric and a magnetic field that travel through space at right angles to each other, electromagnetic radiation is made up of an electromagnetic spectrum, which includes cosmic rays, gamma rays, ultraviolet radiation, visible light, infrared radiation, microwaves, and radiowaves.

Electron (2): A negatively charged particle that orbits the central nucleus. The closer the electron is to the nucleus, the greater its binding energy.

Endogenous radiation (3): Radiation that is produced within or caused by factors within the body.

Energy of the radiation (10): The penetrating power of the x-ray beam.

Entrance skin dose (11): Also referred to as exposure to the skin surface.

Entrance skin exposure (3): Refers to the skin dose.

Equivalent dose (1): The most recent revision to the terminology used in conceptualizing dose limitation was introduced in 1990, when ICRP Publication No. 60 used this term to replace dose equivalent limit. It is the weighted absorbed dose in a tissue or organ and is obtained by weighting the absorbed dose by the radiation factor, W_R.

Erythema dose (1): The amount of radiation needed to produce a reddening of the skin.

Excitation (2): The process by which energy is transferred to the electrons in irradiated material, causing them to move into orbital levels that are farther away from the nucleus.

Exposure (3): The radiation quantity used to measure the amount of ionization produced in a specific mass of air by x or gamma radiation.

Exposure linearity (9): To achieve exposure linearity, the combination of mA and time selections produces constant mAs values that should produce constant output radiation intensities (mR/mAs).

Exposure rate (9): This measurement refers to the amount of radiation exposure to the patient per unit of time at a given point.

Exposure reproducibility (9): There is said to exist exposure reproducibility when the same exposure techniques used repeatedly result in the same output of radiation intensity for all exposures. It is recommended that the output intensity not be greater than ± 5% of the average intensities of a series of 10 exposures.

Exposure-to-dose factors (11): These known factors (sometimes referred to as f-factors) are used to calculate average glandular doses of radiation, because they cannot be measured directly.

Fallout (3): Radiation produced as a result of nuclear testing and chemical explosions in nuclear facilities.

f-factor: See exposure-to-dose factors.

Field size (8): The area covered by the beam falling on the patient. Also called field of view (FOV).

Film badge detector (3): This type of radiation detector was very popular in the past as a monitoring device in personnel dosimetry.

Filters (8): Metal absorbers inserted into the useful beam, before it strikes the patient, for the purposes of removing or absorbing low-energy photons.

Filtration (8): The process by which low-energy photons are absorbed or removed from the useful beam, thereby protecting the patient from exposure to unnecessary radiation. Inherent filtration is accomplished by the x-ray tube itself. Added filtration, on the other hand, is characterized by the addition of a specified thickness of aluminum outside the x-ray tube: Total filtration = Inherent filtration + Added filtration.

Fluoroscopy (8): A diagnostic imaging technique that displays images in real time on a television monitor and is dependent upon continuous x-ray production. Intermittent fluoroscopy, during which the beam is on for short bursts of time rather than continuously, is used to mitigate the effects of high exposures by reducing overall "beam-on" time.

Free radicals (2): This term is used to refer to atoms or molecules that have an unpaired electron in the outermost shell. They are highly reactive chemical species characterized by an ability to combine with other free radicals to form molecules that are potentially toxic to the cell.

Frequency (2): The number of vibrations per second made by a wave.

Fringe field (12): The stray magnetic field that extends beyond the MR scanner.

Genetically significant dose (GSD) (11): To determine the genetic impact of low-dose radiation on a specific population, an average is calculated from the actual gonadal doses received by that population.

Genetic effects (1): These effects occur in the future descendants of those individuals who have undergone radiation exposure.

Glow curve (5): The curve that results when light is plotted as a function of temperature.

Gonadal shielding (5): Shielding the gonads with lead to protect them from radiation.

Gradient coils (12): Electric coils of wire used to produce gradient (slope) magnetic fields.

Gradient magnetic field (12): For frequencies below 1 kHz, the limit is 20 T/s for longer than 0.12 msec. If the pulses are shorter and the frequencies are higher, then higher values are allowed.

Gray (Gy) (3): In SI units, the unit of absorbed dose is called the Gray in honor of the English radiobiologist Louis Harold Gray.

Grid (8): A lead screen fashioned from crisscrossing lead strips that is positioned between the tabletop and the image receptor to absorb radiation scattered from the patient. The absorbed radiation is thus prevented from reaching the film, which results in improved radiographic contrast.

Grid factor (8): See Bucky factor.

Grid frequency (8): The number of lead strips or lines per inch or per centimeter.

Grid ratio (8): The ratio of the height of the lead strip to the distance between the strips.

Half value layer (HVL) (2): This practical measure of attenuation is actually defined as the thickness of the material needed to reduce the intensity of a beam of radiation by 50%.

Health physicist (1): A radiation specialist or engineer who is qualified to engage in the research or teaching of radiation safety, as well as in its operational aspects. This person generally assumes the role of radiation safety officer (RSO), sometimes known simply as a safety officer.

High-level-control (HLC) (8): A feature that allows all state-of-the-art fluoroscopic machines to provide a dose rate higher than that achievable through conventional exposure.

Image receptor (8): The piece of equipment used to capture images of radiation passing through the patient. The sensitivity of the image receptor refers to the speed of the receptor as it relates to both the film speed and the screen speed.

Image receptor sensitivity (8): The speed of the film-screen combination.

Indirect action (2): One of the two classes of radiation interaction that leads to biological responses in living things. In indirect action, an ionizing particle or photon ionizes or excites water to form free radicals, which in turn attack biological macromolecules (e.g., DNA, RNA, or proteins).

Induction of electric currents (12): The strength of the main magnetic field causes, or induces, electric currents in devices that conduct electrical currents. This effect is particularly problematic in pacemakers, which can cause fibrillation, burns, or other serious problems.

Industrial radiation (3): This includes radiation from mining, nuclear power plants, and consumer products.

Integral dose (3): The total amount of energy absorbed by a particular mass of tissue.

Integral exposure (3): The total radiation delivered to a body.

Intermittent fluoroscopy (8): Fluoroscopy occurring at varied intervals.

International System of Units (3): Originally known by its French name (Le Système International d'Unités), this extension of the metric system was adopted by the General Conference of Weights and Measures in 1960 to ensure consistency of measurement across all branches of science.

Interphase (4): The nondividing or intermitotic period between two successive divisions of a cell.

Interspace material (8): This portion of the grid supports the lead strips and ensures that there is an equal amount of space between neighboring strips.

Inverse square law (5): Expressed mathematically as $I = 1/d^2$, this physical law states that the radiation exposure decreases as the distance increases.

Ionization (2): When radiation produces enough energy to completely eject electrons in the exposed material from the atom, it is referred to as ionizing radiation.

Ionization chamber (3): Consisting of an electrode placed in the middle of a gas-filled chamber, this device is useful for measuring x-ray intensity.

Ion pair (2): This results when an ejected electron (negative ion) pairs off with the remaining atom, which is now considered a positive ion because of its loss of the electron.

Justification (5): Reason for the radiation exposure (net–benefit concept).

Kerma (3): An acronym for the **k**inetic **e**nergy **r**eleased in the **ma**terial, the kerma is the unit of measure used to describe the energy transfer that occurs when the photons from the radiation beam interact with the atoms in the exposed patient.

Lambert-Beer law (2): A law in physics, which describes what happens to a beam of radiation as it passes through tissues. It shows that the intensity of the radiation decreases exponentially as it passes through certain thicknesses of material.

Leakage radiation (1): Radiation that penetrates the protective housing of the x-ray tube.

Lethal dose 50 (4): The dose that kills 50% of a population in a given period of time.

Linear attenuation coefficient (2): The value μ in the Lambert-Beer law, which represents the probability that a photon will be attenuated per centimeter (cm^{-1}) of the absorbing material.

Linear energy transfer (LET) (2): Expressed in units of keV per micrometer (μm) of path length (keV/μm), LET is the rate at which an electron or the x-ray photon transfers energy to the tissue surrounding the tissue through which it is traveling.

Luminescence (5): The property by which certain materials emit light when stimulated by a physiological process, a chemical or electrical action, or heat.

Magnetic resonance imaging (MRI) (1): An imaging modality that uses magnetic fields and radiowaves to produce diagnostic images of the human body.

Maximum permissible dose (MPD) (7): The maximum dose of radiation that is expected to produce neither somatic nor genetic responses in the exposed individual. Although the risk associated with MPD is not zero, it is much lower than the risks associated with other exposure doses and is considered reasonable "in light of the benefits derived."

Mean active bone marrow dose (11): Average radiation dose to the entire bone marrow.

Medical exposure (3): Exposure to radiation knowingly incurred as a result of medical diagnosis or treatment.

Metaphase (4): The stage of mitosis in which the chromosomes become aligned on the equatorial plate of the cell with the centromeres mutually repelling each other.

Mitosis (4): The process of cellular reproduction in somatic cells whereby one "parent cell" divides to form two "daughter cells" with the same chromosome number and DNA content as the original "parent cell." Consists of four phases—prophase, metaphase, anaphase, and telophase.

Mitotic death (4): Cell death while attempting to divide.

Multiple scan average dose (MSAD) (11): This is the average dose at the center of a series of adjacent scans.

Neutron (2): An electrically neutral particle in the atomic nucleus.

Nonionizing radiation (2): Any form of radiation that does not have enough energy to eject electrons from atoms.

Nonstochastic effects (6): See deterministic effects.

Nonthreshold models (1): According to this model, there is no threshold below which radiation doses can be considered safe. There is some risk associated with even small doses.

Nucleus (2): This positively charged mass at the center of the atom consists of two particles, protons and neutrons, which are collectively known as nucleons.

Occupancy factor (10): The amount of time (T) individuals occupy areas outside the x-ray room. This factor has three subcategories:

(1) *Full occupancy*—areas normally occupied by individuals (e.g., offices, nursing stations, children's play areas) during the course of a workday. The full occupancy factor for these areas

is 1. This factor applies to all those who are occupationally exposed.

(2) *Partial occupancy*—areas that are occupied only partially during the workday (e.g., washrooms, elevators). The occupancy factor for these areas is ¼.

(3) *Occasional occupancy*—areas such as toilets, stairways, and waiting rooms that are only occasionally occupied during the full workday. The occupancy factor is 1/16.

Occupational dose limits (10): Annual limits of radiation exposure to which radiation workers are exposed.

Occupational exposure (3): Radiation exposures that occur at work.

Oncogene (4): Any gene sequence contributing directly to a malignant change in a cell.

Optimization of radiation protection (5): The use of techniques to keep the radiation dose as low as reasonably achievable.

Overkill effect (2): Deposition of radiation in excess of that needed for cell killing.

Patient-image intensifier distance (P-IID) (8): The distance from the patient to the input screen of the image intensifier tube.

Personnel dosimetry (5): The practice of monitoring individuals who are occupationally exposed to radiation during the course of their work. This monitoring is done with devices such as the film badge, the thermoluminescent dosimeter, and the pocket dosimeter.

Personnel shielding (5): Protection of staff from radiation by using lead to prevent them from being exposed to radiation.

Photographic effect (5): The process by which radiation blackens photographic films.

Pocket dosimeter (5): Another type of personnel radiation detector, this device consists of an ionization chamber with an eyepiece, a transparent scale, a hollow charging rod, and fixed and moveable fibers. It is worn on the pocket.

Positive beam limitation (PBL) (7): Automatic collimation of the beam of radiation emanating from the x-ray tube.

Primary protective barrier (9): A wall to which the primary beam or useful beam from the x-ray tube is exposed.

Primary radiation (1): The useful beam of radiation from the x-ray tube.

Principles of radiation protection (3): In trying to decide if radiation exposure is necessary, three factors must be taken into consideration:

(1) *Justification*—radiation exposure must be of sufficient benefit to the individual to be exposed, or to society at large, in order to *justify* the procedure. In other words, if the net benefit outweighs the potential risks, then radiation exposure should be given.

(2) *Optimization*—the diagnostic or therapeutic effect of radiation exposure should be achieved with doses that are **a**s **l**ow **a**s **r**easonably **a**chievable (ALARA); in other words, the protective measures instituted should be optimized.

(3) *Dose and risk limits*—sources of radiation are determined and then relevant dose limits are set to ensure that risk of harmful biological effects is minimized.

Probability (2): The likelihood or chance of something occurring.

Projectile effect (12): Also known as the missile effect, this refers to the attraction of ferromagnetic objects distant to the MR magnet by the main magnetic field. The attraction is so great that it causes the object to accelerate at great speed (which varies depending on its size) toward the magnet.

Prophase (4): The first stage of mitosis or meiosis consisting of linear contraction and increasing thickness of the chromosomes accompanied by division of the centriole.

Protective barriers (10): These barriers, or lead-lined walls of the radiology department, are classified as primary or secondary depending on the type of radiation striking the wall:

primary protective barrier—if the wall is struck by a useful beam, it is referred to as a primary protective barrier.

secondary protective barrier—if the wall is struck by secondary radiation, which includes leakage from the x-ray tube and scattered radiation from the patient, it is referred to as a secondary protective barrier.

Protective clothing (9): A class of garments including aprons, gloves, and thyroid shields that are generally made of lead-impregnated vinyl and worn during fluoroscopic and some radiographic procedures.

Protons (2): Positively charged particles in the atomic nucleus.

Psychological effects of MRI examinations (12): Claustrophobia, anxiety, panic disorders, and emotional distress have been reported in some patients.

Quality administration (1): The area of quality assurance that ensures that personnel are carrying out QC monitoring functions judiciously.

Quality assurance (QA) (1, 13): Radiology departments that subscribe to this policy strive to obtain optimum diagnostic information at the lowest possible cost and the lowest possible dose to the patient. These conditions are met by periodically or continuously monitoring the performance of both the equipment and personnel in the radiological facility. (See quality control and quality administration.)

Quality control (QC) (1, 13): The portion of quality assurance management that deals with the technical aspects of instrumentation. The quality control technologist is responsible for carrying out all QC test procedures, recording the results, and, in some cases, interpreting those results and making recommendations for remedying any detected shortcomings in technical operations.

Quality factor (3): This factor reflects the effectiveness of a particular type of radiation resulting in the same biological effect as another type of radiation. In calculating the equivalent dose, $H = DQ$, where D is the absorbed dose and Q is the quality factor, which describes the effectiveness of a particular type of radiation.

Quantum level (2): This term refers to one of several fixed distances that correspond to the different levels at which electrons orbit the nucleus. A quantum level is sometimes called a shell because the orbit it describes is three-dimensional. These quantum levels, or shells, are labeled K, L, M, . . . Z, with K representing the innermost shell.

Quantum number (2): The number assigned to each quantum level in addition to its alphabetical label. The K-shell is assigned the number 1.

Quenching (12): In superconducting MRI scanners, helium is used to maintain the superconductivity of the magnetic coils. If this superconductivity is not maintained, the magnet will become resistive and give off heat, which will convert the liquid helium into a gaseous state. This quenching is dangerous because it can escape into the MR scanning room, thus potentially leading to asphyxiation and frostbite.

Rad (3): Traditional unit of absorbed dose.

Radiation (2): A form of energy that is sent through space or matter in the form of waves or particles. Ionizing radiation, the kind used in radiography, causes ionization of atoms resulting in positively and negatively charged ions and has the potential to cause biological damage. It should be noted that there is also a whole spectrum of nonionizing radiation, which encompasses microwaves, radiowaves, and ultraviolet rays among them. These radiations do not cause ionization.

Radiation concentration (3): Described by three fundamental dosimetric quantities—exposure, absorbed dose, and dose equivalent—radiation concentration characterizes the amount of radiation falling on the patient.

Radiation detection devices (5): Devices used to detect radiation.

Radiation dosimeters (5): Instruments used to measure radiation.

Radiation field (3): An area, or field, consisting of an average number of rays that can be shaped or collimated to cover the appropriate area of anatomical interest.

Radiation weighting factor (3): The factor W_R, which is used to express the relationship of the sievert to the gray: Sievert $=$ Gray $\times$ W_R. This radiation weighting factor is selected for the type and energy of radiation directed at the body, and it is used in determining the absorbed dose of tissue or an organ.

Radiofrequency (RF) (12): Radiowaves that have lower energies than microwave radiation. In MRI, the RF energies range from 10 to 100 MHz.

Radiography (8): Technique used to produce images of objects (patient) for the purpose of diagnosis using ionizing (x-ray) radiation.

Radiowaves (12): Radiation on the electromagnetic spectrum having less energy than microwaves.

Radiowaves include those used in commercial broadcast (e.g., AM and FM radio; television; shortwave) and in MRI.

Radon (3): A naturally occurring gas that is the major source of radiation exposure to the general public. Radon gas is of concern because of its association with lung cancer.

Relative biological effectiveness (RBE) (2): This mathematical equation describes the relationship between the effectiveness of the dose of radiation (D_{test}) and the dose of the reference radiation ($D_{reference}$) as

$$RBE = \frac{D_{reference}}{D_{test}}$$

In other words, if test radiation is more effective than reference radiation, the smaller dose is needed to produce the same biological effect and the greater will be the RBE.

Rem (rad equivalent man) (3): Conventional unit of measure used to describe H, the dose equivalent.

Ripple (8): A change in voltage over the period of a cycle. Reported in terms of a percentage.

Roentgen (3): The conventional unit of radiation exposure, first proposed in 1928. The SI unit for this radiation quantity is coulombs per kilogram.

Scattered radiation (1): That which is scattered by the patient as the result of Compton interactions.

Scintillation (5): The property whereby certain crystals can absorb radiation and convert it to light.

Scintillation detector (5): Another type of radiation detector, the scintillation detector is based on the principle that certain crystals (e.g., sodium iodide and cesium iodide) emit light when struck by x-rays or by charged particles.

Secondary protective barrier (10): A wall that is exposed to scattered radiation as well as leakage radiation from the x-ray tube.

Selectivity (8): Characterized as the ratio of primary radiation transmission to scattered radiation transmission, selectivity is just one of the factors that affects patient dose.

Shadow shield (8): Protective shield that is attached to the x-ray tube head and/or collimator; projects a shadow onto the area that receives radiation.

Shell (2): See quantum level.

Shields (8): Appliances used to protect radiosensitive portions of the patient's body from exposure to radiation.

Shielding requirement tables (10): These precalculated values provide a simple method of determining protective barrier thickness.

Sievert (Sv) (3): Named after the Swedish physicist Rolf Maximilian Sievert, this SI unit of measure describes the dose equivalent.

Skin dose (3): Also referred to as the entrance skin dose (ESE), this measure refers to the exposure to the entrance of the skin.

Skin erythema dose (7): A term first introduced by Mutscheller and Sievert, this term refers to the dose of x-rays needed to produce a reddening of the skin within 10–14 days of exposure.

Solar radiation (3): This type of radiation includes protons and helium. See cosmic radiation.

Somatic effects (1): These physical effects appear in the person exposed to radiation.

Source shielding (10): Lead-lined x-ray tube housing to prevent x-ray from leaking through the tube (leakage radiation).

Source-to-film distance (SFD) (9): The distance between the source of radiation and the film on which the radiographic image is to be captured.

Source-to-image receptor distance (SID) (8): The distance from the focal spot to the receptor that holds the film.

Source-to-skin distance (SSD) (9): The distance between the source of radiation and the patient.

Specific absorption rate (SAR) (7): The tissue heating caused by radiowaves is described as the specific absorption rate and is measured in watts per kilogram (W/kg).

Specific area shielding (9): Protecting specific organs and tissues such as the eye, gonads, and breasts from radiation using lead shields.

Spot film camera recording (8): The use of 100-mm or 105-mm cut film or roll film with exposures that occur at a rate of between 6 and 12 frames per second to capture fluoroscopic images.

Static magnetic field (12): The main magnetic field in MRI. The Food and Drug Administration recommends 2.0 T for whole-body exposure.

Stochastic effects (6): Effects for which the probability of occurrence increases with the radiation dose. There is no threshold for stochastic effects.

Strong static external magnetic field (12): Very high stationary magnetic field strength in MRI; also referred to as the primary magnetic field.

Structural shielding (10): Refers to the practice of lining the walls of x-ray rooms with lead to protect the patient from primary scattered and leakage radiation.

Supplementary units (3): One of the two classes of units in the SI system, the supplementary units radian (rad) and steradian (S) are used to measure plane angles and solid angles, respectively.

Surface integral exposure (SIE) (3): This measure, which is the product of exposure and the area of the radiation beam falling on the patient, is described mathematically as follows: SIE = Exposure × area of the radiation beam.

Syndrome (4): A group of signs and symptoms that occur together and characterize a particular abnormality or disease.

Technique factors (1): Kilovoltage (kVp), milliamperes (mA), and exposure time are the three factors that determine the density and contrast of the radiographic image.

Ten-day rule (9): The goal of this rule is to prevent unintentional exposure of the embryo or fetus. This rule recommends that women of childbearing age who need abdominal or pelvic radiography should have the procedure done during the 10 days following menstruation because it is highly unlikely that the woman might be pregnant during this period. This rule is now obsolete.

Thermoluminescent dosimetry (TLD) (5): This type of personnel dosimeter overcomes the shortcomings of film badges, which are susceptible to fogging and not highly sensitive in terms of radiation measurement. The TLD can measure exposures to individuals as low as 1.3 μC/kg (vs. the pocket dosimeter, which cannot measure anything <2.6 μC/kg); and it can withstand a certain degree of heat, humidity, and pressure.

Threshold dose model (1): According to this model, there is a threshold dose below which no effect is observed. It is only when the threshold dose has been reached that we begin to see biological effects.

Time-distance-shielding (5): Another triad of radiation protection:

(1) *Time:* When setting the control panel, the technologist should always try to use short exposure times without sacrificing image quality.

(2) *Distance:* The radiation exposure decreases inversely as the square of the distance the individual moves farther away from the radiation source.

(3) *Shielding:* In this radiation protection action, materials such as lead, concrete, or Clear-Pb are placed between the exposed individual and the radiation source to reduce the intensity of the delivered radiation. There are four types of shielding in diagnostic radiology: gonadal, personnel, room, and x-ray tube shielding.

Time-integrated dose (5): Sum of doses over a period of time.

Tissue weighting factor (3): Because the actual tissue or organ exposed to radiation plays a role in the development of biological effects, the ICRP introduced this factor to account for "the relative contribution of that organ or tissue to the total detriment due to those effects resulting from uniform irradiation of the whole body" (ICRP, 1991, p. 7).

Tolerance dose (7): This term, which was proposed in 1928, refers to the acceptable amount of radiation. It was subsequently replaced by the term maximum permissible dose (MPD), which gave way to the concept of dose equivalent limit, a term introduced in 1977.

Types of exposure (1): Individuals receive radiation doses from one of the following types of exposures: occupational (those related to work activities), medical (as the result of diagnostic procedures), and public (all other sources of radiation, including natural).

Use factor (10): The amount of time the primary beam is pointed to or directed at any of the walls (barriers) of the x-ray room. The factor, denoted by U, is also known as the beam direction factor.

Useful beam (9): This is also referred to as the primary beam. It is the beam of radiation used to image the specific anatomy.

Viewing window (10): Lead-glass window of the control booth, which allows the operator to view the patient during the examination.

Watts per kilogram (7): Unit of exposure to radiowaves.

Wave (2): Essentially a disturbance that carries energy from point to point, a wave is characterized by its velocity, wavelength, and frequency.

Wavelength (2): The distance taken up by one cycle of a wave.

Wave-particle duality (2): The ability of a source of energy to behave in ways that are characteristic of both waves and particles. Electromagnetic radiation is such a source of energy.

Workload (10): The factor (W) that refers to the amount of use of the x-ray unit.

X-ray (2): Discovered by W.C. Roentgen in 1895, these invisible, penetrating rays were characterized as having the following properties: (1) they can affect photographic plates; (2) they are *not* affected by magnetic or electrical fields; (3) they can cause certain materials to fluoresce; (4) they can cause ionization, (5) they can be absorbed by elements that have a high atomic number (e.g., lead); and (6) they can penetrate most substances including soft tissues and bones. The quantity of an x-ray beam is defined as the number of x-ray photons in the beam per unit of energy. The quality of the beam, on the other hand, refers to the "penetrating power" of the beam.

X-ray emission spectrum (2): A plot of the number of x-ray photons per unit energy (intensity) as a function of x-ray energy.

X-ray tube (2): The x-ray tube is made up of two major components: an anode (positive electrode) and a cathode (negative electrode). When high-speed electrons interact with the charged nuclei of target atoms, Bremsstrahlung (Brems) x-rays are produced.

APPENDIX

ORGANIZATIONS THAT PLAY A ROLE IN RADIATION PROTECTION

Atomic Energy Control Board (AECB): A federal agency in Canada that is charged with overseeing the proper functioning of the nuclear industry.

American Association of Physicists in Medicine (AAPM): Society of medical physicists which plays an active role in the application of physicists to problems in medicine and in particular to radiology, in the analysis of equipment, test tools, and radiation protection.

Biological Effects of Ionizing Radiation Committee (BEIR): This committee was formed by the National Research Council, which was itself organized by the National Academy of Sciences (NAS). Each BEIR committee (from the original BEIR I through the most recent BEIR V), advises the U.S. government on the health effects of radiation exposures based on a "comprehensive review of the biological effects of ionizing radiation" (NRC, 1990, p. vi).

Canadian Radiation Protection Association (CRPA): This organization, which was incorporated in 1982, has several objectives regarding radiation protection: to develop scientific knowledge; to encourage research; to promote education; to aid in the development of professional standards; and to support the endeavors of other national and international organizations that have related objectives.

Center for Devices and Radiological Health (CDRH): A division of the Food and Drug Administration of the U.S. Department of Health, Education, and Welfare that supports and encourages the development of quality assurance programs in radiology departments.

Conference of Radiation Control Program Directors (CRCPD): Founded in 1968, this is a nonprofit organization consisting of state and local government members who issue regulations for most state and local radiation protection programs in general radiation protection medicine and the nuclear industry. In medicine, the CRCPD works with the U.S. Food and Drug Administration in two major areas: quality assurance in radiography and mammography and the National Evaluation of X-ray Trends (NEXT) program.

International Atomic Energy Agency (IAEA): Organization that deals with the peaceful uses of atomic energy on a global scale.

International Commission on Radiological Protection (ICRP): Founded in 1928 by the Second International Congress of Radiology as the Radium Protection Committee, this organization's primary activity was originally to promote radiation safety in radiology. In 1950, the organization assumed its present name to reflect its expanded role in radiation protection.

International Commission on Radiological Units and Measurements (ICRU): This organization was established in 1925 to develop and promote international adherence to radiation quantities and units, measurement procedures, and uniformity of reporting.

International Radiation Protection Association (IRPA): This organization includes national organizations from all over the world, the primary goal of which is to make recommendations for nonionizing radiation.

National Council on Radiation Protection and Measurements (NCRP): A nonprofit organization chartered in 1964 to replace the Advisory Committee of X-Ray and Radium Protection (originally established in 1929), the NCRP is made up of a main committee and more than 60 subcommittees. The subcommittees prepare reports on radiation protection issues and then submit them to the main committee for approval and possibly publication.

National Radiological Protection Board (NRPB): The British equivalent of the NCRP was established by the Radiological Protection Act of 1970 to provide the government with advice on radiation protection. This board also was instrumental in establishing guidelines on exposure to the electromagnetic fields used in magnetic resonance imaging.

Radiation Effects Research Foundation (RERF): This group, which is run by the Japanese government and receives half of its funding from the United States, was founded in the 1950s to study the survivors of the atomic bombings of Hiroshima and Nagasaki.

Radiation Protection Bureau (RPB)–Health Canada: One of the two main federal government agencies that deal with radiation protection issues in Canada, the RPB-HC handles X-ray protection, operates the National Dosimetry Service (primarily for thermoluminescent TLDs), and the National Dose Registry, a computer-based system that keeps track of dose to radiation workers.

United Nations Scientific Committee of the Effects of Atomic Radiation (UNSCEAR): This committee was established in 1955 and includes among its members expert radiobiologists from around the world. The chief functions of UNSCEAR are to examine data on all radiation risks to both animals and humans, to assess exposures from both natural and man-made sources of radiation, and to make predictions about the potential ill effects of those exposures on the population.

INDEX

Page numbers followed by an *f* indicate a figure; *t* following a page number indicates tabular material.